Severe Dementia

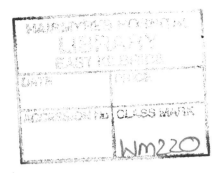

Severe Dementia

Editors

Alistair Burns
Department of Old Age Psychiatry, University of Manchester, UK

Bengt Winblad
Division of Geriatric Medicine, Karolinska Institute, Stockholm, Sweden

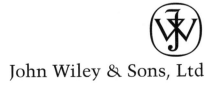

John Wiley & Sons, Ltd

Other Wiley Editorial Offices

John Wiley & Sons, Inc., 111 River Street, Hoboken, NJ 07030, USA

Jossey-Bass, 989 Market Street, San Francisco, CA 94103-1741, USA

Wiley-VCH Verlag GmbH, Boschstr. 12, D-69469 Weinheim, Germany

John Wiley & Sons Australia Ltd, 42 McDougall Street, Milton, Queensland 4064, Australia

John Wiley & Sons (Asia) Pte Ltd, 2 Clementi Loop #02-01, Jin Xing Distripark, Singapore 129809

John Wiley & Sons Canada Ltd, 22 Worcester Road, Etobicoke, Ontario, Canada M9W 1L1

Wiley also publishes its books in a variety of electronic formats. Some content that appears in print may not
be available in electronic books.

Library of Congress Cataloging-in-Publication Data

Severe dementia / editors, Alistair Burns, Bengt Winblad.
      p. ; cm.
      Includes bibliographical references.
      ISBN-10:   0-470-01054-1 (alk. paper)
      ISBN-13:   978-0-470-01054-9 (alk. paper)
      1. Dementia. 2. Dementia–Chemotherapy. 3. Dementia–Treatment.
      [DNLM: 1. Dementia. WM 220 S498 2006]   I. Burns, Alistair S.   II. Winblad, Bengt.
RC524.S48 2006
616.8'3–dc22   2006001098

British Library Cataloguing in Publication Data

A catalogue record for this book is available from the British Library

ISBN-13   978-0-470-01054-9
ISBN-10   0-470-01054-1

Typeset in 9/11 pt Times New Roman by Thomson Press (India) Limited, New Delhi, India.
Printed and bound in Great Britain by T.J. International Ltd, Padstow, Cornwall
This book is printed on acid-free paper responsibly manufactured from sustainable forestry in which at least
two trees are planted for each one used for paper production.

Cover
FDG PET scans show impaired cortical glucose metabolism and MRI scans show brain atrophy. Images were
kindly provided by Karl Herholz, Wolfson Molecular Imaging Centre, University of Manchester, UK

Contents

List of Contributors   vii

Introduction   xi

PART 1   INTRODUCTORY   1

Chapter 1   Assessment and Diagnosis of Severe Dementia   3
Paul Newhouse and Joseph Lasek

Chapter 2   Cholinergic and Serotonergic Systems in Severe Dementia   21
Sally I. Sharp, Paul T. Francis and Clive G. Ballard

Chapter 3   The Molecular Pathology of Severe Dementia   33
Clive Holmes

PART 2   CLINICAL FEATURES OF SEVERE DEMENTIA   41

Chapter 4   Cognitive Functions in Severe Dementia   43
Judith Saxton and François Boller

Chapter 5   Behavioural and Psychological Symptoms of Dementia – Agitation   51
E. Jane Byrne, Deborah Collins and Alistair Burns

Chapter 6   Depression in Severe Dementia   63
Kate Bielinski and Brian Lawlor

Chapter 7   Physical Aspects of Severe Alzheimer's Disease   75
Bruno Vellas

Chapter 8   Clinical Features of Severe Dementia: Staging   83
*Barry Reisberg, Jerzy Wegiel, Emile Franssen, Sridhar Kadiyala,
Stefanie Auer, Liduïn Souren, Marwan Sabbagh and James Golomb*

Chapter 9   Clinical Features of Severe Dementia: Function   117
Serge Gauthier

PART 3   MANAGEMENT   123

Chapter 10   Drug Treatment: Memantine   125
Anton P. Porsteinsson and Pierre N. Tariot

Chapter 11   Drug Treatment: Cholinesterase Inhibitors   131
Michael Woodward and Howard H Feldman

Chapter 12   Drug Treatment: Treatment of Behavioural and Psychological
Symptoms of Dementia with Neuroleptics   151
Peter Paul De Deyn

Contents

Chapter 13   Non-pharmacological Treatment of Severe Dementia:
An Overview   163
Ross Overshott and Alistair Burns

Chapter 14   Non-pharmacological Treatment of Severe Dementia:
the Seattle Protocols   177
Rebecca G. Logsdon, Linda Teri and Sue M. McCurry

Chapter 15   Care by Families for Late Stage Dementia   185
Steven H. Zarit and Joseph E. Gaugler

Chapter 16   Person-centred Care for People with Severe Dementia   193
Murna Downs, Neil Small and Katherine Froggatt

Chapter 17   Palliative Care in Patients with Severe Dementia   205
*Raymond T.C.M. Koopmans, H. Roeline W. Pasman and
Jenny T. van der Steen*

Chapter 18   Narrative Ethics and Ethical Narratives in Dementia   215
Clive Baldwin

Chapter 19   Health Economics of Severe Dementia   227
Anders Wimo and Bengt Winblad

Index   237

List of Contributors

Stefanie Auer
Morbus Alzheimer's Society
Lindaustrasse 28
A 4820 Bad Ischl, Austria

Clive Baldwin
Bradford Dementia Group
School for Health Studies
Unity Building
University of Bradford Bradford
BD5 0BB, UK

Clive G. Ballard
Wolfson Centre for Age Related Diseases
King's College London
Guy's Campus
St. Thomas Street
London SE1 1UL, UK

Kate Bielinski
Martha Whiteway Day Hospital
St. Patrick's Hospital
PO Box 136
James's Street
Dublin 8, Ireland

François Boller
INSERM Unit 549
Centre Paul Broca
2terrue d'Alésia
75014 Paris, France

Alistair Burns
Department of Old Age Psychiatry
University of Manchester
Education and Research Centre
Wythenshawe Hospital
Manchester M23 9Lt, Uk

E. Jane Byrne
Department of Old Age Psychiatry
2nd Floor
Education and Research Centre
Wythenshawe Hospital
Manchester M23 9LT, UK

Deborah Collins
Department of Old Age Psychiatry
2nd Floor

Education and Research Centre
Wythenshawe Hospital
Manchester M23 9LT, UK

Peter Paul De Deyn
Department of Neurology
General Hospital Meddelheim
University of Antwerp
Lindendreef 1
Antwerp 2020, Belgium

Murna Downs
Bradford Dementia Group
School for Health Studies
Unity Building
University of Bradford
Bradford BD5 0BB, UK

Howard H. Feldman
Division of Neurology
University of British Columbia
2329 West Mall
Vancouver V6T 1Z4, Canada

Paul T. Francis
Wolfson Centre for Age Related Diseases
King's College London
Guy's Campus
St. Thomas Street
London SE1 1UL, UK

Emile Franssen
Department of Psychiatry
Aging and Dementia Research Center
NYU Medical Center
550 First Avenue
New York, NY 10016, USA

Katherine Froggatt
Palliative and End of Life Care Research
Group
Sheffield University
Bartolomé House
Winter Street
Sheffield S3 7ND, UK

Joseph E. Gaugler
Department of Behavioral Sciences
University of Kentucky

110 College of Medicine
Lexington, KY 40536-6774, USA

Serge Gauthier
McGill Centre for Studies in Aging
6825 La Salle Boulevard
Verdun
Quebec H4H IR3, Canada

James Golomb
Department of Psychiatry
Aging and Dementia Research Center
NYU Medical Center
550 First Avenue
New York, NY 10016, USA

Clive Holmes
Southampton Community Health Services
Memory Clinic
Thornhill Unit
Moorgreen Hospital
Southampton SO30 3JB, UK

Sridhar Kadiyala
Department of Psychiatry
Aging and Dementia Research Center
NYU Medical Center
550 First Avenue
New York, NY 10016, USA

Raymond Koopmans
Department of Nursing Home Medicine
University Medical Centre Nijmegen
PO Box 9101, code 229 VPHG
6500 HB Nijmegen, The Netherlands

Joseph Lasek
Clinical Neuroscience Research Unit
Department of Psychiatry
University of Vermont College of Medicine
1 South Prospect Street
Burlington, VT 05401, USA

Brian Lawlor
Martha Whiteway Day Hospital
St. Patrick's Hospital
PO Box 136
James's Street
Dublin 8, Ireland

Rebecca G. Logsdon
Department of Psychosocial and
Community Health
University of Washington School of Nursing
Box 357263
Seattle, WA 98195-7263, USA

Sue M. McCurry
Department of Psychosocial and Community
Health
University of Washington School of Nursing

Box 357263
Seattle, WA 98195-7263, USA

Paul Newhouse
Clinical Neuroscience Research Unit
Department of Psychiatry
University of Vermont College of Medicine
1 South Prospect Street
Burlington, VT 05401, USA

Ross Overshott
Department of Old Age Psychiatry
2nd Floor
Education and Research Centre
Wythenshawe Hospital
Manchester M23 9LT, UK

H. Roeline W. Pasman
VU University Medical Center
Institute for Research in Extramural Medicine
Department of Public and Occupational Health
Van der Boechorststraat7
1081 BT Amsterdam, The Netherlands

Anton P. Porsteinsson
University of Rochester School of Medicine &
Dentistry
Monroe Community Hospital
435 East Henrietta Road
Rochester, NY 14620, USA

Barry Reisberg
Department of Psychiatry
Aging and Dementia Research Center
NYU Medical Center
550 First Avenue
New York, NY 10016, USA

Marwan Sabbagh
The Cleo Roberts Center for Clinical
Research
Sun Health Research Institute
Sun City, AZ, USA

Judith Saxton
Department of Neurology
University of Pittsburgh
Kaufmann Medical Building, Suite 811
3471 Fifth Avenue
Pittsburgh, PA 15213, USA

Sally I. Sharp
Wolfson Centre for Age Related Diseases
King's College London
Guy's Campus
St. Thomas Street
London SE1 1UL, UK

Neil Small
Primary and Community Care
School of Health Studies

University of Bradford
The Unity Building, 25 Trinity
Bradford, West Yorkshire BD5 0BB, UK

Liduïn Souren
Department of Psychiatry
Aging and Dementia Research Center
NYU Medical Center
550 First Avenue
New York, NY 10016, USA

Pierre N. Tariot
Psychiatry Unit
Monroe Community Hospital
435 East Henrietta Road
Rochester, NY 14620, USA

Linda Teri
Department of Psychosocial and Community
Health
University of Washington School of Nursing
Box 357263
Seattle, WA 98195-7263, USA

Jenny T. van der Steen
VU University Medical Center
Institute for Research in Extramural Medicine
Department of Public and Occupational Health
Van der Boechorststraat7
1081 BT Amsterdam, The Netherlands

Bruno Vellas
Department of Internal Medicine and Clinical

Gerontology
170 Avenue de Casselardit
31300 Toulouse, France

Jerzy Wegiel
Institute for Basic Research
Staten Island
New York, USA

Anders Wimo
HC Bergsjo
Box 16
S-82070 Bergsjo, Sweden

Bengt Winblad
Karolinska Institute
Neurotec B 84
Karolinska University Hospital
SE-14186 Stockholm, Sweden

Michael Woodward
Aged & Residential Care CSU
Austin
Heidelberg Repatriation Hospital
PO Box 5444
Heidelberg West, Victoria, Australia

Steven H. Zarit
Department of Human Development and
Family Studies
211 Henderson Bldg. South
Penn State University
University Park, PA 16802-6505, USA

Introduction

Importance of severe dementia

Dementia, regardless of its cause, is a progressive condition with deterioration inevitable in all domains whether they be neuropsychological, neuropsychiatric or neurofunctional. The course of the illness may be gradual (classically seen in Alzheimer's disease) punctuated by episodes of sudden deterioration (as in vascular dementia, possibly representing transient ischaemic attacks), episodic confusion (as in Lewy body dementia) or insidious personality change (as in fronto-temporal dementia).

Severe dementia is relatively neglected. Much clinical attention and research effort is directed towards early diagnosis and mild and moderate stages of the illness (with the emphasis on cholinergic therapies which have been licensed for these earlier stages) and even prodromal stages as with Mild Cognitive Impairment (MCI). The later stages of the disease are as important, if not more important, than the earlier stages because they harbour unique characteristics and events which occur affecting the lives of patients and their carers.

The later stages of the illness require special attention for four main reasons. First, many of the impairments in dementia become more apparent later on in the illness and begin to have a real and significant impact on carers. For example, functional disabilities mean that carers have to take over more practical tasks such as bathing and toileting which give rise to a more physical burden of care. Second, behavioural problems become more pronounced with agitation and aggression more commonly occurring than in early illness. Third, issues surrounding admission to care are prominent – for carers, presiding over the admission of a loved one to care is often accompanied by feelings of guilt and these are only partly offset by the benefits (potentially for both patients and carers) of admission to a nursing home. Fourth, there are special considerations of palliative care, ethics issues of terminal care and management of terminal illness along with physical problems.

The special circumstances of severe dementia and its relative neglect were the principal stimulus for the creation of this book which aims to bring together key aspects of dementia that are unique to the later stages.

Definition

Definitions of severe dementia vary from those which use a specific cut-off on a cognitive scale such as the Mini Mental State Examination (Folstein *et al.*, 1975, less than 10 often indicating severe impairment) or a global assessment such as the Clinical Dementia Rating (Morris, 1993) or the Global Deterioration Scale (Reisberg *et al.*, 1982). Many use a more holistic approach defining it as the situation where someone's ability to live independently is compromised and help is needed with basic activities of daily living such as dressing, bathing and toileting (Reisberg and his colleagues Chapter 8). These clinical ratings of the severe stages of the illness have been correlated with neuropathological findings. The molecular pathology and the neurochemistry drive many of the advances in research and are respectively described in detail by Holmes (Chapter 3) and Sharp and colleagues (Chapter 2). In people with a diagnosis of dementia, about a third would have severe dementia at any one time (Helmer *et al.*, 2003).

Assessment

Evaluation need not be a complicated process and follows the fundamentals of history, examination and investigations. It should be comparatively rare for a person to present for the first time in the later stages of dementia because of all the current clinical emphasis on early diagnosis and treatment. Newhouse and Lasek (Chapter 1) describe six axes of evaluation. Assessment scales for the measurement of dementia include the Severe Impairment Battery and the Mini Mental State Examination (although this has a floor effect in patients with severe disease), global scales include the Clinical Dementia Rating and Global Deterioration Scale, activities of daily living scales which assess basic functions (Bucks *et al.*, 1996), and the Neuropsychiatric Inventory (Cummings *et al.*, 1994) which assesses Behavioural and Psychological Symptoms (BPSD).

Behavioural and psychological symptoms (BPSD)

The majority of people, by the time they have reached the severe stages of dementia will have experienced one or more of a cluster of psychological/psychiatric symptoms known collectively as BPSD. Agitation is one of the commonest of these and is particularly distressing to patients and their carers (Byrne, Collins and Burns, Chapter 5). A variety of drug (DeDeyn, Chapter 12) and other treatments are available (Overshott and Burns, Chapter 13). The diagnostic difficulties of detecting treatable depression in dementia are well described by Bielinski and Lawlor (Chapter 6). There is a particular diagnostic challenge in people with severe dementia as the inability to communicate the phenomenology of affective disorder is often significantly impaired. Diagnostic criteria following the diagnosis of depression in dementia have been established with particular emphasis on the behavioural and neurovegetative aspects.

Cognitive function

Saxton and Boller (Chapter 4) summarise this important area where traditional methods of assessment have questionable applicability and validity but assessments of cognitive loss are important. By using appropriate and sensitive assessments, these can be carried out successfully.

Functional abilities

The specific aspects of function have been described by Gauthier (Chapter 9) emphasising the use of scales to measure activities of daily living and beginning to tease out motivation and ability in the carrying out of practical tasks. Physical changes occur with the onset of severe dementia which have to be assessed and managed (Vellas, Chapter 7).

Special considerations in care

Challenges of care for people with severe dementia are varied. Koopmans and colleagues (Chapter 17) describe a palliative care approach, Downs and colleagues (Chapter 16) remind us of the importance of person-centred care and Baldwin provides an insight into ethical issues (Chapter 18). Family carers of people with severe dementia are reviewed by Zarit and Gaugler (Chapter 15).

Treatment

Severe dementia often attracts therapeutic nihilism but there is compelling evidence that the cholinesterase inhibitors are effective even although they are primarily licensed for mild to moderate Alzheimer's disease (Woodward and Feldman, Chapter 11). The only drug licensed for severe dementia, memantine, is reviewed by Porsteinsson and Tariot (Chapter 10). Drug treatments can also be directed towards BPSD and De Deyn (Chapter 12) provides an overview of treatment in this field. Logsdon, Teri and McCurry (Chapter 14) summarise the work of their group with protocols for the management of behaviours and problems particularly common to severe dementia. Treatment always brings with it the matter of cost-effectiveness and the economics of the later stages of the illness are dealt with by Wimo and Winblad (Chapter 19).

We are grateful to the contributors for submitting manuscripts on time, to our assistants Barbara Dignan and Gunilla Johansson and to the publishers at John Wiley who have given unstinting support.

References

Bucks RS, Ashworth Dl, Wilcock GK, Siefried K (1996) Assessment of Activites of Daily Living in Dementia: Development of the Bristol Activities of Daily Living Scales. *Age and Ageing*, 25:113–20.

Cummings J *et al.* (1994) The Neuropsychiatric Inventory. *Neurology*, 44:2308–14.

Folstein MF, Folstein SE, McHugh PR (1975) Mini Mental State: A practical method of grading the cognitive state of patients for the clinician. *Journal of Psychiatric Research*, 12:189–98.

Helmer *et al.* (2003) Epidemiology of severe dementia. In *Severe Dementia Research and Practice in Alzheimer's disease*, Vol. 8. Servier, Paris.

Morris J (1993) The CDR: current version and scoring rules. *Neurology*, 43:2412–3.

Reisberg B, Ferris S, DeLeon M, Crook T (1982) The global deterioration scale (GDS) for the assessment of primary degenerative dementia. *American Journal of Psychiatry*, 139:1136–9.

Alistair Burns, *Manchester*
Bengt Winblad, *Stockholm*

Introductory

1

Assessment and Diagnosis of Severe Dementia

Paul Newhouse and Joseph Lasek

Introduction

When presented with a patient who appears to have moderate to severe cognitive impairment, differential diagnosis is often difficult. The physician may be confronted with a patient in a clinical situation that is not amenable to comprehensive or leisurely diagnostic procedures. Such patients are not typically brought to standard Memory Disorders clinics but may be found in clinical situations that require rapid assessment and management. Typical clinical scenarios for the differential diagnosis and assessment of patients with severe dementia include more complex clinical settings where patient management may be more urgent and becomes the focus of the clinical intervention. Most diagnostic criteria for the differential diagnosis of the various dementias are predicated on mild cases with a clear history of progression from an asymptomatic state. This is often lacking in the patient who presents with severe dementia for clinical ascertainment.

Typical clinical scenarios for the differential diagnosis of severe dementia might include: (1) a clinician is referred a patient who is now behaviourally agitated and/or disruptive. The patient has never been formally diagnosed with a dementia and is now severely impaired prompting admission to long-term care; (2) a patient is referred by a general practitioner who has been managing his/her care but without a formal workup ever having been performed; (3) the specialist is referred a problematic patient for whom severe behavioural disturbances have begun to develop in the community prompting the threat of institutionalisation; (4) a patient presents in the hospital with delirium – as the patient's delirium clears it becomes evident that the patient is severely demented in addition. It is still the case that the vast majority of patients with dementia do not have specific diagnostic workups or evaluation when they are in the mild to moderate stages. Many patients will progress through their entire illness without a formal evaluation or diagnosis, necessitating a diagnostic evaluation in later stages of illness.

For a comprehensive approach to the differential diagnosis of dementia in general, the reader is referred to several excellent reviews in standard textbooks (e.g. Eastley and Wilcock, 2000). For the rapid assessment and diagnosis of severe dementia, the approach recommended here consists of examining six Axes of Evaluation (Table 1). Evaluating these axes will help the clinician get a complete picture of the patient's illness, improve the likelihood of successful diagnosis, and to aid in treatment planning, which is the primary purpose of a diagnostic assessment at this stage of illness. The specific axes are discussed in some detail. We then review some specific features of common dementias that may be helpful in distinguishing more severe cases, and finally structured assessment instruments are reviewed with an eye toward their applicability to the severely impaired patient.

Severe Dementia. Edited by A. Burns and B. Winblad.
Copyright © 2006 John Wiley & Sons, Ltd.   ISBN 0-470-01054-1

Table 1.   Axes of Evaluation for Severe Dementia

Historical
Cognitive
Motor
Behavioural
Functional
Medical

Axes of evaluation
Axis of evaluation: historical
Aspects of the history of the disorder, if obtainable, may provide significant clues to the patient's underlying diagnosis or diagnoses. These include the length of illness, if known, the time from first onset of cognitive and/or behavioural impairment to the present time, and characteristics of the patient's course of illness. Potential types of illness course include steady deterioration, step-wise deterioration with periods of stabilisation, periods of worsening and then improvement, and whether particular medical or historical events are temporally related to alterations in the severity of the disorder or specific symptomatology (Eastley and Wilcock, 2000). Families commonly underestimate the length of illness and multiple informants are best to corroborate and correct the history. Certain structured instruments discussed later in the chapter may be particularly helpful in obtaining information from multiple informants.

The course of associated features discussed below is particularly important in discerning the particular underlying illness. For example, did behaviour or memory problems begin to occur first? If motor problems developed, did they precede or follow the memory disorder? If language problems became prominent, what was the temporal relationship between the development of language difficulties and other cognitive impairments such as learning and memory deficits? For example, the development of behavioural disturbances prior to the recognition by informants of significant learning and memory or language deficits may tend to suggest a fronto-temporal dementia as the primary underlying cause (Perry and Hodges, 2000).

The history of any response to treatment may be helpful. If the patient has been exposed to an acetylcholinesterase inhibitor, whether the patient responded with stabilisation versus a relentless deterioration may be helpful in understanding whether there is an underlying cholinergic deficit. Cognitive stabilisation, particularly if confirmed by cognitive testing scores, may tend to suggest cholinergic pathology which is particularly characteristic of Alzheimer's disease, Lewy body dementia, and/or vascular dementia. Lack of response to cholinergic agonist drugs, particularly taken together with early onset of behavioural disturbances, may suggest non-Alzheimer pathology such as Pick's disease or other types of fronto-temporal dementia.

If behavioural symptoms and disturbances have developed as part of the patient's course of illness, the particular characteristics and historical trajectory may be helpful in ascertaining the nature of the underlying pathology. Affective disturbances, the development of severe anxiety, impairment of insight and judgement and the development of psychosis all have specific implications for particular diagnostic entities. For example, the early development of visual hallucinations in the context of relatively mild learning and memory impairment may be particularly suggestive of Lewy body dementia (McKeith, 2000). Disinhibited behaviour, odd obsessions, and early impairment of insight and judgement all may be consistent with Pick's disease or other fronto-temporal dementias (De Deyn, Engelborghs *et al.*, 2005). Affective disturbances may be particularly common early in the course of vascular dementia (Reed and Goetz, 2004).

Axis of evaluation: cognitive

Many patients who present for evaluation with severe dementia may have such severe deficits that full cognitive assessment will be difficult or impossible, at least with standard instruments. As with behaviour, the history of a cognitive deficit development may be very helpful if there is a knowledgeable informant. For example, the development of early language dysfunction may be suggestive of primary progressive aphasia (Harvey, Tyrrell *et al.*, 2000), whereas early loss of verbal declarative memory is particularly characteristic of Alzheimer's disease (Walker, Meares *et al.*, 2005). It would be highly unusual for procedural memory skills to be the earliest and/or primary cognitive symptom in a patient with Alzheimer's disease. Orientation difficulties and navigational impairments are also quite characteristic of Alzheimer's disease and would be commonly cited as part of the patient's history. Whether cognitive impairment developed abruptly or gradually is often useful. If the history is consistent with an abrupt onset of cognitive difficulties a particular medical event should be sought, such as the occurrence of surgery, evidence of a cerebral vascular event, etc. The particular type of course of cognitive impairment should be ascertained if possible. If the cognitive course is found to be staccato or punctuated, this may be more suggestive of underlying vascular pathology. Also characteristic of vascular impairments are periods of cognitive improvement. This may also occur following a particular event such as a hypoxic episode secondary to surgery, etc. Periods of improvement are extremely unlikely to be consistent with Alzheimer's disease unless the improvement is secondary to medication.

Attention to particular cognitive domains is helpful in ascertaining a cognitive profile. There has been significant research focusing on the particular cognitive profiles characteristic of early dementia patients with a variety of different underlying neuropathology. There have been relatively few or no studies of the characteristics of these cognitive domains in late-stage dementia. Nonetheless, careful characterisation of impairments in a variety of domains may be very helpful.

Language impairments may be one of the most valuable features in the later-stage dementia patient to help the clinician make a diagnostic assessment. The characteristics of the particular language dysfunction, if present, can be helpful. Does the patient have an anomia or fluent aphasia versus a non-fluent aphasia? Is echolalia present, suggesting frontal lobe pathology? Stereotypic phrases, especially repetitive, are also characteristic of patients with Pick's disease. Coarsening of the patient's language, the use of expletives or other language not characteristic of the premorbid personality of the patient may be also seen in disorders with impaired frontal functioning. Fluent aphasias are particularly characteristic of Alzheimer's disease (Kirshner, 1994). Loss of language functioning without prominent learning and memory impairments may suggest specific syndromes such as primary progressive aphasia (Kirshner, Tanridag *et al.*, 1987).

Attention, learning and memory

Before considering the assessment of these cognitive domains, the clinician must ensure that the patient's hearing and vision are optimised. Poor sensory input will make patients appear more impaired than they actually are and may contribute to the appearance of severe cognitive impairment when in fact such impairment does not exist or at least is much milder than would be the case if not for sensory loss. This can be very difficult to ascertain in the severely demented patient and may contribute significantly to the overall cognitive picture. The use of hearing aids and glasses and correction of very poor vision or hearing to the extent possible may produce significant improvements in cognitive performance.

Particular impairment of attention may be an indication of delirium, especially if it appears to be the primary cognitive symptom (Rabinowitz, Murphy *et al.*, 2003). Delirium should be suspected as a primary problem if the patient is unable to attend to the examiner or if behavioural agitation is so severe as to preclude assessment. Large doses of psychotropic drugs will render an assessment of the patient's particular cognitive impairments difficult or impossible owing to attentional impairment and must be accounted for in the clinical assessment. Specific defects in spatial attention, for example, left hemi-spatial neglect, may point to lesions secondary to vascular dementia (e.g. right parietal CVA) (Erkinjuntti, 2000). Assessment of hemi-spatial neglect or spatial attentional impairments must be done only after the clinician satisfies him- or herself that the patient's visual fields are intact.

Impairment of episodic memory is characteristic of medial temporal lobe-related dementias such as Alzheimer's, Lewy body dementia and vascular dementia. If such impairment is not present, consider fronto-temporal dementia, Pick's disease, and/or specific vascular lesions. Praxis and motor skill loss are generally associated with cortical dementia such as Alzheimer's disease and frontal lobe or fronto-temporal dementias (Perry and Hodges, 2000). If these functions are not lost then this may suggest subcortical disorders such as AIDS dementia, Huntington's disease, etc. (Eastley and Wilcock, 2000).

Loss of recognition, particularly of loved ones is a cortical sign, suggestive of Alzheimer's or vascular dementia. Impairments of orientation to time, place or person are particularly characteristic of cortical dementias and are unlikely to be seen in subcortical dementias such as Huntington's disease or Parkinson's disease (Chua and Chiu, 2000).

Axis of evaluation: motor

The presence of a motor disorder, either hyper- or hypokinetic, particularly if it began relatively early in the course of the patient's illness is strongly suggestive of underlying subcortical pathology (Assal and Cummings, 1994).

Hypokinetic, i.e. bradykinesia or Parkinsonian-type, symptoms suggest Parkinson's disease, multisystem atrophy, cortical basal degeneration, depression-associated dementia, progressive supranuclear palsy or AIDS. Hyperkinetic motor problems including chorea and myoclonus are particularly suggestive of Huntington's disease, Wilson's disease, or rarely Creutzfeldt–Jakob disease (Assal and Cummings, 1994). Gait impairment or abnormalities may be particularly characteristic of normopressure hydrocephalus (along with other associated features). Parkinson's disease, multisystem atrophy, cortico-basal degeneration and progressive supranuclear palsy all have characteristic gait impairments which are often associated with a history of falls relatively early in the course of the patient's illness.

Patients with cortical dementia will develop subcortical motor symptoms in some cases. For example, from 10% to 80% of patients (depending on the study) with Alzheimer's disease will develop some evidence of extrapyramidal system dysfunction at some point in their illness (Corey-Bloom, 2000). Stereotypic or compulsive movements or ritualistic motor behaviour may suggest fronto-temporal or frontal lobe dementia. Examples might include repetitive picking at the skin of the patient or other repetitive motor movements.

Some apparent motor dysfunction may in fact, represent difficulty in translating intention to movement. Such impairments represent an apraxia rather than a true movement disorder or impairment and may be more commonly seen in patients with cortical dementia such as Alzheimer's disease. Development of extrapyramidal signs and symptoms early in the course of dementia may lead to a diagnosis of Lewy body dementia; conversely late-appearing extrapyramidal dysfunction may suggest the development of secondary Parkinsonism, etc., which can be unrelated to the primary underlying diagnosis of cortical dementia.

Axis of evaluation: behavioural

Of all the axes, behavioural manifestations of severe dementia may be the most helpful in differentiating the various illnesses. While all of the dementias can produce behavioural disturbances, some particular behavioural signs and symptoms are more characteristic of certain disorders (see Chapter 5 in this volume).

As has been suggested earlier, the development of severe behavioural pathology prior to the onset of significant learning and memory impairments is particularly characteristic of frontal lobe and/or fronto-temporal dementias (Binetti, Growdon *et al.*, 1998; Levy, Miller *et al.*, 1998). Such behavioural disturbances are often mistaken for other psychiatric illnesses and are often misdiagnosed, even quite late in the disease process, unless significant learning impairment has become manifest. Patients may be diagnosed as hypomanic if they exhibit poor judgement, there may be a diagnosis of obsessive-compulsive disorder entertained if the patient shows prominent obsessive-compulsive symptoms, and perhaps most commonly a misdiagnosis of major depression may be made if the patient shows increasing apathy and decline in self-care. In frontal or fronto-temporal dementias these types of behavioural abnormalities will often progress to include bizarre obsessions and compulsions, hyper-orality, counting rituals, eating and food ritualistic behaviour, etc. (Binetti, Growdon *et al.*, 1998). The development of Klüver–Bucy type symptoms may occur late in the disorder and may be a helpful differential diagnostic feature (Levy, Miller *et al.*, 1998), for example placing inedible objects in the mouth.

The development of psychotic symptoms is also helpful diagnostically. The most common associated psychotic symptom may be paranoid ideation or delusions, which appears to be connected to memory loss. Occasionally the patient's course may be characterised by the apparent development of late-life delusional disorder prior to a more severe dementia becoming manifest. Such development of paranoid delusions or ideation is thought to be more characteristically associated with Alzheimer's disease and/or vascular dementia (Mirea and Cummings, 2000).

Early onset of psychosis by history, particularly if the symptoms include visual hallucinations may indicate Lewy body dementia (McKeith, 2000; Ballard, O'Brien *et al.*, 2001). Visual hallucinations are often of people or animate creatures. While this may be associated particularly with Lewy body dementia, such hallucinatory experiences may be seen in later or severe stages in Alzheimer's disease and vascular dementia (Ballard, O'Brien *et al.*, 2001). Such visual hallucinations need to be distinguished from hallucinosis without concomitant delusions which may be seen in such syndromes and such disorders as Charles Bonnet Syndrome, related to macular degeneration (Ffytche, 2005). Auditory hallucinations are somewhat rarer and may be initially musical in nature, particularly associated with hearing loss and therefore may be essentially cases of auditory Charles Bonnet Syndrome (Wengel, Burke *et al.*, 1989).

Affective disturbances
While full depressive illness (e.g. major depressive disorder) is relatively rare in patients with underlying dementia, depressive symptoms are common in Alzheimer's disease and other cortical and subcortical dementias. It is not unusual for patients with fairly severe frontal lobe syndromes to be mistaken for depression especially with patients who show decline in self-care and loss of functioning. Antidepressant treatment and even electroconvulsive therapy has been used in a generally futile attempt to improve the patient's symptoms. Manic symptoms are perhaps less common early in the course of the patient's illness but if they occur are particularly associated with frontal lobe dementia. Later, in severe dementia, manic-like agitation is common, particularly in Alzheimer's disease and mixed Alzheimer's/vascular dementias but less so in frontal lobe dementia or fronto-temporal dementia and subcortical disorders (Neary, 2000).

Apathy, or the lack of goal-directed behaviour is often mistaken for depression in patients with severe dementia but is not identical. The development of profound apathy may be one of the most common behavioural symptoms and is particularly related to the deterioration of certain frontal circuits (Cummings, 2000). The early development of profound apathy in patients may be helpful in distinguishing cortical from subcortical disorders. It is important not to mistake apathy for hypokinesia. Overall mood dysregulation may be more frequent as dementia progresses, at least through the mid stages. Late stages of dementia tend to show lesser affective disturbances.

Anxiety/agitation

The development of anxiety symptoms in the moderately to severely demented patient is generally non-specific and can occur in many types of cortical dementias (Teri, Larson *et al.*, 1988). Anxiety tends to correlate with fear or psychosis in moderately demented patients (especially paranoia) but the correlation in severely demented patients is less clear. Motor restlessness can sometimes be mistaken for anxiety as well as the inverse. Obsessive-compulsive behaviours, particularly repetitive ritualistic behaviours, are particularly characteristic of frontal lobe dementias or fronto-temporal dementias (Snowden, Neary *et al.*, 2002). Such ritualistic behaviour is often of a bizarre nature and includes features such as counting rituals, odd oral habits, or ritualistic oral behaviour as well as odd and bizarre eating habits. In Alzheimer's disease, patients may develop significant apraxia associated with eating but are less likely to develop odd, obsessive, or ritualistic eating behaviours.

Axis of evaluation: functional

Changes in functional abilities may provide clues to the underlying diagnosis. Functional abilities can be assessed by a variety of instruments including ADL (Activities of Daily Living) scales, physical self-maintenance scales, and newer instruments such as the Older Adult Behavior Checklist (OABCL) (Achenbach, Newhouse *et al.*, 2004). However the use of such instruments has not been systematically tested diagnostically in severe dementia, thus particular profiles are not yet fully characterised. In general, loss of function is closely tied to overall cognitive impairment. More specifically, cognitive deficits and apraxias will lead to particular functional impairments. Loss of functional abilities that depend on specific cognitive domains will be affected by cognitive loss and/or behavioural disturbances.

In frontal lobe dementia or fronto-temporal dementia loss of drive or motivation to perform tasks may be present even when the patient retains the ability to perform the task (Neary, 2000). Obsessive rituals may preclude task accomplishment in frontal lobe dementia. In Parkinson's disease and other subcortical dementias executive dysfunction (probably from damage to frontal-striatal circuits) may lead to difficulty in organising and sequencing task performance (Cummings, 1988). For example, a patient with Parkinson's disease and dementia was able to describe how to fix a door but took so long to organise the tools necessary, that his ability to actually complete the task was severely impaired.

In contrast, loss of specific motor skills, i.e. dyspraxias, are particularly characteristic of cortical dementias such as Alzheimer's disease and mixed Alzheimer's disease/vascular states (Sjögren, Wallin *et al.*, 1994).

Axis of evaluation: medical

Medical evaluation will provide ancillary clues or direct confirmation of the underlying diagnosis. In patients with either cortical or subcortical dementias the presence of peripheral vascular disease, diabetes or organ-related vascular disorders such as atherosclerotic cardiovascular disease or vascular-related renal impairment will be strongly suggestive of vascular dementia or mixed Alzheimer's disease–vascular dementia. In the younger patient rapid onset of severe dementia may suggest an infectious cause such as AIDS, Creutzfeldt–Jakob disease, a neoplastic process such as cerebral lymphoma, or unusual metabolic derangements. Head trauma and/or anoxia may initiate cognitive dysfunction that may be stable or progressive and may lead to a very severely demented patient over a relatively short period of time secondary to haematoma formation, hydrocephalus, and perhaps progressive damage (Eastley and Wilcock, 2000).

In alcoholism, Wernicke's encephalopathy may present abruptly and may have persisting cognitive deficits especially in patients with additional cerebral pathology or continued alcohol consumption (so-called 'alcoholic dementia') (Joyce, 2000).

Patients who meet criteria for major depressive disorder who have a history of recurrent affective disorders appear to be at higher risk for the development of dementia. The presence of depression in the mildly demented patient may reproduce a picture of severe dementia (double disability) but may be at least partially reversible (Emery and Oxman, 1994). There continues to be controversy as to whether patients with late-onset psychosis such as late-onset schizophrenia or delusional disorder do progress to dementia, but patients with a history of schizophrenia or psychotic disorder will tend to show more severe deficits if psychotic symptoms are present (Howard and Almeida, 2000). Schizophrenia itself produces cognitive impairment but it does not appear to be progressive. Thus severe dementia symptoms or signs in a patient with a history of schizophrenia or another chronic psychotic disorder are likely to be secondary to other underlying cerebral pathologies rather than the major psychiatric illness (Sachdev and Reutens, 1994).

Aspects of severe dementia in common dementia disorders

There are many potential causes of severe dementia (Table 2). The reader is referred to standard textbooks on dementia for a fuller discussion all of these disorders. Whether they can be accurately distinguished at late stages of severe dementia is unclear. We discuss here four major diagnostic subgroups for which substantial clinical information is available on the severe stages and for which there is evidence that remaining clinical, behavioural, and biomedical characteristics may help in diagnostic separation.

Vascular dementia/mixed vascular dementia–Alzheimer's disease
Clinical description

Vascular dementia is usually thought to result from any combination of multiple infarcts secondary to large and small artery vessel disease, cardiac embolic events, and intracranial haemorrhages (Pirttilä, Erkinjuntti *et al.*, 1994). Also included are arteriopathies, small vessel disease leading to ischaemic white matter disease, etc. Vascular dementia, therefore, reflects the interactions between vascular lesions, risk factors, host factors and cognition (Erkinjuntti, 2000). So-called cortical vascular dementia or traditionally called multi-infarct dementia may include classical cortical symptoms such as aphasia, apraxia, agnosia, visuospatial impairment, and executive dysfunction and can be seen in a variety of combinations and courses. The course is occasionally characterised by abrupt onset and fluctuating course with periods of stability and even occasional improvement. Associated symptoms that may aid in diagnosis include focal neurological symptoms and signs including upper motor neuron signs and gait impairment.

So-called strategic infarct dementias may be related to particular infarcts in critical areas such as the thalamus (Kirshner, 1994). Severe memory impairment, fluctuating consciousness, and confusion are observed in many patients and may be confused with delirium (Rabinowitz, Murphy *et al.*, 2003). Apathy, perseveration and mild dysphasia may also be characteristic of strategic infarct dementia (Pirttilä, Erkinjuntti *et al.*, 1994).

Subcortical vascular dementia represents a more homogeneous subgroup than other vascular dementia subtypes (Erkinjuntti, 1987). The cognitive syndrome of subcortical vascular dementia is characterised by a dysexecutive syndrome with slowed information processing. The memory deficit in subcortical vascular dementia is said to be different from that seen in Alzheimer's disease with less episodic memory dysfunction (Assal and Cummings, 1994; Erkinjuntti, 2000; Schmidtke and Hüll, 2002). The course is often characterised by a slow, less abrupt onset with slow progression. In cortical vascular dementia or so-called multi-infarct dementia, the course is traditionally considered stepwise but this may be difficult to discern in practice. Periods of stabilisation and even improvement support the diagnosis of cortical vascular dementia. Patients with small vessel disease may have a more insidious course that is more gradually progressive. In combination

Table 2. Causes of severe dementias

Potentially reversible/arrestable dementias and exacerbating states

Psychiatric
  delirium
  depression
  schizophrenia
  cancer syndrome
  malingering

Toxic
  drugs
  alcohol and Wernicke–Korsakoff syndrome
  chemical poisoning (heavy metals
    [lead, manganese, mercury, arsenic],
    organic compounds, CO)
  substance-induced persisting dementia

Metabolic
  azotaemia
  hyponatraemia
  volume depletion
  hypo/hyperglycaemia
  hepatic encephalopathy
  hypothyroidism
  hyperparathyroidism
  Addison's disease
  Cushing syndrome
  Wilson's disease
  acute intermittent porphyria
  metachromatic a leukodystrophy
  adrenoleukodystrophy
  adult polyglucosan body disease
  ceroid lipofuscinosis (Kopf's disease)
  Leigh's disease
  Hallervorden–Spatz syndrome
  choreoacanthocytosis

Inflammatory
  collagen vascular disease
    Bechet syndrome
    Sjögren syndrome

systemic lupus erythematosus
vasculitides
  granulomatous angiitis
  lymphomatoid granulomatosis
  polyarteritis nodosa
  Wagener's granulomatosis

Anoxic
  anaemia
  congestive heart failure
  chronic obstructive pulmonary disease

Vitamin deficiencies (B12, folic acid, thiamine, niacin)

Vascular
  ischaemic or haemorrhagic stroke, ischaemic/hypoxic brain lesions

Trauma
  acute or chronic subdural haematoma
  post-concussion syndrome
  dementia pugilistica

Infections
  bacterial: meningitis, encephalitis, brain abscess
  viral: HIV and opportunistic infections, meningitis/encephalitis, HSV, progressive multifocal leukoencephalopathy, encephalitis lethargica (sleeping sickness), subacute sclerosing panencephalitis
  spirochaetal: neurosyphilis, Lyme disease
  fungal: meningitis, encephalitis, brain abscess
  prion: Subacute spongiform encephalopathy, CJD, nvCJD

Neoplasm
  primary or metastatic, paraneoplastic syndromes

Irreversible dementias

cerebral autosomal dominant arteriopathy
  with subcortical infarcts and
  leukoencephalopathy (CADASIL)
cerebral amyloid angiopathy
Binswanger's disease
Cortical dementias
  Alzheimer's disease
  Mixed dementia
  Dementia with Lewy bodies
  Fronto-temporal dementia (Pick's disease)

primary progressive aphasia
Subcortical dementias
  Huntington's disease
  progressive supranuclear palsy
  Parkinson's disease
  corticobasal degeneration
  multiple sclerosis
Vascular dementia
  large vessel or small vessel stroke
  multiple lacunar infarcts

with the above cognitive features, other symptoms suggestive of vascular dementia include gait disturbance, unsteadiness and falls, urinary frequency, mood impairment, and personality changes (Pirttilä, Erkinjuntti *et al.*, 1994; Erkinjuntti, 2000). While none of these signs and symptoms is specific for vascular dementia, the combination, especially with a history of associated vascular pathology in non-CNS tissues or a known specific CNS event is highly suggestive.

Neuroimaging may be helpful even in the severe patient. Bilateral lesions seen on CT or MRI, multiple lesions, deep white matter pathology, lesions located in the dominant hemisphere and limbic structures all are consistent with vascular dementia (Varma, Adams *et al.*, 2002).

In moderate to severe dementia patients with vascular dementia, abrupt worsening of cognition, if not due to a transient disorder such as infection, may well be secondary to new-onset vascular lesions. As patients with other dementias progress, the likelihood of a vascular pathology mixed with the primary underlying disorder increases.

Psychiatric and behavioural disturbances   Disinhibited behaviour, especially sexually disinhibited or aggressive behaviour disturbances, may be more common in vascular dementia, consistent with damaged frontal and supraorbital circuits (Erkinjuntti, 2000). Affective disturbances, including psychomotor retardation, emotional bluntness, emotional lability, and incontinence, are also generally believed to be more common in vascular dementia and may aid in the differential diagnosis even in the severely impaired patient.

Alzheimer's disease
Clinical description
Cognitive   In severe Alzheimer's disease (AD), all cognitive functions are markedly impaired. At this stage, all memory systems are affected. Episodic memory, recollection of one's past, semantic and linguistic memory, and general knowledge, are profoundly impaired. Short-term memory, the ability to store and recollect a limited number of items within a very limited time delay, is relatively preserved, although more impaired than in earlier stages of the disease. Some aspects of implicit memory, those not involved in semantic processing, may be relatively spared in severe dementia. Emotional signals may be received and reciprocated even after language function has largely been lost. Over-learned skills, habits and expression of memory are relatively spared until the very late stages of the disease (Corey-Bloom 2000).

As dementia advances, language is greatly affected with loss of fluency, echolalia, perseveration or verbal stereotypies, and nonverbal utterances. In contrast, auditory discrimination and repetition may be spared until relatively late in the course of illness. Mutism may ultimately occur, but this is less common. The language disorder of severe dementia differs from global aphasia in that demented patients are generally unable to use nonverbal communication to supplement their verbal deficits (Kirshner, 1994).

Other domains of cognition such as executive function, praxis and visuospatial behaviour are very severely impaired in later stages and are difficult to assess in most instances.

Psychiatric and behavioural disturbances   These may be conceptualised as falling into three groups: psychomotor disturbances (pacing and agitation); psychiatric disturbances (hallucinations, delusions, depression, anxiety); behavioural disturbances (aggressiveness, inappropriate verbalisation and incontinence).

Pathological, inappropriate pacing has prevalence rates in late stage Alzheimer's disease anywhere from 10% to 61% (Merriam, Aronson *et al.*, 1988; Teri, Larson *et al.*, 1988; Mirea and Cummings, 2000). Patients may be attempting to return home or wandering without a precise goal. One must consider akathisia related to side effects of medication as a possibly related factor. Studies of agitation show prevalence rates anywhere from 18% to 75% (Eastwood and Reisberg, 1996;

Verny *et al.*, 1998). The wide variability in prevalence may be accounted for by lack of clear criteria as to what constitutes agitation. Agitation may be driven by anxiety and mild–moderate dementia and by psychosis in moderate–severe dementia (Mirea and Cummings, 2000).

Hallucinations may occur on average in 28% of cases (Wragg and Jeste, 1989). It may be difficult to assess hallucinations in more severely demented patients because of the inability to verbally report them. There may be a relationship between visual hallucinations and visual acuity. Delusions are relatively common during the course of severe dementia with frequencies reported between 13% and 73% (Binetti, Padovani *et al.*, 1995). Delusions tend to commonly be paranoid or persecutory in nature. As with hallucinations, verbal reporting of delusions may decrease as dementia progresses (Corey-Bloom, 2000; Mirea and Cummings, 2000).

Depression prevalence ranges between 17% and 35% in severe dementia, though higher rates have been reported (Lazarus, Newton *et al.* 1987; Teri, Larson *et al.*, 1988; Wragg and Jeste, 1989; Zubenko, 1994; Lebert, Pasquier *et al.*, 1996). Depression may have an atypical presentation in the severely demented with sleep changes, aggressiveness, irritability or agitation. Scales such as the Dementia Mood Assessment Scale (Sunderland, Alterman *et al.*, 1988) may be useful in assessing depression in severe dementia. Anxiety may also be found in patients with dementia but may be difficult to assess in severely ill people who lack verbal expression.

Aggressiveness toward others is a behaviour seen in severe Alzheimer's disease that is poorly tolerated by family and staff members and nursing homes. Its frequency has been estimated to be between 30% and 55% (Patel and Hope, 1993). Various authors have found that a correlation exists with depression, hallucinations and delusions, loss of self-care, impaired verbal skills, and limited self-expression.

Screaming episodes are a troublesome aspect of severe dementia, and is estimated to occur in up to 25% of cases (Eastwood, 1994). Studies have shown them to be associated with the most severe cases of dementia and may be associated with pain and discomfort or hallucinations. Others have found associations with impairment in ADLs, multiple medical problems, physical restraints and taking psychotropic medications. Patients who scream have more hearing impairment, cognitive impairment, and greater dependency in daily living compared to patients who can express themselves verbally. Studies have suggested that up to a quarter of patients who scream frequently die within six months (Sloane, Davidson *et al.*, 1999).

While incontinence is found in earlier stages in fronto-temporal dementia and dementia with Lewy bodies, approximately 25% of patients with severe Alzheimer's suffer from incontinence.

Motor disorders and neurological signs   In patients with Alzheimer's, prevalence of extrapyramidal signs has been estimated between 23% and 65% of patients (Franssen, Kluger *et al.*, 1993). Parkinsonism has been found to be related to greater severity of dementia and presence of primitive reflexes. Parkinsonian signs and symptoms are usually of moderate intensity with predominance of akinesia over tremor and are inversely correlated with Mini Mental State Examination (MMSE) scores.

The percentage of patients with severe dementia who are confined to bed ranges from 20% to 41% and contractures are present in 16% of cases (Auer, Sclan *et al.*, 1994). Myoclonus has been estimated to occur in 10% of cases and is believed to be related to severe dementia (Mayeux, Stern *et al.*, 1985). Myoclonus in severe dementia must be differentiated from transient, reversible symptoms seen in conditions which affect global cerebral function such as metabolic disorders or infections. Studies have found that falls occur in 29% to 44% of patients with severe dementia (Teri, Larson *et al.*, 1988; Ousset, Vellas *et al.*, 1994; Vellas, Gillette-Guyonnet *et al.*, 2000). Significant relationships between frequency of falls and severity of dementia have also been noted.

Severe dementia with Lewy bodies

Overview

Dementia with Lewy bodies (DLB) is the second most common neurodegenerative dementia in older people, accounting for 10–15% cases at autopsy resulting from an abnormal aggregation of the synaptic protein alpha-synuclein (McKeith, 1996). Diagnosing DLB is of clinical importance because patients with this affliction tend to respond quite well to cholinesterase inhibitors, but they are extremely sensitive to the parkinsonian side effects of neuroleptic medications (Ballard, Grace *et al.*, 1998). DLB has been known by several names in the past and shares clinical and pathophysiological similarities with dementia associated with Parkinson's disease (PDD). A 12-month period has been arbitrarily assigned to discriminate DLB from PDD; onset of dementia within 12 months of onset of Parkinsonism qualifies for a diagnosis of DLB, after 12 months meets criteria for PDD. These criteria are arbitrary, however, and the presentations share more similarities than differences.

Clinical features

Cognitive The cognitive presentation typically consists of recurrent, episodic confusion in the context of gradual progressive decline (McKeith, 2000). There is a combination of cortical and subcortical impairment with attentional deficits and profound fronto-subcortical and visuospatial dysfunction. These symptoms help distinguish early DLB from AD, though in later stages of DLB, more global dysfunction makes these comparisons in neuropsychological function more difficult. Levels of attention and alertness may fluctuate over minutes, hours or days in up to 75% of individuals.

Psychiatric The common psychiatric manifestations of DLB, including visual hallucinations, delusions, apathy, depression and anxiety, tend to appear early in the course of the illness and persist into more advanced stages. The visual hallucinations (VH) are similar to those seen in PD and Charles Bonnet syndrome. They are vivid, colourful and three-dimensional, and are usually mute images of animate objects provoking emotions ranging from fear to amusement to indifference. Relative insight into the unreality of these hallucinations is usually maintained after the episode is over. Their persistence helps discriminate them from VH seen in other dementias or delirium. They occur in 46% of DLB cases during the course of illness. Of clinical note, some investigators have noted that the presence of visual hallucinations may predict a better response to cholinesterase inhibitors (Wesnes, 2002). Delusions are seen in 65% of cases at some point in their illness. The quality of delusions is usually complex and bizarre and based on hallucinatory content. This contrasts with blander and less well-formed delusions usually seen in AD. Depression is seen in up to half of DLB cases and is sufficiently more common than in AD to be considered an aid in differential diagnosis.

Neurological Extrapyramidal signs (EPS) are present in 25–50% of DLB patients at time of diagnosis and most will develop these signs by the late stages of the illness. Parkinsonism may not be present in all cases, however, and autopsy cases confirm that up to 25% of patients with DLB had no recorded EPS (McKeith, 2000). The pattern of EPS in DLB and PDD are different from those generally seen in Parkinson's disease without dementia. In DLB, there is an axial pattern with more postural instability, gait difficulty and facial flatness with fewer tremors. This is consistent with more non-dopaminergic neuronal involvement than is seen in Parkinson's without dementia.

Sleep Rarely seen in AD, REM sleep disorders with vivid and frightening dreams and simple or complex motor behaviour is frequently seen in DLB. Other sleep disorders seen in DLB include REM sleep behaviour disorder, daytime somnolence and cataplexy; as such this may resemble primary narcolepsy (Arnulf, 2000).

Autonomic dysfunction   Orthostatic hypotension and carotid-sinus hypersensitivity are more common in DLB than in AD. DLB often presents with symptoms of dizziness, pre-syncope, syncope and falls. Urinary incontinence is also seen earlier in the course than is seen in AD.

Differential diagnosis   Main differential diagnoses are AD, vascular dementia, PDD, atypical parkinsonian syndromes including progressive supranuclear palsy (PSP), multiple system atrophy and cortico-basal degeneration and Creutzfeldt–Jakob disease. Retrospective and prospective studies have looked at predictive accuracy of clinical criteria and found variable sensitivity but generally high specificity (McKeith, Galasko *et al.*, 1996; McKeith, 2000).

Investigations   EEG may show early slowing, epoch-by-epoch fluctuation and transient temporal slowing. On MRI, there is generally preservation of hippocampal and medial temporal lobe volume. SPECT shows occipital hypoperfusion and dopaminergic SPECT shows transporter loss in the caudate and putamen. A sensitivity of 83% and specificity of 100% has been reported for SPECT when compared to autopsy in one study (Varma, Adams *et al.*, 2002; Walker, 2002).

Severe fronto-temporal dementia
Clinical features
Fronto-temporal dementia is a form of primary degenerative dementia, affecting people in middle-age, accounting for up to 20% of cases. Dementia onset usually occurs between 45 and 65 years of age though some cases have been reported before age 30 as well as in the elderly. There is an equal incidence in men and women. The mean duration of illnesses is eight years, ranging from two to 20 years, and a family history of dementia is present in about half of cases (Binetti, Growdon *et al.*, 1998; Levy, Miller *et al.*, 1998).

While functions of perception, spatial skills, praxis and memory are relatively preserved, there is an early and profound disruption in character and social conduct. Current consensus diagnostic criteria include several behavioural features. Core features include insidious onset and gradual progression, early decline in social and personal conduct, early impairment in regulation of personal conduct, early emotional blunting and early loss of insight. Worsening social conduct includes poor interpersonal etiquette, tactlessness, and disinhibition. Impairment in regulation of personal conduct includes passivity as well as overactivity, pacing, and wandering. Emotional blunting includes difficulty in expressing primary emotions such as happiness, sadness, and fear as well as social emotions such as embarrassment and empathy. Worsening insight includes disruption in cognitive awareness of symptoms as well as emotional unawareness with lack of concern or distress even in the face of difficulty.

Supportive features of a diagnosis of fronto-temporal dementia include behavioural features, speech and language alterations, physical signs and salient investigational data. Specific patterns of deficits have been found to distinguish fronto-temporal dementia from Alzheimer's disease, but the applicability of these criteria to severe dementia is uncertain (Perry and Hodges, 2000; Grossi, Fragassi *et al.*, 2002; De Deyn, Engelborghs *et al.*, 2005).

Cognitive and behavioural problems   There is a notable decline in personal hygiene and grooming noted early on in the disorder that progresses as patients become more severely demented. Frontal lobe deficits lead to mental concreteness and inflexibility as well as attentional problems, distractibility, and impersistence. Dietary changes include overeating and preference for sweet food. Perseverative and stereotyped behaviours include simple repetitive behaviours such as humming, head-rubbing, and toe-tapping as well as more complex behavioural routines. These behaviours might include compulsive behaviours such as clock-watching, adhering to fixed routines, or superstitious rituals. Visual perception is relatively spared with preserved visual recognition, naming of pictures, and use of objects. However, utilisation behaviour may be observed. This is a term coined to represent stimulus-induced behaviour in which patients touch and utilise objects in their visual fields when such use is inappropriate, e.g. drinking from an empty cup (Levy, Miller *et al.*, 1998). While patients have memory impairment, this impairment may be improved with more direct questioning and cues and being given multiple choices.

Speech and language problems   Multiple abnormalities in speech and language occur, including lack of spontaneity of speech as well as pressure of speech. Echolalia and perseveration may be featured prominently. Verbal stereotypies include repeated words, phrases or more complex themes. As dementia progresses into the more severe stages, mutism ultimately occurs. While language is severely affected later in the illness, reading aloud may be preserved, though comprehension may be diminished (Kirshner, 1994).

Physical signs   While primitive reflexes are usually present, other neurological signs may be relatively absent early on in the disease. Parkinsonian signs of akinesia, tremor, and rigidity develop as the disease progresses and may become severe (Neary, Snowden *et al.*, 1998; Hodges, 2000; Neary, 2000). Hypotension and labile blood pressure may be present and, in conjunction with other neurological dysfunction, may increase risk of falls. Urinary incontinence may also be a sign of more severe illness.

Investigations   Routine EEG is almost always normal. Brain imaging may show abnormalities and atrophy in the fronto-temporal areas bilaterally, but sometimes asymmetrically. MRI is more sensitive than CT. Functional imaging such as SPECT scans are most sensitive to changes (Varma, Adams *et al.*, 2002). Neuropsychological testing reveals significant impairment on frontal lobe tests without marked amnesia, aphasia or visuospatial disturbances (Slachevsky, Villalpando *et al.*, 2004).

Subtypes of fronto-temporal dementia   Several subtypes have been identified that are believed to be related to regional differences in pathological involvement (Neary, 2000). Patients with prominent disinhibition, purposeless overactivity, distractibility, social inappropriateness and lack of concern have pathological changes in orbitofrontal and anterior temporal cortex. Patients on the other end of the spectrum display apathy, lack of volition, mental rigidity and perseveration. These patients tend to have pathological changes throughout the frontal lobes and the dorsolateral frontal cortex. Finally, there is a subtype characterised by stereotypical, ritualised behaviour with changes in the striatum as well as prominent temporal lobe involvement (Kirshner, 1994).

Differential diagnosis   The most important features in differentiating fronto-temporal dementia from other causes of dementia are the severe changes in character and behaviour noted early in the course of the illness. In comparing fronto-temporal patients with AD patients, the behavioural features of loss of social awareness, hyper-orality, stereotyped and perseverative behaviour, paucity of speech, and preserved spatial orientation best discriminate the two groups with good sensitivity and excellent specificity (Perry and Hodges, 2000). Other studies have verified that dietary changes, repetitive behaviours, generalised blunting of emotions, loss of social emotions, and disordered social behaviour are valuable in differentiating fronto-temporal patients from AD patients and vascular dementia patients.

Assessment instruments – clinical assessment tools

Clinical assessment instruments developed for dementia patients have generally focused on evaluation and tracking of patients in the mild to moderate stages of severity. Only recently have tools been designed or previously developed instruments have been extended to enable utilisation in the severely demented patient. We review instruments here that may be of particular applicability to the clinical assessment, staging, and/or management of patients with severe dementia.

Two tools are commonly used to stage dementia. The Clinical Dementia Rating scale (CDR) and the Global Deterioration Scale (GDS). The CDR is based on caregiver and patient interviews. Although it was not designed initially to be sensitive to severe dementia, an extended version shows correlation with increasing functional impairment, decreased independence and long-term care (Dooneief, Marder et al., 1996). A score of 0 to 5 is given in six different cognitive areas including memory, orientation, judgement and problem-solving, community affairs, home and hobbies and personal care (Heyman, Wilkinson et al., 1987). Ratings consistent with profound (Stage IV) and terminal (Stage V) have been shown to predict shortened survival (Ferris and Yan, 2003).

The GDS system consists of the GDS, the Brief Cognitive Rating Scale (BCRS), and the Functional Assessment Staging (FAST). The GDS is a seven-stage rating system based on clinical, patient, and informant interview (Reisberg, Ferris et al., 1982). The BCRS is a semi-structured clinical assessment to evaluate cognitive parameters such as concentration, recent memory, remote memory, and orientation. The FAST is informant-interview-based and examines five to 10 successive stages through which patients with dementia will pass (Sclan and Reisberg, 1992). This scale may be useful for patients with more severe dementia impairment because Stages VI and VII contain several substages that describe the level of impairment in a specific way (Ferris and Yan, 2003). Usefulness of this scale diagnostically is somewhat unclear.

Cognitive evaluation

As patients with severe dementia are generally too impaired to complete the more typical instruments used at early stages such as the Alzheimer's Disease Assessment Scale – Cognitive subscale (ADAS-Cog), MMSE or other batteries, the Severe Impairment Battery (SIB) was designed to give a way to assess patients below the level of conventional instruments (Schmitt, Ashford et al., 1997). The SIB is a clinician-rated, performance-based evaluation with 40 questions. It describes nine areas of function to assess including social interaction, memory, orientation, language, attention, praxis, visuospatial ability, construction, and orientation. Items are presented as single words or one-step commands combined with gestural cues and can be repeated. The SIB has shown utility in severe dementia patients (MMSE < 10) and has been successfully used in drug treatment trials to show treatment-related improvement (Tariot, Farlow et al., 2004).

Behavioural Disturbances

Several structured interview-based instruments are widely used for behavioural assessment including the Neuropsychiatric Inventory (NPI) and the BEHAVE-AD.

The NPI is based on a clinician interview of the caregiver (Cummings, Mega et al., 1994). The caregiver is asked to rate the frequency and severity of behavioural pathology in 10 domains including delusions, hallucinations, agitation/aggression, dysphoria, anxiety, euphoria, apathy, disinhibition, irritability/lability, and aberrant motor behaviour. In addition, caregivers are asked to assess the impact of each symptom on themselves. A frequency × severity score is then calculated and totals are obtained across all the domains. The NPI has proved to be useful in assessing development of behavioural pathology and in judging the impact of treatment on those problems. A nursing home version is available.

The BEHAVE-AD is also interview-based with the caregiver and is designed to assess behavioural pathology (Reisberg, Auer et al., 1996). Twenty-five symptoms are grouped into seven categories. Recently a frequency rating has been added to the basic scale (Monteiro, Boksay et al., 2001), similar to the NPI.

Functioning

The Alzheimer's Disease Cooperative Study – Activities of Daily Living Scale (ADCS-ADL) uses information from caregivers to rate performance of 19 daily activities. Performance is rated 0–1 or 0–5 depending on the question (Galasko, Bennett et al., 1997). The scale is best utilised for community dwelling patients as questions are not geared to nursing home residents. The Disability Assessment in Dementia (DAD scale) assesses 10 domains of instrumental and basic activities of daily living (Feldman, Gauthier *et al.*, 2001).

Multi-informant caregiver-based assessment

A new approach to dementia assessment is represented by the Older Adult Self-Report (OASR) and the Older Adult Behavior Checklist (OABCL) (Achenbach, Newhouse *et al.*, 2004). These instruments are designed for the caregiver, family members, and other informants to complete about the patient. For milder patients there is a self-completed version (OASR); however, for more severe patients it is presumed that only the informant versions will be utilised (OABCL). This 127-item scale is completed without input from the clinician and requires no clinician involvement except to ensure completion of the forms. It provides multi-informant ratings of function, psychopathology and behaviour. Self-administered in 15–20 minutes, the OABCL obtains informant reports of diverse aspects of adaptive functioning and problems. The OABCL can be utilised by a spouse, partner, family members, friends, caregivers, home health aides, residential staff, and health care providers. The OASR/OABCL are scored on profiles that make it easy to see similarities and differences between self-reports and reports by other people. The profiles display scale scores in relation to gender- and age-specific norms. Clinical staff can score profiles by hand in 5–10 minutes or by computer in about two minutes.

The OABCL produces a comprehensive picture of seven syndrome subscales including anxious/depressed, worries, somatic complaints, thought problems, functional impairment, memory/cognition problems, and irritable/disinhibited. These are factor-analytically derived syndrome subscales based on large elderly normative populations along with elders receiving treatment. Scores are plotted as *t*-scores allowing rapid assessment of normal and abnormal ranges for each syndrome subscale. These allow comparison of self-ratings (in mild cases) and multiple informants for more severe cases.

Preliminary data suggests that the OABCL exhibits excellent correlation with diagnosis of dementia in the Memory Clinic and high correlations with NPI subscales in patients with behavioural disturbances (Newhouse, Brigidi *et al.*, 2004). Though no studies in severe dementia have yet been done, this instrument shows considerable promise as a tool for comprehensive assessment and tracking as well as the effects of treatment. Test/re-test reliability has been excellent and similar instruments have been shown to be sensitive to treatment effects in other populations. Extensive information regarding the utilisation of this scale is now available for research and clinical use (Achenbach, Newhouse *et al.*, 2004).

Conclusion

Despite advances in the understanding of the nature of the various dementias and the availability of sophisticated diagnostic evaluation and pharmacological treatments, many patients will present for management with severe dementia having never been evaluated previously. The diagnosis of such patients can be quite challenging as many of the distinguishing clinical features of the various dementing disorders that may have been present early in the course of the illness have now disappeared and many of the neuropsychological and the biomedical distinguishing characteristics may also no longer be present. Nonetheless, careful attention to the axes of evaluation described here and armed with a knowledge of the clinical characteristics of the major dementia groups, clinicians and investigators may still be able to arrive at a differential diagnosis or a diagnostic formulation was some degree of confidence. While relatively few studies have been performed attempting to diagnose, characterise or treat severe dementia, such studies may be forthcoming in the future, particularly with the advance of increased efficacy of treatments for late stage dementing illness. As the efficacy of treatments, both pharmacological and psychosocial, enable more dementia patients to survive longer periods of time, the challenge of managing severe dementia patients will only increase.

References

Achenbach T, Newhouse P *et al.* (2004) Manual for the ASEBA Older Adult Forms and Profiles. USA, Library of Congress.

Arnulf I, (2000) Hallucinations, REM sleep and Parkinson's disease: a medical hypothesis. *Neurology* 281–288.

Assal F, Cummings JL (1994) Cortical and Frontosubcortical Dementias: Differential Diagnosis. *Dementia*, V. O. B. Emery and T. E. Oxman. Baltimore, Johns Hopkins University Press: 239–262.

Auer S, Sclan S *et al.* (1994) The neglected half of Alzheimer's disease: cognitive and functional concomitants of severe dementia. *Journal of the American Geriatric Society*, 42:1266–1272.

Ballard C, Grace J *et al.* (1998) Neuroleptic sensitivity in dementia with Lewy Bodies and Alzheimer's Disease. *Lancet*, 351:1032–1033.

Ballard CG, O'Brien JT *et al.* (2001) The natural history of psychosis and depression in dementia with Lewy bodies and Alzheimer's disease: persistence and new cases over 1 year of follow-up. *Journal of Clinical Psychiatry*, 62:46–49.

Binetti G, Growdon JH *et al.* (1998) Pick's Disease. *The Dementias*. Growdon JH and Rossor MN. USA, Butterworth-Heinemann, 7–44.

Binetti G, Padovani A *et al.* (1995) Delusions and dementia: clinical and CT correlates. *Acta Neurologica Scandinavica*, 91:271–275.

Chua P, Chiu E (2000) Huntington's Disease. *Dementia*. O'Brien J, Ames D and Burns A. New York, Oxford University Press, 827–844.

Corey-Bloom J (2000) The natural history of Alzheimer's disease. *Dementia*. O'Brien J, Ames D and Burns A. New York, Oxford University Press, 405–415.

Cummings JL (1988) Intellectual impairment in Parkinson's disease: clinical, pathologic, and biochemical correlates. *Journal of Geriatric Psychiatry and Neurology*, 1:24–36.

Cummings J (2000) Cognitive and behavioural heterogeneity in Alzheimer's disease: Seeking the neurobiological basis. *Neurobiology of Aging*, 21:845–861.

Cummings JL, Mega M *et al.* (1994) The Neuropsychiatric Inventory: comprehensive assessment of psychopathology in dementia. *Neurology*, 44(12):2308–2314.

De Deyn PP, Engelborghs S *et al.* (2005) The Middleheim Frontality Score: a behavioural assessment scale that discriminates frontotemporal dementia from Alzheimer's disease. *International Journal of Geriatric Psychiatry*, 20:70–79.

Dooneief G, Marder K *et al.* (1996) The Clinical Dementia Rating scale: community-based validation of 'profound' and 'terminal' stages. *Neurology*, 46(6):1746–1749.

Eastley R, Wilcock G (2000) Assessment and differential diagnosis of dementia. *Dementia*. O'Brien J, Ames D and Burns A. New York, Oxford University Press, 41–47.

Eastwood M (1994) Abnormal behaviour associated with dementia. *International Psychiatry Today*, 4:8–10.

Eastwood R, Reisberg B (1996) Mood and behaviour. *Clinical Diagnosis and Management of Alzheimer's Disease*. S. Gauthier. London, Martin Dunitz, 175–189.

Emery VOB, Oxman TE (1994) Depressive dementia: a 'prepermanent intermediate-stage dementia' in a long-term disease course of permanent dementia? *Dementia*. Emery VOB and Oxman TE. Baltimore, Johns Hopkins University Press, 361–397.

Erkinjuntti T (1987) Types of multi-infarct dementia. *Acta Neurologica Scandinavica*, 75:391–399.

Erkinjuntti T (2000) Vascular dementia: an overview. *Dementia*. O'Brien J, Ames D and Burns A. New York, Oxford University Press, 623–634.

Feldman H, Gauthier S *et al.* (2001) A 24-week, randomized, double-blind study of donepezil in moderate to severe Alzheimer's disease. *Neurology*, 57(11):613–620.

Ferris SH, Yan B (2003) Differential diagnosis and clinical assessment of patients with severe Alzheimer disease. *Alzheimer Disease and Associated Disorders*, 17(Supplement 3):S92–S95.

Ffytche DH (2005) Visual hallucinations and the Charles Bonnet syndrome. *Current Psychiatry Reports*, 7:168–179.

Franssen E, Kluger A *et al.* (1993) The neurologic syndrome of severe Alzheimer's disease. Relationship to functional decline. *Archives of Neurology*, 50:1029–1039.

Galasko D, Bennett D *et al.* (1997) An inventory to assess activities of daily living for clinical trials in Alzheimer's disease: the Alzheimer's Disease Cooperative Study. *Alzheimer Dissease and Associated Disorders*, 11(Suppl 2):33–39.

Grossi D, Fragassi NA *et al.* (2002) Do visuospatial and constructional disturbances differentiate frontal variant of frontotemporal dementia and Alzheimer's disease? An experimental study of a clinical belief. *International Journal of Geriatric Psychiatry*, 17:641–648.

Harvey RJ, Tyrrell PJ *et al.* (2000) Progressive aphasia and other focal syndromes. *Dementia*. O'Brien J, Ames D and Burns A. New York, Oxford University Press, 779–786.

Heyman A, Wilkinson WE *et al.* (1987) Early-onset Alzheimer's disease: clinical predictors of institutionalisation and death. *Neurology*, 37(6):980–984.

Hodges J (2000) Pick's disease: its relationship to progressive aphasia, semantic dementia and frontotemporal dementia. *Dementia*. O'Brien J, Ames D and Burns A. New York, Oxford University Press: 747–758.

Howard R, Almeida O (2000) Cognitive changes in schizophrenia, late-onset schizophrenia and very late-onset schizophrenia-like psychoses. *Dementia*. O'Brien J, Ames D and Burns A. New York, Oxford University Press Inc., 821–825.

Joyce E (2000) Dementia associated with alcoholism. *Dementia*. O'Brien J, Ames D and Burns A. New York, Oxford University Press, 799–811.

Kirshner HS (1994) Progressive aphasia, frontotemporal dementia, and other 'focal dementias'. *Dementia*. Emery VOB and Oxman TE. Baltimore, Johns Hopkins University Press, 156–176.

Kirshner HS, Tanridag O *et al.* (1987) Progressive aphasia without dementia: two cases with focal spongiform degeneration. *Annals of Neurology*, 22:527–532.

Lazarus L, Newton N *et al.* (1987) Frequency and presentation of depressive symptoms in patients with primary degenerative dementia. *American Journal of Psychiatry*, 144:41–45.

Lebert F, Pasquier F *et al.* (1996) Evaluation comportementale dans la démence de type Alzheimer par le questionnaire de dyscontrole comportemental. *Presse Médicale*, 25:665–667.

Levy ML, Miller BL *et al.* (1998). Frontal and Frontotemporal Dementia. *The Dementias*. Growdon JH and Rossor MN. USA, Butterworth-Heinemann, 45–65.

Mayeux R, Stern Y *et al.* (1985) Heterogeneity in dementia of the Alzheimer type: evidence of subgroups. *Neurology*, 35(4):453–461.

McKeith I (1996) Consensus guidelines for the clinical and pathological diagnosis of dementia with Lewy Bodies: Report of the consortium on DLB international workshop. *Neurology*, 47:1113–1124.

McKeith I (2000) Dementia with Lewy bodies: a clinical overview. *Dementia*. O'Brien J, Ames D and Burns A. New York, Oxford University Press, 685–697.

McKeith IG, Galasko D *et al.* (1996) Consensus guidelines for the clinical and pathologic diagnosis of dementia with Lewy bodies. *Neurology*, 47:1113–1124.

Merriam A, Aronson M *et al.* (1988) The psychiatric symptoms of Alzheimer's disease. *Journal of the American Geriatric Society*, 36:7–12.

Mirea A, Cummings J (2000) Neuropsychiatric aspects of dementia. *Dementia*. O'Brien J, Ames D and Burns A. New York, Oxford University Press, 61–79.

Monteiro IM, Boksay I *et al.* (2001) Addition of a frequency-weighted score to the Behavioral Pathology in Alzheimer's Disease Rating Scale: the BEHAVE-AD-FW. Methodology and reliability. *European Psychiatry*, 16(Suppl 1):5–24.

Neary D (2000) Frontotemporal dementia. *Dementia*. O'Brien J, Ames D and Burns A. New York, Oxford University Press, 737–746.

Neary D, Snowden JS *et al.* (1998) Frontotemporal lobar degeneration: a consensus on clinical diagnostic criteria. *Neurology*, 51:1546–1554.

Newhouse P, Brigidi B *et al.* (2004) The Older Adult Self Report and Older Adult Behavior Checklist: development and initial dementia discrimination study. 8th International Montreal/Springfield Symposium on Advances in Alzheimer Therapy.

Ousset PJ, Vellas B *et al.* (1994) Typologie des démences vasculaires et de type Alzheimer: résultats de l'évaluation gérontologique de 178 patients. *L'année Gérontologique*, 8:133–142.

Patel V, Hope T (1993) Aggressive behaviour in elderly people with dementia: a review. *International Journal of Geriatric Psychiatry*, 8(6):457–472.

Perry PJ, Hodges JR (2000) Differentiating frontal and temporal variant frontotemporal dementia from Alzheimer's disease. *Neurology*, 54:2277–2284.

Pirttilä T, Erkinjuntti T *et al.* (1994) Vascular dementias and Alzheimer disease: differential diagnosis. *Dementia*. Emery VOB and Oxman TE. Baltimore, Johns Hopkins University Press, 306–335.

Rabinowitz T, Murphy KM *et al.* (2003) Delirium: pathophysiology, recognition, prevention and treatment. *Expert Rev. Neurotherapeutics*, 3(3):343–355.

Reed BR, Goetz CG (2004) Vascular dementia. *Archives of Neurology*, 61(3):433–435.

Reisberg B, Auer SR *et al.* (1996) Behavioral pathology in Alzheimer's disease (BEHAVE-AD) rating scale. *International Psychogeriatrics*, 8(Suppl 3):301–308.

Reisberg B, Ferris SH *et al*. (1982) The Global Deterioration Scale for assessment of primary degenerative dementia. *American Journal of Psychiatry*, 139(9):1136–1139.

Sachdev PS, Reutens S (1994) The Nondepressive Pseudodementias. *Dementia*. Emery VOB and Oxman TE. Baltimore, Johns Hopkins University Press, 417–443.

Schmidtke K, Hüll M (2002) Neuropsychological differentiation of small vessel disease, Alzheimer's disease and mixed dementia. *Journal of the Neurological Sciences*, 203–204:17–22.

Schmitt FA, Ashford W *et al*. (1997) The severe impairment battery: concurrent validity and the assessment of longitudinal change in Alzheimer's disease: the Alzheimer's Disease Cooperative Study. *Alzheimer Dissease and Associated Disorders*, 11(Suppl 2):S51–56.

Sclan SG and Reisberg B (1992) Functional assessment staging (FAST) in Alzheimer's disease: reliability, validity, and ordinality. *International Psychogeriatrics*, 4(Suppl 2):55–69.

Sjogren M, Wallin A *et al*. (1994) Clinical subgroups of Alzheimer disease. *Dementia*. Emery VOB and Oxman TE. Baltimore, Johns Hopkins University Press, 139–155.

Slachevsky A, Villalpando JM *et al*. (2004) Frontal Assessment Battery and differential diagnosis of fronto-temporal dementia and Alzheimer disease. *Archives of Neurology*, 61:1104–1107.

Sloane PD, Davidson S *et al*. (1999) Severe disruptive vocalizers. *Journal of the American Geriatric Society*, 47:439–445.

Snowden JS, Neary D *et al*. (2002) Frontotemporal dementia. *British Journal of Psychiatry*, 180:140–143.

Sunderland T, Alterman IS *et al*. (1988) A new scale for the assessment of depressed mood in demented patients. *American Journal of Psychiatry*, 145:955–959.

Tariot P, Farlow M *et al*. (2004) Memantine treatment in patients with moderate to severe Alzheimer's disease already receiving donepezil. *Journal of the Americam Medical Association*, 291(3):317–324.

Teri L, Larson E *et al*. (1988) Behavioral disturbances in dementia of Alzheimer's type. *Journal of the American Geriatric Society*, 36:1–6.

Varma AR, Adams W *et al*. (2002) Diagnostic patterns of regional atrophy on MRI and regional cerebral blood flow change on SPECT in young onset patients with Alzheimer's disease, frontotemporal dementia and vascular dementia. *Acta Neurologica Scandinavica*, 105:261–269.

Vellas B, Gillette-Guyonnet S *et al*. (2000) Falls, frailty and osteoporosis in the elderly: a public health problem. *Rev Med Interne*, 21:608–613.

Verny M, KM *et al*. (1998) Démence à un stade très évolué. *Demences et Longévité*. Forette F, Christen Y and Boller F. Paris, Fondation Nationale de Gérontologie, 135–153.

Walker (2002) Differentiation of dementia with Lewy Bodies from Alzheimer's disease using a domaminergic presynnaptic ligand. *Journal of Neurology, Neurosurgery and Psychiatry*, 73:134–140.

Walker AJ, Meares S *et al*. (2005) The differentiation of mild frontotemporal dementia from Alzheimer's disease and healthy aging by neuropsychological tests. *International Psychogeriatrics*, 17(1):57–68.

Wengel SP, Burke WJ *et al*. (1989) Musical hallucinations. The sounds of silence? *Journal of the American Geriatrics Society*, 37(2):163–6.

Wesnes K (2002) Predicting responses to rivastigmine in DLB. *European Neuropsychopharmacology*, s373.

Wragg R, Jeste D (1989) Overview of depression and psychosis in Alzheimer's disease. *American Journal of Psychiatry*, 146:577–587.

Zubenko GS (1994) Neurobiology of major depression in Alzheimer disease. *Dementia*. Emery VOB and Oxman TE. Baltimore, Johns Hopkins University Press, 444–460.

2

Cholinergic and Serotonergic Systems in Severe Dementia

Sally I. Sharp, Paul T. Francis and Clive G. Ballard

Introduction

Severe dementia is associated with frequent psychiatric and behavioural disturbances in addition to marked cognitive and functional deficits. Research to determine a neurochemical understanding of dementia over the last three decades has generated therapeutic strategies which improve patient's cognition and activities of daily living. Different key dementia syndromes have been shown to have distinct neurotransmitter biochemical pathology, with important implications for therapy. Given space limitations, the current review focuses on cholinergic and serotonergic excitatory neurotransmitter systems implicated in severe dementia.

Disease Severity

Alzheimer's disease (AD) accounts for more than 50% of late-onset dementias. Neuropathological staging shows a characteristic pattern of progressive accumulation of insoluble fibrous extracellular β-amyloid, Aβ, surrounded by dystrophic and degenerative neuritic processes as well as reactive microglia and astrocytes, forming neuritic plaques and neurofibrillary tangles (NFT), in pyramidal nerve cell soma, extending into dendrites of the neocortex and hippocampus. Subcortical nuclei, including nucleus basalis of Meynert, locus coeruleus (LC) and raphe nuclei, which project into the cortex, suffer cell loss. Atrophy is closely correlated with neuritic plaque and NFT formation and is usually most marked in the hippocampus and cortex of AD patients. Prefrontal cortical synapses are not susceptible to pathological changes until later stages of disease. Acetylcholine (ACh), glutamate, serotonin (5-HT) and noradrenaline (NA) are the neurochemical transmitter systems showing the greatest loss in AD, with relative sparing of dopamine (DA), gamma-aminobutyric acid (GABA) and most peptides.

Other common late-onset dementias include dementia with Lewy bodies (DLB), Parkinson's disease dementia (PDD) and vascular dementia (VaD). The neurochemical and neuropathological correlates of dementia severity are less well established in these patient groups, although α-synuclein pathology appears to be associated with the severity of impairment in DLB and PDD (Harding et al., 2002), and recent evidence has shown significant correlations between increased staging of pathology (Aβ, Lewy bodies, Lewy neurites and NFT) in Parkinson's disease (PD) and increased cognitive dysfunction in this patient group (Braak et al., 2005). However, the severity of microvascular disease is probably of particular importance in VaD (Esiri et al., 1997). Concurrent pathological changes of AD are probably important in all groups. It is evident that cholinergic deficits are severe and associated with key cognitive and psychiatric symptoms in DLB and PDD (Ballard et al., 2000), whilst the neurochemical profile of VaD and how it relates to the different key

Severe Dementia. Edited by A. Burns and B. Winblad.
Copyright © 2006 John Wiley & Sons, Ltd.   ISBN 0-470-01054-1

vascular substrates and disease severity has not been established (Perry *et al.*, 2005). Changes in the two of the main excitatory neurotransmitter systems associated with dementia severity in these syndromes will be discussed here.

Neurochemistry of Dementia Severity
Cholinergic Neurotransmission
Global Cholinergic Changes in AD

Primary degenerative dementia is accompanied by a progressive loss of cholinergic function in the CNS (Davies and Maloney, 1976). Cholinergic neurotransmission in the cerebral cortex is severely impaired in AD and the loss of neurons from the cholinergic nucleus of Meynert is well documented. There appears to be at least some subtle loss of neocortical cholinergic innervation in the early stages, namely Braak stages I and II, of AD (Beach *et al.*, 2000), with a reduction in functional cholinergic markers where ACh synthesis and choline uptake exceeded the reduction in choline acetyltransferase (ChAT) activity (Francis *et al.*, 1985). Thalamic cholinergic activity is relatively unchanged in AD (Perry *et al.*, 1998) and similarly, the striatum is relatively spared, although a reduction in striatal nicotinic receptors, particularly the putamen, compared to control has been reported (Court *et al.*, 2000). However, of particular relevance to the current chapter, it is also evident that the greatest reduction in cholinergic markers occurs between moderate and severe disease, with little change between people without dementia and early AD. This is illustrated clearly from the work of Davis and colleagues, in a pivotal study which linked the severity of cholinergic deficit to the stage of dementia, defined using the Clinical Dementia Rating (CDR) Scale. No significant difference in ChAT and acetylcholinesterase (AChE) activity was identified in any of the nine neocortical brain regions examined from people without dementia, with questionable dementia or in the mild stages of disease, but individuals with severe AD showed significantly lower ChAT and AChE (Figure 1) (Davis *et al.*, 1999). These findings are supported by further work identifying a significant loss of ChAT activity in frontal and temporal cortical regions in autopsy material from people with AD. In this study, ChAT levels were strongly correlated with the severity of cognitive impairment at the last interview before death, evaluated using the Mini Mental State Examination (MMSE), with a mean MMSE score at death of 4.3 in this patient group (Minger *et al.*, 2000). Additional findings have shown an AD patient group with severe cognitive impairment, indicated by a significantly greater mean Blessed Information-Memory-Concentration (BIMC) score of 23.6 prior to death, had a significantly lower mean ChAT activity in the mid-frontal cortex compared to a control group with a BIMC score of 1.3 (Sabbagh *et al.*, 1998).

Global Cholinergic Changes in DLB and VaD

There is a more significant loss of neocortical presynaptic cholinergic neurons and ChAT activity in DLB compared with AD. In addition, there are greater losses of cholinergic activity in the basal ganglia, including the striatum, and in the pedunculopontine pathway that projects to areas such as the thalamus in these individuals compared to people with AD (Francis *et al.*, 2005).

The literature regarding VaD is less consistent. Several autopsy studies have suggested greater cholinergic deficits in people with VaD compared to age-matched controls, although the only study to quantify concomitant AD changes indicates that cholinergic deficits are only evident in individuals with concurrent AD pathology (Perry *et al.*, 2005).

Nicotinic Cholinergic Receptors

Changes in nicotinic acetylcholine receptor (nAChR) expression in neuropsychiatric disorders appear to be brain region and subtype specific and have been shown in some instances to be associated with pathology and symptomatology (Graham *et al.*, 2002). Several post-mortem studies show a more consistent loss of nAChRs compared to muscarinic acetylcholine receptor (mAChR) in AD

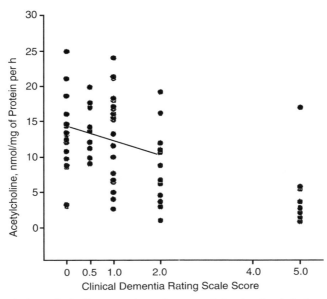

Figure 1. Correlation of choline acetyltransferase activity in the inferior temporal gyrus (Brodmann area 20) with Clinical Dementia Rating Scale scores. Regression line depicts correlation ($r = 0.58$ and $P < 0.001$). From Davis *et al.* (1999) Cholinergic markers in elderly patients with early signs of Alzheimer disease. JAMA 281:1401–1406. Copyright, the American Medical Association.

(e.g. Nordberg and Winblad, 1986). Selective loss of nAChR protein expression rather than loss of the nAChR-expressing neurons suggests loss of the $\alpha 4$ receptor subunit (Martin-Ruiz *et al.*, 1999). A significant loss of the $\alpha 4$ subunit in the entorhinal cortex, the temporal cortex and the dentate gyrus is documented in both AD and DLB compared to age-matched controls (Teaktong *et al.*, 2004). There is also a highly significant reduction in $\alpha 4$ nAChRs in the reticular nucleus of the thalamus in DLB patients. However, of some interest, the highest Lewy bodies density in the parahippocampal gyrus did not correlate with the greatest nAChR loss in DLB, yet, conversely, receptor levels were actually higher in this region in DLB patients. In AD, the selective loss of high-affinity nAChRs in key cortical areas such as the temporal cortex parallels the loss of ChAT and AchE (Perry *et al.*, 1995). Surprisingly, despite greater reductions in ChAT, nicotinic receptor loss appears to be less pronounced in DLB than in AD (Martin-Ruiz *et al.*, 2000). In contrast, expression of the low-affmity $\alpha 7$ nAChR subunit was decreased in the subiculum of AD and DLB and the entorhinal cortex of DLB only (Teaktong *et al.*, 2004), although a more severe loss is reported in DLB compared to age-matched controls (Reid *et al.*, 2000).

Primary histopathological changes are closely associated with nAChR abnormalities, including dopaminergic cell loss in PD and DLB and amyloid plaques and tangles in subicular and entorhinal areas in AD (Perry *et al.*, 2000). β-amyloid binds with high affinity to the $\alpha 7$ nAChR, thus cholinergic function through $\alpha 7$ may be compromised because of high levels of (soluble) peptide with advancing AD pathology (Wang *et al.*, 2000). Contradicting this, a reduction of nAChR activity in AD or DLB does not appear to be related to plaques or NFTs in mid-frontal cortex compared to controls (Sabbagh *et al.*, 2001), and further mechanistic studies are required to clarify the situation.

In both PD and DLB, nicotine binding is significantly reduced in the substantia nigra (Perry *et al.*, 1995) compared to age-matched controls, although, unlike in DLB, neuronal loss accounts for most of the nAChR reduction in PD. There is a 70% and 40% loss of neurons in PD and DLB respectively and a 70% decrease in nicotine binding in both diseases. In PD, the loss of striatal nAChR closely parallels the loss of nigrostriatal dopaminergic markers, probably because the majority of nAChRs are located on dopaminergic neurons in these areas. However, it also suggests a relationship between the loss of nAChRs and more severe nigrostriatal pathological changes (Martin-Ruiz et al., 2000a). Similarly, reduced striatal $\alpha 4\beta 2$ nAChR subtype in AD patients, defined as Braak stage V and VI, has been demonstrated, while no significant loss in striatal nAChRs was seen in mild AD (Braak stage $\leqslant$ III) compared to controls, possibly related to cortical atrophy and subsequent loss of striatal inputs in these patients. These reported reductions of nAChRs observed in AD, DLB and PD are not apparent in VaD (Pimlott et al., 2004) with relative preservation of nAChRs (Martin-Ruiz et al., 2000b). Alterations in vascular nAChR expression may be important in other neurodegenerative diseases (Graham et al., 2002).

As well as neuropathological changes in AD and DLB, the relationship between the loss of nAChR and cognitive decline has also been investigated. A significant loss of the high-affinity $\alpha 4$ nAChR was reported in the mid-frontal cortex from an AD patient group with severe cognitive impairment assessed by a significantly greater mean BIMC score 23.6 before death than controls with BIMC score 1.3 (Sabbagh et al., 1998). This is supported by a significant inverse correlation with reduced $\alpha 4$ binding in the temporal cortex of AD and DLB patient brains and increasing severity of dementia according to the Clinical Dementia Rating score, but with a subtle loss of receptor subtypes even in the groups with mildest cognitive impairment (CDR 0.5) compared to age-matched controls (Perry et al., 2000). However, using BIMC, MMSE, and total Mattis Dementia Rating Scale (DRS) scores at the end of life (22.2, 10.6, 74.0 scores for AD respectively; 27.1, 5.5, 51.9 for DLB respectively; and 1.3, 29.1, 137.2 for controls respectively), the severity of impairment in cognitive function did not significantly correlate with a loss of nAChR in the frontal cortex of either AD or DLB (Sabbagh et al., 2001).

Muscarinic Cholinergic Receptors

Most M2 mAChRs located presynaptically on cholinergic terminals in the hippocampus and cerebral cortex are known to mediate autoinhibition of ACh release. Compared to controls, M2 receptors are reduced in AD in the hippocampus (Rinne et al., 1989), frontal cortex (Lai et al., 2001) and cerebral cortex (Mash et al., 1985) yet preserved in the striatum (Piggott et al., 2003) and the temporal cortex, implying this receptor subtype is present on non-cholinergic neurons or upregulated on surviving terminals (Lai et al., 2001). Decreasing M2 mAChR in the frontal cortex of AD patients has also been correlated with reductions in ChAT (Araujo et al., 1988). However, one study reported that the M2 receptor number was unchanged in the frontal cortex of AD brains compared to controls (Rinne et al., 1989).

The postsynaptic cholinergic system (usually present upon glutamatergic neurons) appears to be less affected, with relative preservation of postsynaptic M1 mAChRs in AD (Flynn et al., 1995). However, M1 has also been shown to be reduced late in the disease process when dementia was most severe in AD patients studied post mortem (Rodriguez-Puertas et al., 1997) and there may be a degree of functional uncoupling from the intracellular cascade in AD (Flynn et al., 1995). In the hippocampus, uncoupling of M1 receptors does occur in areas most affected by Aβ plaques and NFT formation, indicating a link between disruption of muscarinic function and the severity of AD pathology. Interestingly, increased striatal M1, M2 and M4 mAChRs correlated with Alzheimer-type pathology in an AD group, which had significantly higher mean plaque and NFT counts as well as mean Braak stage (5.4) than in controls (2.3) and DLB, PD (both 1.6) and PDD (2.6) disease groups (Piggott et al., 2003).

As with nAChRs, expression of muscarinic receptors appears to be brain region and subtype specific. A significant loss of striatal M1 mAChRs was observed in DLB and PDD compared to controls, AD and PD, which significantly correlated with increased cortical Lewy body pathology. This supports evidence of 'mis-regulation' of striatal neurons containing the M1 subtype in DLB

(Piggott *et al.*, 2003). In comparison with AD, post-mortem studies have shown M1 receptors not only to be preserved but elevated in temporal and parietal cortices in DLB patients, but appeared to be reduced in the hippocampus in both DLB and AD (Ballard *et al.*, 2000). Preserved cortical mAChRs are, however, associated with increased Lewy bodies pathology in the cortex (Piggott *et al.*, 2003).

Postsynaptic mAChRs, however, remain more functionally intact in DLB than in AD. Signal transduction is maintained in DLB, unlike in AD, with unchanged M1 mAChR coupling to second messengers, which is probably explained by the lower density of plaque and tangle pathology in these patients (Perry *et al.*, 1998). Preservation of M1 receptor number and function in the temporal cortex in DLB may partially explain why these patients respond very well to cholinergic agents, such as acetylcholinesterase inhibitors (AChEI) (McKeith *et al.*, 2000).

By contrast, M2 mAChR number was unaltered in the hippocampus from PD patients and higher in the frontal and temporal cortices in PD than in control. The total number of cortical mAChRs in PDD negatively associated with ChAT activity and surprisingly positively correlated with increased dementia severity (Rinne *et al.*, 1989). Evidence of cognitive performance deficits in a passive avoidance test in M2 knockout mice suggests dysregulation of synaptic ACh release contributes to cognitive deficits (Seeger *et al.*, 2004). However, there was no correlation between M1 and M2 mAChR expression with dementia severity in AD as measured by (1) the mean of last five MMSE scores of cognition, (2) MMSE scores in the last interview before death, and (3) average decline in MMSE score per year from recruitment into study until death (Lai *et al.*, 2001).

Activation of cholinergic receptors is thought to influence the metabolism of amyloid precursor protein (APP), one of the two key proteins involved in AD, diverting metabolism away from the formation of Aβ (Francis *et al.*, 1999). This is supported by evidence that muscarinic M1 agonists reduced CSF concentrations of Aβ in man (Hock *et al.*, 2000). Furthermore, nAChR stimulation is associated with reduced plaque densities in human brain (Court *et al.*, 1998). Cholinergic neurotransmission may also beneficially modulate the generation of NFT via reduced phosphorylation of tau protein (the second key protein involved in AD pathology) and may be a specific target for Aβ, which reduces both choline uptake and ACh release *in vitro* (Auld *et al.*, 1998).

Cholinesterases

Acetylcholinesterase, one of the key enzymes responsible for the breakdown of ACh, is reduced in AD, possibly related to the loss of cholinergic terminals, while butyrylcholinesterase (BuChE) activity increases. The function of BuChE is not yet fully understood, but it is present in extrasynaptic areas and plaques, and hence increases together with the severity of the plaque pathology. Recent studies indicate that BuChE may contribute to the breakdown of ACh in some important brain areas such as the hippocampus and thalamus (Darvesh and Hopkins, 2003), may accelerate plaque maturation (Mesulam and Geula, 1994) and is associated with an accelerated rate of cognitive decline, specifically in people with more severe dementia in later stages of AD (O'Brien *et al.*, 2003; Holmes *et al.*, 2005). Interestingly, AD patients carrying the K allele of BuChE, with baseline MMSE scores of less than or equal to eight points, showed a slower rate of cognitive decline than patients with a baseline MMSE score above eight points (Holmes *et al.*, 2005). Similarly, AD and DLB individuals with Ala^{539}Thr allele mutations in BuChE (causing reduced BuChE enzyme activity) had a significantly slower rate of cognitive decline, measured by annual decline in Cambridge Cognitive Examination (CAMCOG) score averaged over two to three years (mean 9.6-point decline) versus a mean of 16.5-point decline in patients with the wild-type gene. Patients carrying the BuChE gene mutations also showed a trend towards a later age of dementia onset than those with the wild-type (O'Brien *et al.*, 2003). Further work needs to investigate the mechanism of these important associations, and to determine whether they are mediated through cholinergic or other mechanisms.

Serotonergic Neurotransmission
Global Serotonergic Changes in AD

In AD, serotonergic neurotransmission is decreased, with a loss of dorsal and median raphe neurons which innervate the forebrain. The association between serotonin (5-HT) and NFT formation in the dorsal raphe nucleus (Chen *et al.*, 2000) emphasises a link between serotonergic changes and disease pathology, and indicates that these changes are likely to become more pronounced as the disease becomes more severe and in particular as the tangle pathology in the dorsal raphe nucleus becomes more marked. One study, without reported evaluations of AD pathology, demonstrated that 5-HT levels in the frontal cortex correlated negatively with increased disease severity, determined by the mean annual rate of MMSE (4.0 points) decline in AD subjects with a mean MMSE at recruitment of 14.0 score (Lai *et al.*, 2002). Both the 5-HT transmitter and its major metabolite 5-hydroxy-indoleacetic acid (5-HIAA), were reduced in the neocortex of AD subjects, although neither of these serotonergic parameters correlated with severity of dementia, as determined by MMSE score (Palmer *et al.*, 1987a). However, half of the cortical areas in the AD brain at autopsy showed no evidence for a selective reduction in presynaptic 5-HT activity (Palmer *et al.*, 1988) thus a serotonergic deficit in AD is probably not widespread (Francis *et al.*, 1993). This is consistent with the preservation of 5-HIAA in CSF from AD patients both with and without extrapyramidal signs (Kaye *et al.*, 1988), where the 5-HT turnover rate appears to be elevated compared to controls, although the same is not apparent in lumbar CSF with decreased 5-HIAA concentration in AD compared to control (Palmer *et al.*, 1984). Dementia severity was not associated with 5-HIAA in CSF from AD subjects with extrapyramidal signs with a lower mean MMSE score than the AD group without (Kaye *et al.*, 1988).

Global Serotonergic Changes in DLB, PDD and VaD

In DLB, Lewy bodies occur in the dorsal raphe nucleus and marked reductions of 5-HT levels have been reported in the striatum, neocortex and frontal cortex. There is also evidence to show a loss of 5-HT metabolism in VaD patient brains. In several reports the concentration of 5-HT was reduced in the hypothalamus and caudate nucleus in VaD compared to controls. Importantly, in these patients, decreasing concentration of 5-HIAA is significantly correlated with the severity of subcortical symptomatology (Wallin *et al.*, 1989). There are no reported changes in 5-HT receptors in PDD although a number of studies have identified reduced 5-HIAA concentration in the CSF of PD patients (Kuhn *et al.*, 1996).

Serotonergic Receptors

The $5-HT_{1A}$ receptors function as presynaptic autoreceptors in the raphe nuclei and postsynaptic receptors in other forebrain areas. However, it is less clear whether $5-HT_{1A}$ density is affected in AD compared to age-matched controls (Lai *et al.*, 2003) with a report of a significant loss of $5-HT_{1A}$ (Middlemiss *et al.*, 1986), although to a lesser extent than $5-HT_{2A}$ receptors (Cross *et al.*, 1988). Similarly, the literature is contradictory regarding possible changes in $5-HT_{2A}$ receptors. Reductions in postsynaptic $5-HT_{2A}$ receptors in AD have been identified (Reynolds *et al.*, 1984), while Dewar and colleagues (1990) showed no difference in the number of $5-HT_{2A}$ receptors in frontal cortex and hippocampus compared to age-matched controls (Dewar *et al.*, 1990). Clinico-pathological studies indicate that the mean of the last five MMSE scores measured during life inversely correlated with $5-HT_{1A}$ density in the temporal cortex (Francis *et al.*, 1992a). Similarly, the number of $5-HT_{1A}$ receptors in the frontal cortex positively correlated with the mean annual rate of MMSE decline in AD (4.0 score), although the ratio of 5-HT to $5-HT_{1A}$ more strongly predicted the rate of MMSE cognitive decline than either 5-HT or $5-HT_{1A}$ individually, suggesting that antagonism of inhibitory $5-HT_{1A}$ may protect against accelerated cognitive impairment in AD (Lai *et al.*, 2002). In AD, there was also a reported loss of $5-HT_{1B/1D/6}$ receptor subtypes in both the frontal and temporal cortices compared to control patients. The reduction in $5-HT_{1B/D}$ receptor subtypes in the frontal cortical area was also significantly positively correlated with mean MMSE decline in AD (10.0 points), defined as the difference between maximum scoring and last MMSE score before death (Garcia-Alloza *et al.*, 2004). The ratio of ChAT levels to both these receptor subtypes 1B and 1D as well as the concentration of 5-HT in this frontal brain region of AD subjects was negatively associated with the final MMSE score (average MMSE 5.0 points before death) (Garcia-Alloza *et al.*, 2005). However, the 5-HT_6 receptor loss in these patients was unrelated to cognitive status before death (Garcia-Alloza *et al.*, 2004). Interestingly, both 5-HT_{1A} and 5-HT_{2A} postsynaptic receptors are increased in the neocortex of PD patients (Chen *et al.*, 1998), although no interaction with neuropathology or cognitive decline in these patients was investigated.

Serotonergic Transporter
There is a reported loss of cortical 5-HTT in the temporal cortex in AD (Chen *et al.*, 1996) but this loss has not been associated with dementia severity measured by MMSE score (Palmer *et al.*, 1987).

Conclusion

The current chapter provides a review of the relationship between dementia severity and neurochemical dysfunction in two key systems involved in the pathogenesis of the primary dementias (summarised in Table 1). As the mean level of cognitive impairment at post mortem is severe in most studies, there is a particular focus on neurochemical disturbances in severe dementia. Although alterations in cholinergic function have been well described, there are a number of inconsistencies in the literature regarding other neurotransmitter systems, and very little data regarding most of these systems in non-AD dementias. Of particular interest, a number of post-mortem studies have been able to identify associations between the rate of cognitive decline during life and brain neurochemistry, highlighting that undertaking further neurochemical studies to clarify key issues still holds tremendous potential as a tool for developing and improving treatment approaches.

Table 1. Alterations in neurotransmitter systems in severe dementia

Neurotransmitter system	Location	Alterations in severe dementia[a]	Dementia severity index[b]
Cholinergic	Cerebral cortex	↓ ChAT – AD	↑ Severity according to CDR (Davis *et al.*, 1999)
	Frontal and temporal cortices	↓ ChAT – AD	↓ MMSE 4.3 before death (Minger *et al.*, 2000)
	Frontal cortex	↓ ChAT – AD	↑ BIMC 23.6 before death (vs. 1.3 in CT) (Sabbagh *et al.*, 1998)
	Cerebral cortex	↓ AChE – AD	↑ Severity according to CDR (Davis *et al.*, 1999)
	Genotype	BuChE wild-type gene – AD	↑ Severity according to CAMCOG 16.5 decline (vs. 9.6 mutant carriers) (O'Brien *et al.*, 2003)
	Striatum	↓ α4 nAChR – AD	↑ Braak stage 5.0/6.0; → Braak stage ≤ 3 (Pimlott *et al.*, 2004)
	Frontal cortex	↓ α4 nAChR – AD	↑ Severity according to BIMC 23.6 before death (vs. 1.3 in CT) (Sabbagh *et al.*, 1998)

(Continued)

Table 1. (*Continued*)

Neurotransmitter system	Location	Alterations in severe dementia[a]	Dementia severity index[b]
		– AD/DLB	→ BIMC/MMSE/Total Mattis DRS (Sabbagh *et al.*, 2001)
	Temporal cortex	↓ α4 nAChR – AD/DLB	↑ Severity according to CDR vs. controls (Perry *et al.*, 2000)
	Frontal and temporal cortices	→ M1 mAChR – AD	→ MMSE (Lai *et al.*, 2001)
	Striatum	↓ M1mAChR – DLB	↑ LB cortical pathology (Piggott *et al.*, 2003)
	Frontal cortex	↓ M2 mAChR – AD	→ MMSE (Lai *et al.*, 2001)
	Temporal cortex	→ M2 mAChR – AD	→ MMSE (Lai *et al.*, 2001)
	Striatum	↑ M1, M2 and M4 mAChR – AD	↑ NFT/plaque count; ↑ Braak stage 5.4 (vs. CT, DLB, PD, PDD Braak stage 2.0) (Piggott *et al.*, 2003)
Serotonergic	Frontal cortex	↓ 5-HT – AD	↑ Severity according to MMSE 4.0 annual decline (Lai *et al.*, 2002)
	Cerebral cortex	↓ 5-HT/5-HIAA – AD	→ MMSE (Palmer *et al.*, 1987a)
	Frontal and temporal cortices	↓ 5-HIAA – AD	↑ NFT count (Palmer *et al.*, 1987a; Palmer *et al.*, 1987b)
	Temporal cortex	↑ 5-HT$_{1A}$ – AD	↑ Severity according to last five MMSE scores (Francis *et al.*, 1992a; Francis *et al.*, 1992b)
	Frontal cortex	↑ 5-HT$_{1A}$ – AD	↑ Severity according to MMSE 4.0 annual decline (Lai *et al.*, 2002)
		↑ 5-HT: 5-HT$_{1A}$ ratio – AD	↓ MMSE (Lai *et al.*, 2002)
		↓ 5-HT$_{1B/D}$ – AD	↑ Severity according to MMSE 10.0 annual decline (Garcia-Alloza *et al.*, 2004)
		↑ 5-HT$_{1B/D}$:ChAT / 5-HT:ChAT ratios – AD	↑ Severity according to MMSE 5.0 before death (Garcia-Alloza *et al.*, 2004; Garcia-Alloza *et al.*, 2005)
		↓ 5-HT$_6$ – AD	→ MMSE (Garcia-Alloza *et al.*, 2004)
	Temporal cortex	↓ 5-HTT – AD	→ MMSE (Palmer *et al.*, 1987a)

[a]AD, Alzheimer's disease; CT, control; DLB, dementia with Lewy bodies.

[b]All values quoted in this table are mean scores of dementia severity. CDR, Clinical Dementia Rating; MMSE, Mini Mental State Examination; BIMC, Blessed Information–Memory–Concentration; CAMCOG, Cambridge Cognitive Examination; Total Mattis DRS, Dementia Rating Scale; LB, Lewy body; NFT, neurofibrillary tangles.

Correlations between neurochemical alterations described in column 3 and dementia severity scores in column 4 are indicated as follows: arrows in the same direction show a positive correlation; arrows in opposite directions show a negative correlation; and → arrows show no correlation.

References

Araujo DM, Lapchak PA, Robitaille Y, Gauthier S, Quirion R (1988) Differential alteration of various cholinergic markers in cortical and subcortical regions of human brain in Alzheimer's disease. J Neurochem 50:1914–1923.

Auld DS, Kar S, Quirion R (1998) Beta-amyloid peptides as direct cholinergic neuromodulators: a missing link? Trends Neurosci 21:43–49.

Ballard C, Piggott M, Johnson M, Cairns N, Perry R, McKeith I, Jaros E, O'Brien J, Holmes C, Perry E (2000) Delusions associated with elevated muscarinic binding in dementia with Lewy bodies. Ann Neurol 48:868–876.

Beach TG, Kuo YM, Spiegel K, Emmerling MR, Sue LI, Kokjohn K, Roher AE (2000) The cholinergic deficit coincides with Abeta deposition at the earliest histopathologic stages of Alzheimer disease. J Neuropathol Exp Neurol 59:308–313.

Braak H, Rub U, Jansen Steur EN, Del TK, de Vos RA (2005) Cognitive status correlates with neuropathologic stage in Parkinson disease. Neurology 64:1404–1410.

Chen CP, Alder JT, Bowen DM, Esiri MM, McDonald B, Hope T, Jobst KA, Francis PT (1996) Presynaptic serotonergic markers in community-acquired cases of Alzheimer's disease: correlations with depression and neuroleptic medication. J Neurochem 66:1592–1598.

Chen CP, Alder JT, Bray L, Kingsbury AE, Francis PT, Foster OJ (1998) Post-synaptic 5-HT1A and 5-HT2A receptors are increased in Parkinson's disease neocortex. Ann N Y Acad Sci 861:288–289.

Chen CP, Eastwood SL, Hope T, McDonald B, Francis PT, Esiri MM (2000) Immunocytochemical study of the dorsal and median raphe nuclei in patients with Alzheimer's disease prospectively assessed for behavioural changes. Neuropathol Appl Neurobiol 26:347–355.

Court JA, Lloyd S, Thomas N, Piggott MA, Marshall EF, Morris CM, Lamb H, Perry RH, Johnson M, Perry EK (1998) Dopamine and nicotinic receptor binding and the levels of dopamine and homovanillic acid in human brain related to tobacco use. Neuroscience 87:63–78.

Court JA, Piggott MA, Lloyd S, Cookson N, Ballard CG, McKeith IG, Perry RH, Perry EK (2000) Nicotine binding in human striatum: elevation in schizophrenia and reductions in dementia with Lewy bodies, Parkinson's disease and Alzheimer's disease and in relation to neuroleptic medication. Neuroscience 98:79–87.

Cross AJ, Slater P, Perry EK, Perry RH (1988) An autoradiographic analysis of serotonin receptors in human temporal cortex: changes in Alzheimer-type dementia, Neurochem Int 11:89–96.

Darvesh S, Hopkins DA (2003) Differential distribution of butyrylcholinesterase and acetylcholinesterase in the human thalamus. J Comp Neurol 463:25–43.

Davies P, Maloney AJ (1976) Selective loss of central cholinergic neurons in Alzheimer's disease. Lancet 2:1403.

Davis KL, Mohs RC, Marin D, Purohit DP, Perl DP, Lantz M, Austin G, Haroutunian V (1999) Cholinergic markers in elderly patients with early signs of Alzheimer disease. JAMA 281:1401–1406.

Dewar D, Graham DI, McCulloch J (1990) 5 HT2 receptors in dementia of Alzheimer type: a quantitative autoradiographic study of frontal cortex and hippocampus. J Neural Transm Park Dis Dement Sect 2:129–137.

Esiri MM, Wilcock GK, Morris JH (1997) Neuropathological assessment of the lesions of significance in vascular dementia. J Neurol Neurosurg Psychiatry 63:749–753.

Flynn DD, Ferrari-DiLeo G, Mash DC, Levey AI (1995) Differential regulation of molecular subtypes of muscarinic receptors in Alzheimer's disease. J Neurochem 64:1888–1891.

Francis PT, Palmer AM, Sims NR, Bowen DM, Davison AN, Esiri MM, Neary D, Snowden JS, Wilcock GK (1985) Neurochemical studies of early-onset Alzheimer's disease. Possible influence on treatment. N Engl J Med 313:7–11.

Francis PT, Pangalos MN, Pearson RC, Middlemiss DN, Stratmann GC, Bowen DM (1992a) 5-HydroxytryptaminelA but not 5-hydroxytryptamine2 receptors are enriched on neocortical pyramidal neurones destroyed by intrastriatal volkensin. J Pharmacol Exp Ther 261:1273–1281.

Francis PT, Pangalos MN, Bowen DM (1992b) Animal and drug modelling for Alzheimer synaptic pathology. Prog Neurobiol 39:517–545.

Francis PT, Sims NR, Procter AW, Bowen DM (1993) Cortical pyramidal neurone loss may cause glutamatergic hypoactivity and cognitive impairment in Alzheimer's disease: investigative and therapeutic perspectives. J Neurochem 60:1589–1604.

Francis PT, Palmer AM, Snape M, Wilcock GK (1999) The cholinergic hypothesis of Alzheimer's disease: a review of progress. J Neurol Neurosurg Psychiatry 66:137–147.

Francis PT, Perry EK, Piggott MA, Duda JE (2005) The neurochemical pathology. In: Dementia with Lewy Bodies (O'Brien J, McKeith IG, Ames D, Chiu E, eds). Third edition, Taylor and Francis Group publishers.

Garcia-Alloza M, Hirst WD, Chen CP, Lasheras B, Francis PT, Ramirez MJ (2004) Differential involvement of 5-HT(1B/1D) and 5-HT6 receptors in cognitive and non-cognitive symptoms in Alzheimer's disease. Neuropsychopharmacology 29:410–416.

Garcia-AUoza M, Gil-Bea FJ, ez-Ariza M, Chen CP, Francis PT, Lasheras B, Ramirez MJ. (2005) Cholinergic–serotonergic imbalance contributes to cognitive and behavioral symptoms in Alzheimer's disease. Neuropsychologia 43:442–449.

Graham AJ, Martin-Ruiz CM, Teaktong T, Ray MA, Court JA (2002) Human brain nicotinic receptors, their distribution and participation in neuropsychiatric disorders. Curr Drug Targets CNS Neurol Disord 1:387–397.

Harding AJ, Broe GA, Halliday GM (2002) Visual hallucinations in Lewy body disease relate to Lewy bodies in the temporal lobe. Brain 125:391–403.

Hock C, Maddalena A, Heuser I, Naber D, Oertel W, von der KH, Wienrich M, Raschig A, Deng M, Growdon JH, Nitsch RM (2000) Treatment with the selective muscarinic agonist talsaclidine decreases cerebrospinal fluid levels of total amyloid beta-peptide in patients with Alzheimer's disease. Ann N Y Acad Sci 920:285–291.

Holmes C, Ballard C, Lehmann D, David SA, Beaumont H, Day IN, Nadeem KM, Lovestone S, McCulley M, Morris CM, Munoz DG, O'Brien K, Russ C, Del ST, Warden D (2005) Rate of progression of cognitive decline in Alzheimer's disease: effect of butyrylcholinesterase K gene variation. J Neurol Neurosurg Psychiatry 76:640–643.

Kaye JA, May C, Daly E, Atack JR, Sweeney DJ, Luxenberg JS, Kay AD, Kaufman S, Milstien S, Friedland RP, et al. (1988) Cerebrospinal fluid monoamine markers are decreased in dementia of the Alzheimer type with extrapyramidal features. Neurology 38:554–557.

Kuhn W, Muller T, Gerlach M, Sofic E, Fuchs G, Heye N, Prautsch R, Przuntek H (1996) Depression in Parkinson's disease: biogenic amines in CSF of 'de novo' patients. J Neural Transm 103:1441–1445.

Lai MK, Lai OF, Keene J, Esiri MM, Francis PT, Hope T, Chen CP (2001) Psychosis of Alzheimer's disease is associated with elevated muscarinic M2 binding in the cortex. Neurology 57:805–811.

Lai MK, Tsang SW, Francis PT, Keene J, Hope T, Esiri MM, Spence I, Chen CP (2002) Postmortem serotoninergic correlates of cognitive decline in Alzheimer's disease. Neuroreport 13:1175–1178.

Lai MK, Tsang SW, Francis PT, Esiri MM, Keene J, Hope T, Chen CP (2003) Reduced serotonin 5-HT1A receptor binding in the temporal cortex correlates with aggressive behavior in Alzheimer disease. Brain Res 974:82–87.

Martin-Ruiz CM, Court JA, Molnar E, Lee M, Gotti C, Mamalaki A, Tsouloufis T, Tzartos S, Ballard C, Perry RH, Perry EK (1999) Alpha4 but not alpha3 and alpha7 nicotinic acetylcholine receptor subunits are lost from the temporal cortex in Alzheimer's disease. J Neurochem 73:1635–1640.

Martin-Ruiz CM, Piggott M, Gotti C, Lindstrom J, Mendelow AD, Siddique MS, Perry RH, Perry EK, Court JA (2000a) Alpha and beta nicotinic acetylcholine receptors subunits and synaptophysin in putamen from Parkinson's disease. Neuropharmacology 39:2830–2839.

Martin-Ruiz C, Court J, Lee M, Piggott M, Johnson M, Ballard C, Kalaria R, Perry R, Perry E (2000b) Nicotinic receptors in dementia of Alzheimer, Lewy body and vascular types. Acta Neurol Scand Suppl 176:34–41.

Mash DC, Flynn DD, Potter LT (1985) Loss of M2 muscarine receptors in the cerebral cortex in Alzheimer's disease and experimental cholinergic denervation. Science 228:1115–1117.

McKeith IG, Grace JB, Walker Z, Byrne EJ, Wilkinson D, Stevens T, Perry EK (2000) Rivastigmine in the treatment of dementia with Lewy bodies: preliminary findings from an open trial. Int J Geriatr Psychiatry 15:387–392.

Mesulam MM, Geula C (1994) Butyrylcholinesterase reactivity differentiates the amyloid plaques of aging from those of dementia. Ann Neurol 36:722–727.

Middlemiss DN, Palmer AM, Edel N, Bowen DM (1986) Binding of the novel serotonin agonist 8-hydroxy-2-(di-*n*-propylamino) tetralin in normal and Alzheimer brain. J Neurochem 46:993–996.

Minger SL, Esiri MM, McDonald B, Keene J, Carter J, Hope T, Francis PT (2000) Cholinergic deficits contribute to behavioral disturbance in patients with dementia. Neurology 55:1460–1467.

Nordberg A, Winblad B (1986) Reduced number of [3H]nicotine and [3H]acetylcholine binding sites in the frontal cortex of Alzheimer brains. Neurosci Lett 72:115–119.

O'Brien KK, Saxby BK, Ballard CG, Grace J, Harrington F, Ford GA, O'Brien JT, Swan AG, Fairbairn AF, Wesnes K, Del ST, Edwardson JA, Morris CM, McKeith IG (2003) Regulation of attention and response to therapy in dementia by butyrylcholinesterase. Pharmacogenetics 13:231–239.

Palmer AM, Sims NR, Bowen DM, Neary D, Palo J, Wikstrom J, Davison AN (1984) Monoamine metabolite concentrations in lumbar cerebrospinal fluid of patients with histologically verified Alzheimer's dementia. J Neurol Neurosurg Psychiatry 47:481–484.

Palmer AM, Francis PT, Benton JS, Sims NR, Mann DM, Neary D, Snowden JS, Bowen DM (1987a) Presynaptic serotonergic dysfunction in patients with Alzheimer's disease. J Neurochem 48:8–15.

Palmer AM, Wilcock GK, Esiri MM, Francis PT, Bowen DM (1987a) Monoaminergic innervation of the frontal and temporal lobes in Alzheimer's disease. Brain Res 401:231–238.

Palmer AM, Stratmann GC, Procter AW, Bowen DM (1988) Possible neurotransmitter basis of behavioral changes in Alzheimer's disease. Ann Neurol 23:616–620.

Perry EK, Morris CM, Court JA, Cheng A, Fairbairn AF, McKeith IG, Irving D, Brown A, Perry RH (1995) Alteration in nicotine binding sites in Parkinson's disease, Lewy body dementia and Alzheimer's disease: possible index of early neuropathology. Neuroscience 64:385–395.

Perry E, Court J, Goodchild R, Griffiths M, Jaros E, Johnson M, Lloyd S, Piggott M, Spurden D, Ballard C, McKeith I, Perry R (1998) Clinical neurochemistry: developments in dementia research based on brain bank material. J Neural Transm 105:915–933.

Perry E, Martin-Ruiz C, Lee M, Griffiths M, Johnson M, Piggott M, Haroutunian V, Buxbaum JD, Nasland J, Davis K, Gotti C, Clementi F, Tzartos S, Cohen O, Soreq H, Jaros E, Perry R, Ballard C, McKeith I, Court J (2000) Nicotinic receptor subtypes in human brain ageing, Alzheimer and Lewy body diseases. Eur J Pharmacol 393:215–222.

Perry E, Ziabreva I, Perry R, Aarsland D, Ballard C (2005) Absence of cholinergic deficits in 'pure' vascular dementia. Neurology 64:132–133.

Piggott MA, Owens J, O'Brien J, Colloby S, Fenwick J, Wyper D, Jaros E, Johnson M, Perry RH, Perry EK (2003) Muscarinic receptors in basal ganglia in dementia with Lewy bodies, Parkinson's disease and Alzheimer's disease. J Chem Neuroanat 25:161–173.

Pimlott SL, Piggott M, Owens J, Greally E, Court JA, Jaros E, Perry RH, Perry EK, Wyper D (2004) Nicotinic acetylcholine receptor distribution in Alzheimer's disease, dementia with Lewy bodies, Parkinson's disease, and vascular dementia: in vitro binding study using 5-[(125)i]-a-85380. Neuropsychopharmacology 29:108–116.

Reid RT, Sabbagh MN, Corey-Bloom J, Tiraboschi P, Thai LJ (2000) Nicotinic receptor in dementia with Lewy Bodies: comparisons with Alzheimer's disease. Neurobiol Aging 21:741–746.

Reynolds GP, Arnold L, Rossor MN, Iversen LL, Mountjoy CQ, Roth M (1984) Reduced binding of [3H]ketanserin to cortical 5-ht2 receptors in senile dementia of the Alzheimer type. Neurosci Lett 44:47–51.

Rinne JO, Lonnberg P, Marjamaki P, Rinne UK (1989) Brain muscarinic receptor subtypes are differently affected in Alzheimer's disease and Parkinson's disease. Brain Res 483:402–406.

Rodriguez-Puertas R, Pascual J, Vilaro T, Pazos A (1997) Autoradiographic distribution of Ml, M2, M3, and M4 muscarinic receptor subtypes in Alzheimer's disease. Synapse 26:341–350.

Sabbagh MN, Reid RT, Corey-Bloom J, Rao TS, Hansen LA, Alford M, Masliah E, Adem A, Lloyd GK, Thai LJ (1998) Correlation of nicotinic binding with neurochemical markers in Alzheimer's disease. J Neural Transm 105:709–717.

Sabbagh MN, Reid RT, Hansen LA, Alford M, Thai LJ (2001) Correlation of nicotinic receptor binding with clinical and neuropathological changes in Alzheimer's disease and dementia with Lewy bodies. J Neural Transm 108:1149–1157.

Seeger T, Fedorova I, Zheng F, Miyakawa T, Koustova E, Gomeza J, Basile AS, Alzheimer C, Wess J (2004) M2 muscarinic acetylcholine receptor knock-out mice show deficits in behavioral flexibility, working memory, and hippocampal plasticity. J Neurosci 24:10117–10127.

Teaktong T, Graham AJ, Court JA, Perry RH, Jaros E, Johnson M, Hall R, Perry EK (2004) Nicotinic acetylcholine receptor immunohistochemistry in Alzheimer's disease and dementia with Lewy bodies: differential neuronal and astroglial pathology. J Neurol Sci 225:39–49.

Wallin A, Blennow K, Gottfries CG (1989) Neurochemical abnormalities in vascular dementia. *Dementia*, 1:120–130.

Wang HY, Lee DH, Davis CB, Shank RP (2000) Amyloid peptide Abeta(1-42) binds selectively and with picomolar affinity to alpha7 nicotinic acetylcholine receptors. J Neurochem 75:1155–1161.

3

The Molecular Pathology
of Severe Dementia

Clive Holmes

Alzheimer's disease

At post mortem severe Alzheimer's Disease (AD) is characterised at the microscopic level by the presence of large numbers of classic (neuritic) senile plaques and neurofibrillary tangles (NFTs) (Figure 1). These pathological changes are also associated with neuroinflammation and widespread neuronal cell loss.

Senile plaques

Characteristics

In AD, senile plaques (SPs) can be broadly classified into two main categories, diffuse and classic (neuritic) plaques.

Diffuse plaques are large (10–100 μm) areas of poorly defined Aβ deposition, detected using antibodies against Aβ. These deposits take a variety of forms and include subpial, vascular, granular, diffuse, stellar and compact deposits. A laminar pattern of Aβ deposits in the neocortex of AD patients has been described with concentrations in layers II, III and V. In addition, Aβ deposits have also been reported in peripheral tissues such as skin and gut in AD. Aβ deposits in diffuse plaques are found uniformly throughout the neocortex and hippocampus and do not appear to correlate well with the neuropathological stages in AD (Braak and Braak, 1991) and are present in mild and severe cases of AD. In addition, diffuse plaques are found in the neocortex of non-demented elderly individuals without any neurofibrillary changes, suggesting that they precede neurofibrillary formation. The hypothesis that Aβ deposition is an early event in the pathogenesis of AD has been given further support by the lack of association of diffuse plaques with any neuritic change or astrocytic involvement.

Classical neuritic plaques are larger (50–200 μm) and most clearly present in severe AD. They consist of an amyloid core with radiating amyloid fibrils and are associated with a corona of neuritic processes, glial cell processes, astrocytes and microglial cells. Amyloid fibrils are composed of 5–10 nm filaments, principally composed of Aβ protein, between 40 and 43 amino acids in length. Neuritic processes are often dystrophic and contain paired helical filaments. The distribution of neuritic plaques varies widely from individual to individual and between neocortical layers. Neuritic plaques are more numerous in the associative areas of the neocortex than in the sensory areas and are also largest in those laminae characterised by large pyramidal neurons. In conventional silver staining preparations classical neuritic plaques appear to show three types of histology: 'primitive', 'mature' and 'burnt-out'. On the basis of light and electron microscopic studies, a three-stage evolution of SPs has been proposed. The first stage is the 'primitive plaque', composed

Severe Dementia. Edited by A. Burns and B. Winblad.
Copyright © 2006 John Wiley & Sons, Ltd.   ISBN 0-470-01054-1

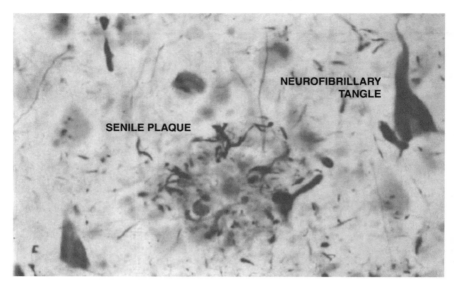

Figure 1.   Neuropathological hallmarks of Alzheimer's disease.

of a small number of distorted neurites, largely presynaptic in origin with few amyloid fibres, astrocytic processes and the occasional microglial cell. The second stage is the 'mature' plaque with a dense amyloid core with a halo of dystrophic neurites, astrocytic processes and cell bodies and the occasional microglial cell. The final sequence is the 'burnt-out' plaque consisting of a dense core of amyloid. In severe AD all forms of neuritic plaques are apparent. The association between the more condensed Aβ with increasing neuritic change, reactive astrocytosis and microglial infiltration implies that classical plaque formation and the aggregation of Aβ is responsible for the damage in the surrounding neuropil as the disease becomes increasingly severe.

Classic neuritic plaque frequency does not correlate well with dementia severity. This may be because plaque frequency increases with severity up to a maximum point, regardless of plaque type, but then reaches a steady state or even decreases (Thal *et al.*, 1997). Thus, the generation of Aβ plaques may cease when the neuronal degeneration and synaptic loss is completed and astrogliosis takes place.

Pathogenesis

The pathological changes described above necessarily describe the findings of severe Alzheimer's disease since most studies have been done on patients with end-stage disease. Although, *in vivo* imaging is becoming increasingly sophisticated, it has not been possible, as yet, to truly visualise the time course of the pathological events in AD. Molecular genetics has, however, offered a route to an understanding of the aetiology of AD which is independent of pathology. The evidence from these genetic studies suggests that the formation of plaques is fundamental to the development of AD and that plaques have a central role to play in the instigation of the other pathological features found in AD. This idea has been termed the amyloid cascade hypothesis (Hardy and Higgins, 1992) and it has also received support from other related diseases. Thus, in Down's syndrome, where AD inevitably occurs (as a result of subjects having three copies of chromosome 21 and hence the amyloid precursor protein (APP) gene) it has been shown that the earliest microscopic pathology is the diffuse deposition of amyloid which precedes tangle formation (Mann *et al.*, 1989). In addition,

Gene	Chromosome	How common	Mutations cause
APP	21	About 15 families in world	Autosomal dominant
Presenilin 1	14	30 – 50 % of young onset autosomal dominant	Autosomal dominant
Presenilin 2	1	<10 % of young onset autosomal dominant	Autosomal dominant
ApoE-E4	19	15 % population 1 copy, 1 % population 2 copies	Risk factor 1 copy × 3–4 2 copies × 10

Figure 2. Genes associated with Alzheimer's disease.

mutations in tau (the main constituent of NFTs) have been shown to give rise to a form of dementia (fronto-temporal dementia with Parkinsonism), which is characterised by neuronal loss and tangle formation, but which has no evidence of amyloid plaque deposition. All of these findings support the idea that the deposition of amyloid plaques is the primary event in the development of AD. Molecular genetics has also enabled a greater understanding of how plaque formation arises.

To date, four genes have been identified and confirmed as contributing to the genetic aetiology of AD. APP (chromosome 21), Presenilin 1 (chromosome 14), Presenilin 2 (chromosome 1) and Apolipoprotein E (APOE) (chromosome 19). Mutations in APP, presenilin 1 and presenilin 2 give rise to rare forms of AD that are predominately of early onset and appear to have a largely autosomal dominant inheritance pattern. Common genetic variation in ApoE (the E4 allele) gives rise to an early, but still largely late-onset, form of AD (Holmes, 2002) (Figure 2).

APP produces a transmembrane protein that is found in most cell types including neuronal and glial cells. APP undergoes proteolytic cleavage by α, β and γ secretase activity to produce Aβ protein of varying lengths (Figure 3). α-secretase cleavage is the non-amyloidogenic pathway, cutting

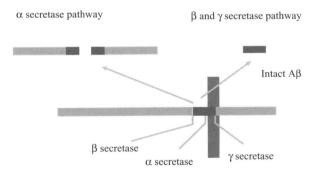

Figure 3. Processing of amyloid precursor protein. Amyloid (Aβ) is formed from a small segment of the parent amyloid precursor protein. The α secretase pathway results in cleavage of the amyloid itself, whilst the β and γ secretase pathway results in intact amyloid.

the Aβ peptide in half between amino acids 16 and 17 resulting in a soluble fragment (sAPPα) and a membrane-bound APP fragment. Under normal circumstances the α secretase pathway accounts for 95% of APP processing.

Cleavage by β secretase at the N terminus of Aβ between amino acids 671 and 672 in addition to cleavage at the C terminus of Aβ by γ secretase yields Aβ and a non-amyloidogenic fragment (sAPPβ). γ secretase cleavage can occur after the 40, 42 or 43 amino acid of the Aβ peptide to generate the shorter Aβ40 or the longer Aβ42 or Aβ43, respectively. The Aβ42 or Aβ43 moieties are considered to be more fibrillogenic and are deposited early in disease compared with the shorter Aβ40. All of the known pathological mutations in APP occur close to the major APP cleavage sites, suggesting that these mutations alter the processing of APP. Thus mutations close to the β secretase site are thought to enhance the production of both Aβ40 and Aβ42, while mutations close to the α secretase site cause impaired α secretase activity with an increase in β and γ secretase activity, and a consequent increase in secreted Aβ. Mutations next to the γ secretase site lead to a selective increase in Aβ42 over the Aβ40 isoform.

Presenilin 1 protein is a transmembrane protein expressed in many tissues including the brain where it is enriched in neurons. Over 40 different mutations have been found in presenilin 1, which account for around 30–50% of all presenile familial AD. Presenilin is thought to be a co-factor for γ secretase and appears to alter APP processing. Thus, presenilin mutations have been shown to increase the ratio of Aβ42 to Aβ40 in transfected cell lines and transgenic mice expressing mutant forms of PS1. The other member of the presenilin family, presenilin 2, is highly homologous to presenilin 1. However, in comparison to presenilin 1 mutations the frequency of presenilin 2 mutations is very low.

Apolipoprotein E is a plasma protein involved in cholesterol uptake, storage, transport and metabolism. The ApoE gene has three allele types, E2, E3 and E4. In the Caucasian population the presence of one E4 allele approximately doubles the risk of AD, while two E4 alleles (E4/E4) increases the risk 10–15-fold compared to E3/E3 genotype. The mode of action of ApoE as a risk factor for AD is unclear. However, current theories suggest that the various isoforms affect the clearance of Aβ or tau, thereby affecting the formation of senile plaques and neurofibrillary tangles. Whilst being a clear risk factor for the development of early AD there is little evidence to suggest that the presence of ApoE E4 leads to a more severe or more rapidly progressive form of AD.

In vitro structural studies of Aβ using synthetic peptides have demonstrated their spontaneous assembly into amyloid-like fibres. Fibrillogenesis is a two-step process involving an initial slow, lag period that reflects the thermodynamic barrier to the formation of nucleation 'seed' followed by a rapid fibril aggregation. Fibril aggregation is modulated by several factors which, in addition to the length of the Aβ fragment, includes the interaction with other elements including small metal ions (copper, iron and zinc) and other proteins including proteoglycans (McLaurin *et al.*, 2003).

Neurofibrillary tangles

Characteristics

Neurofibrillary tangles (NFTs) are the other major histological hallmark of AD. Like SPs, they are not specific to AD and occur in normal ageing, as well as in other neurodegenerative diseases, including Down's syndrome, post-encephalitic Parkinsonism and fronto-temporal lobe dementia with Parkinsonism. NFTs are neuronal inclusions, and are composed mainly of paired helical filaments which are formed by two filaments wound round each other with a periodic twist every 18 nm resulting in a typical double helix. Paired helical filaments are chiefly composed of the microtubule associated protein tau, which is involved in microtubule assembly and stabilisation, and is in a hyperphosphorylated state in NFTs. NFTs also contain other proteins including actin and ubiquitin.

The distribution of NFTs does not appear to closely correlate to that of SPs. NFTs are found throughout the neocortex and are common in the medial temporal structures, in the hippocampus, amygdala and parahippocampal gyrus. In addition they are also found in the deep grey matter, including the nucleus basilis of Meynert, substantia nigra, locus coeruleus, and the raphe nuclei of the brainstem.

While NFTs are intracytoplasmic neuronal inclusions, they may become extracellular after the neuron that contained them has died. These extraneuronal NFTs are most often seen in the hippocampus and entorhinal cortex in severe disease and appear to be chiefly composed of straight, not paired, helical filaments.

The sequential deposition of NFTs appears to closely correlate with dementia severity in AD. The staging method developed by Braak and Braak (Braak and Braak, 1991) postulates that the NFT pathology of AD evolves in a relatively predictable sequence across the medial temporal lobe structures, subcortical nuclei, and neocortical areas of the brain in six stages. These six stages can be reduced to three anatomical stages. In the transentorhinal stage (stages I and II), the neurofibrillary pathology is essentially confined to the transentorhinal and entorhinal cortex with mild involvement of the CA1/CA2 sections of the hippocampus. The limbic stage (stages III and IV) involves severe involvement of the entorhinal areas, moderate tangles in the hippocampus, and spread to the amygdala, thalamus, hypothalamus and basal forebrain. Finally, the neocortical stage (stages V and VI) involves abundant NFT pathology in the neocortex. Initial clinical characterisation of these stages suggested that the transentorhinal stage was 'clinically silent'; the limbic stages represented the first clinical signs of AD and the neocortical stage represented fully developed moderate to severe AD. However, it is increasingly clear that whilst the overall correlation between NFT pathology and ante-mortem cognitive score is good (Spearman rank coefficient = 0.57, $p < 0.0001$) (Riley et al., 2002) there is a degree of individual variability. Thus, some patients in the transentorhinal stage do, in fact, have identifiable memory impairment and some patients with Braak stages IV or higher may have only mild cognitive impairment ante mortem. Variation between individuals outside the expected may be explained by a number of other factors including age, the presence of cerebral atherosclerosis and the degree of cerebral atrophy.

Pathogenesis

The exact route by which aggregated Aβ results in the development of NFTs is unclear. A number of mechanisms have been proposed but the most likely model at present suggests that Aβ fibrils are involved in the phosphorylation of critical residues of tau. The phosphorylation of these residues results in tau being less able to bind to microtubules rendering the microtubules less stable and more likely to depolymerise. Since microtubules are critical in sustaining axonal transport and for cytoskeletal structure, the loss of microtubule stability is thought to be a key factor in neuronal cell death. Aggregated Aβ has also been shown to act as a stimulus for microglia activation. The activation of microglia leads to the generation of the pro-inflammatory cytokine interleukin-1 which has been hypothesised to have a pivotal role in perpetuating an inflammatory cascade by increasing the deposition of Aβ as well as contributing to tau phosphorylation (Griffin et al., 1998). Tau can be phosphorylated by several kinases including GSK-3β, cdk5, MAP kinase and MARK. To date, most attention has focused on the role of GSK-3β. Thus, animal models have shown that overexpression of GSK-3β leads to abnormalities of both axonal transport and long-term potentiation.

Neuronal loss

Neuronal loss in severe AD is predominantly of the large pyramidal neurons from layers three and five of the neocortex. Neocortical loss is most evident in the temporal and frontal lobes whilst the parietal and occipital lobes are less involved. There is also a substantial loss of large pyramidal neurons in the hippocampus, the nucleus basilis of Meynert, the locus coeruleus, and the raphe nuclei.

Notably, whilst this pattern of neuronal loss correlates well with the distribution of tangle-bearing cells, neuronal cell loss exceeds the number of NFTs. This suggests that the tangle-bearing neurons are removed and/or some neurons die without forming tangles.

The death of populations of neurons in the brain regions affected in severe AD occurs over a prolonged period of time of many years, which suggests that a relatively small number of neurons are dying at any one time. Such spatio-temporal pattern of cell death is characteristic of a form of programmed cell death called apoptosis and contrasts with necrosis in which cells die *en masse*.

Inflammation

In the normal brain microglia have a highly characteristic morphology with a small cell soma and thin straight processes. However, in the severe AD brain, microglia are activated, becoming enlarged with elongated tortuous processes, and they congregate around amyloid plaques and degenerating neurons. Whereas many of the changes in glial cells in AD may promote neuronal degeneration, some of the changes may represent adaptive responses aimed at promoting neuronal plasticity and survival. Thus, microglia may also remove $A\beta$ as well as producing toxins and cytokines that contribute to the neurodegenerative process.

Vascular dementia

The development of severe vascular dementia is usually the cumulative effect of multiple focal brain lesions with accumulating loss of neurons or axons. Less commonly a severe dementia may arise from a single focal strategic lesion, diffuse anoxic or ischaemic damage or haemorrhage.

The main reason for cerebrovascular damage is substrate shortage, i.e. an inadequate supply of oxygen or glucose either due to a failing heart or lung function or due to obstruction from stenosis or the occlusion of blood vessels. Occlusion occurs in the carotid artery, in the circle of Willis and its main vessels, including the meningeal main arterial branches (large vessels) and in the intracerebral arteries (small vessels). In larger vessels, emboli and arteriosclerotic changes with thrombosis dominate, resulting in large infarcts, whereas fibrohyaline arteriosclerosis, collagen disease and hypertensive angiopathy are more common when multiple smaller vessels are occluded, resulting in smaller infarcts.

Multi-infarct dementia is defined as resulting from occlusions of large vessels leading to large infarcts. It has been stated that an infarct size of 100 ml is required to produce dementia (Tomlinson, 1980) although the location and bilaterality is also important. An infarct may also be small and still cause a severe dementia if it is strategically placed. Thus, bilateral thalamic infarcts result in a sudden onset severe dementia with frontal traits. Occlusions in the intracerebral vessels results in lacunar infarcts that do not usually exceed 10 mm in diameter. The smallness of the lacunae in combination with the variability in completeness of the infarcts leads to a more gradual, possibly, stepwise, progression into severe dementia.

Haemorrhage as a cause of severe dementia is much less common than infarction. However, the immediate impact on cognitive function can be dramatic with only 20% of patients with intracerebral haemorrhage surviving the acute phase.

Mixed AD and vascular dementia

The proportion of patients with mixed pathology varies according to the strictness of the criteria utilised. Thus, the proportion of cases seen as having mixed dementia may quoted to be as little as 3–5% (Jellinger, 2002) or up to 60–90% (Kalaria, 2000). Few and small vascular lesions may be of little consequence of themselves. However, there is increasing evidence to show that in combination with AD pathology the severity of the dementia is greater than anticipated than if we considered either lesion in isolation. Thus, the Nun study (Snowden *et al.*, 1997) found that less Alzheimer pathology was required to produce dementia if cerebrovascular disease is also present.

Dementia with Lewy bodies

Dementia with Lewy bodies (DLB) has a variable burden of Alzheimer-type pathology, together with Lewy bodies in both the cortical and subcortical regions. However, even when plaque counts are high, DLB cases have mild or insignificant neocortical tau pathology. Lewy bodies are also present in other conditions including Down's syndrome and familial early Alzheimer's disease but are characteristically associated with idiopathic Parkinson's disease (PD).

Subcortical Lewy bodies were originally described in the pigmented monoaminergic and catecholaminergic neurons of the diencephalon and upper brainstem. In these neurons Lewy bodies stood out as rounded intracytoplasmic inclusions characterised by a dense eosinophilic core with a surrounding pale halo. Studies in PD have extended the range for these well-delineated Lewy bodies considerably to include areas of the temporal cortex, limbic cortex, locus coeruleus, nucleus basalis of Meynert and raphe. In the past decade it has also been recognised that Lewy bodies are present in the cortex that lack the intense eosinophilia and peripheral lucency of their subcortical counterparts although these were undoubtedly overlooked in early pathological studies.

A spectrum of Lewy body disease has been proposed which is categorised into three types (brainstem, transitional and diffuse), and this concept is the basis for the categories defined by the Consensus guidelines on the diagnosis of DLB (McKeith *et al.*, 1996). However, whilst in AD, as already described, there is evidence that tangle pathology follows a hierarchic evolution this is not the case for the spectrum of Lewy body disease. Thus, individuals can present clinically with PD but do not develop a dementing illness and are found at autopsy to have brainstem Lewy bodies with few cortical Lewy bodies. Likewise, some individuals may present with dementia alone and never develop PD and at autopsy are found to have cortical Lewy bodies alone with minimal brainstem disease.

Most recently it has been demonstrated that a major component, possibly the core filamentous constituent, of subcortical or cortical Lewy bodies is the protein α-synuclein. α-synuclein is a presynaptic protein that exists in two alternatively spliced forms, with no recognisable secondary structures. While it is clear that point mutations in α-synuclein are associated with the development of autosomal dominant familial Parkinson's disease the mechanism by which α-synuclein leads to DLB is unclear although it may be due to abnormal interaction with neurofilaments or due to the self-aggregation of α-synuclein in an analogous fashion to tau and tangle formation.

In addition to Lewy bodies DLB patients have neuronal degeneration in the substantia nigra that, in terms of severity, is between that seen in PD and normal control individuals of the same age. The mechanism of neuronal loss is unknown but evidence, like in AD, supports apoptosis.

Fronto-temporal dementia

Fronto-temporal dementia (FTD) is characterised by cerebral atrophy, principally in the cerebral hemispheres involving mostly the frontal, anterior parietal, cingulated, insular and temporal regions. All of the variable clinical and pathological phenotypes share, to a greater or lesser degree, a non-Alzheimer-type histological profile. This is characterised by cerebral cortical neuronal loss, gliosis and microvacuolar change due to shrinkage of nerve cell bodies and their processes. In addition, neuronal inclusions including Pick's bodies and neurofibrillary tangles may or may not be present.

A number of familial forms of FTD have been identified. Sequencing of the tau gene has now shown that many of these familial forms bear mutational changes in tau, either relating to missense or deletion mutations within coding (exonic) regions or within regulatory (intronic) regions. Most of the missense mutations appear to reduce the ability of tau protein to interact with microtubules whereas the exonic mutations lead to an increase in the four repeat tau isoforms that leads to its assembly into twisted ribbons. In addition, some tau exonic mutations have been shown to lead to a neuropathology that includes Pick's body inclusions.

The molecular pathology of other fronto-temporal lobe dementias such as semantic dementia and primary progressive aphasia have been less clearly defined, although the patterns of histology would appear identical and the tendency for these conditions to overlap with increasing severity of the disease would suggest that common underlying mechanisms will be found.

References

Braak H, Braak E (1991) Neuropathological staging of Alzheimer related changes. *Acta Neuropathol*, 82:239–59.

Cohen P, Goedert M, GSK3 inhibitors (2004) Development and therapeutic potential. *Nature Reviews. Drug Discovery*, 3:479–87.

Griffin WS, Sheng JG, Royston MC *et al.* (1998) Glial-neuronal interactions in Alzheimer's Disease: the potential role of a 'cytokine cycle' in disease progression. *Brain pathology*, 8:65–72.

Hardy JA and Higgins GA (1992) Amyloid deposition as the central event in the aetiology of Alzheimer's Disease. *Trends Pharm Sci*, 12:383–8.

Holmes C (2002) Genotype and Phenotype in late onset Alzheimer's Disease. *Br J Psychiatry*, 180:131–4.

Jellinger KA. Alzheimer's Disease and cerebrovascular pathology: an update. *J Neural Transm*, 2002; 109:813–36.

Kalaria JN (2000) The role of cerebral ischaemia in Alzheimer's Disease. Neurobiology of Aging 21:321–30.

Mann DM, Brown A, Prinja D *et al.* (1989) An analysis of the morphology of senile plaques in Down's syndrome patients of different ages using immunocytochemical and lectin histochemical techniques. *Neuropath Appl Neurobiol*, 15:317–29.

McLaurin J, Go M, Kierstead M *et al.* (2003) Factors regulating amyloid-b fibril formation and their potential for therapeutic intervention in plaque deposition. In K. Iqbal and B Winblad eds Alzheimer's Disease and Related Disorders: Research Advances, Ch 48. 541–547.

McKeith IG, Galasko D, Kosaka K *et al.* (1996) Consensus guidelines for the clinical and pathologic diagnosis of dementia with Lewy bodies (DLB): report of the consortium on DLB international workshop. *Neurology*, 47(5):1113–24.

Riley KP, Snowdon DA, Markesbery WR (2002) Alzheimer's neurofibrillary pathology and the spectrum of cognitive function: findings from the Nun Study. *Ann Neurol*, 51:567–77.

Snowden DA, Greiner LH, Mortimer JA *et al.* (1997) Brain infarction and the clinical expression of Alzheimer's Disease. The Nun study. *JAMA*, 277:813–17.

Thal DR, Glas A, Schneider W *et al.* (1997) Differential pattern of β amyloid, amyloid precursor protein and apolipoprotein E expression in cortical senile plaques. *Acta Neuropathol*, 94:255–65.

Tomlinson BE (1980) The structural and quantitative aspects of dementias. Roberts, PJ (ed) Biochemistry of Dementia. New York: Wiley, 15–52.

Further reading

Brun A (2000) Vascular dementia: pathological findings. Chapter 50. Dementia 2nd ed. O'Brien, Ames and Burns Arnold.

Parihar MS, Hemnani T (2004) AD pathogenesis and therapeutic interventions. *J Clin Neuroscience* 11:456–7.

Clinical Features of Severe Dementia

4

Cognitive Functions in Severe Dementia

Judith Saxton and François Boller

Introduction

Most studies of cognition in dementia, and Alzheimer's disease (AD) in particular, have dealt with the mild to moderate stages of the disorder. However, because of the very nature of the disease, all AD patients who live long enough, progress to a stage of profound cognitive and functional decline in which the individual is totally dependent on another for their care. The number of patients with severe dementia is unclear but in general it is estimated that, at any one time, one-third of demented individuals will be in the severe stages (Fratiglioni *et al.*, 1994; Dartigues *et al.*, 2002); thus, in the United States, it can be estimated that as many as 1.3 million individuals are severely demented. Despite the size of this population, it is only recently that individuals with severe dementia have become a focus of research interest (Boller *et al.*, 2002).

The small amount of research reviewed in this chapter applies mostly to AD. There is hardly any factual information about the advanced stages of other forms of dementia. And yet, there may be different characteristics in the late stages of other dementias. In particular, vascular and mixed dementia, as well as Parkinson's disease and dementia with Lewy bodies may have different behavioural symptoms and added physical disabilities and neurological signs due to strokes and extrapyramidal features. Similarly, in the case of fronto-temporal dementia, behavioural symptoms may continue to dominate the picture (Florence Pasquier, personal communication, 2001). The last stages of the various forms of dementia will be better known when more widespread use of cognitive batteries specifically designed for the assessment of severe dementia, coupled with the use of behavioural scales and observations, is applied on a longitudinal basis for populations of known aetiologies.

Definition of severe dementia

Severe dementia is operationally defined based on scores on global rating scales completed by observation of subjects' residual abilities and interview with the patient's caregiver. Thus, severe dementia has been defined as a score of 6 or 7 on the Global Deterioration Scale (GDS) (Reisberg *et al.*, 1982); or a score of 3 or higher on the Clinical Dementia Rating (CDR) scale (Hughes *et al.*, 1982); or categories 6a to 7f of the Functional Assessment Staging Test (FAST) (Reisberg, 1988). The Mini Mental State Examination (MMSE) (Folstein *et al.*, 1975) is typically used to identify the presence of severe cognitive dysfunction and a score of 10 or less is generally agreed to represent severe dementia Reisberg *et al.*, 1994; Feldman *et al.*, 2001; Gauthier *et al.*, 2002; Schmitt *et al.*, 1997; Reisberg *et al.*, 2003; Tariot *et al.*, 2004).

Severe Dementia. Edited by A. Burns and B. Winblad.
Copyright © 2006 John Wiley & Sons, Ltd.   ISBN 0-470-01054-1

Description of the cognitive deficit

The cognitive impairment seen in severe dementia is characterised by significant deficits in all cognitive domains, even though not all are affected to the same extent. Thus, the patient with advanced dementia exhibits markedly impaired language functions. The deficits in comprehension are evident in the individual's inability to follow even simple, one-step commands. Expressive speech is also impaired, but there may be echolalia, palilalia, perseverations (e.g. 'help me', 'help me') and/or nonverbal utterances (e.g. groaning, barking). Surprisingly, repetition and simple reading aloud, without comprehension, may be spared well into the late stages of AD. The differential diagnosis between the language disorder of AD and the aphasias that follow focal lesions relies, of course, on history and on accompanying signs. The language disorder of AD differs from that of global aphasia due to focal lesions in that, contrary to many patients with aphasia, demented individuals are often unable to use nonverbal gestures, mimics, or intonations to bypass their language impairment and to express meaning.

Memory decline is the hallmark of AD and all memory systems are affected to a greater or lesser degree in severe dementia. Episodic memory, i.e. the ability to remember episodes that happened in the individual's life, such as the last time they had lunch with their daughter, already impaired in the early stages of the disease become most impaired and actually barely testable in the severe stages. This is evident in some patients who constantly repeat the same question over and over again. Semantic memory, i.e. linguistic and general knowledge about the world, only mildly impaired in the early stages is also profoundly impaired by the late stages. In contrast to episodic and semantic memory, immediate or short-term memory, i.e. the ability to repeat a short sentence or a short string of digits immediately after hearing them, is relatively preserved. Although tests such as digit spans show clear impairment in the early stages of the disease, it is almost as if the loss of other faculties is released and whatever inhibited performance on this test previously is no longer present and the more demented patient is now able to repeat a relatively long string of meaningless digits.

Some aspects of implicit memory, namely those in which semantic processing are not involved, are relatively spared even into the severe stages of dementia. Overlearned skills, habits and implicit expression of memory for perceptually encoded items may be relatively spared until the very last stages. Preserved perceptual priming among AD patients may explain why some institutionalised patients with AD learn the fastest 'escape' route out of the nursing home and, furthermore, why they can reliably repeat this behaviour and thus become labelled as a 'flight risk'. Newly institutionalised patients also frequently develop emotional attachments, both positive and negative, to specific care aides or residents. Such attachments can be made very quickly, sometimes after only one or two interactions, and occasionally may be viewed as inappropriate relationships by family or staff. These friendships sometimes involve a relationship that a spouse or adult child may find difficult to accept. Occasionally severely demented patients may develop a dramatic dislike of a particular individual, sometimes an individual who was present during an emotionally charged situation such as, for some patients, bathing. It is likely that some form of implicit memory is involved in this 'emotional learning'.

Autobiographic memory, i.e. the conscious recollection of events from one's own past, sometimes relatively spared in the early stages of the disorder, is lost by the time the individual reaches the later stages.

Other domains of cognition such as executive functions, praxis and visuospatial abilities are very severely impaired and are in fact difficult to test in most instances. Cases of unilateral spatial neglect have been reported in the late stages of AD (Venneri *et al.*, 1998). If data obtained in patients with moderate dementia can be extrapolated to severe dementia, there are reasons to believe that emotional behaviour (which probably involves some implicit learning as discussed above) is often relatively preserved (Roudier *et al.*, 1998).

Assessment tools for severe dementia

One reason for the paucity of data on cognitive functions in AD has been the lack of standardised neuropsychological tests with the range of sensitivity at the lower end of the scale to evaluate severely impaired patients. Historically, patients beyond the moderate stages of dementia were labelled 'untestable' because these patients typically perform at floor level on traditional neuropsychological tests. Assessment of severely demented patients was restricted to caregiver rating scales that provide a global assessment of functioning. Cognitive scales that allow a direct, performance-based assessment were limited to the brief assessment allowed by the MMSE (Folstein *et al.*, 1975) or a somewhat broader evaluation offered by mental status scales such as the Mattis Dementia Rating Scale (Mattis, 1988). However, in recent years a number of scales have been developed that offer the opportunity to obtain direct, performance-based assessments of patients in the late stages of dementia.

The Severe Impairment Battery (SIB) is a test of cognition developed specifically to allow the reliable assessment of severely demented patients (Saxton and Swihart, 1989; Saxton *et al.*, 1990; Schmitt *et al.*, 1996). The SIB was designed as a research tool having the attributes of a standard neuropsychological test battery, that is, having the power to assess a range of cognitive domains, while being brief enough to be completed by even very impaired individuals. The SIB takes into account the behavioural and cognitive deficits associated with severe dementia. It is brief, taking approximately 20 minutes to administer. Clinical experience suggests that most severely demented patients can maintain attention for around 30 minutes. The SIB is designed to be well-structured and psychometrically reliable but to appear to the patient more as an interview than as a test. Presentation of the items is intended to be performed in a smoothly flowing manner, drawing out a response naturally or automatically. It is composed of simple, one-step commands presented in conjunction with gestural cues and allows credit for nonverbal and partially correct responses. These attributes are essential because of the extent of the comprehension and language production deficits seen in severe dementia. Any assessment device intended for use with severely demented individuals should take such deficits into account and allow for nonverbal responses while maintaining verbal presentation of material with the addition of gestural cues. Any other method of presentation creates an artificial and somewhat novel environment to which the severely demented patient will have difficulty adapting. The use of familiar social, contextual and nonverbal cues in well-structured situations provides the optimum environment for the valid assessment of severely demented patients. The procedure used in the administration of the SIB draws on automatic or overlearned responses.

The SIB is divided into six scorable subscales, each of which yields scores that are 'downward' extensions of instruments used to assess mild to moderate dementia. The six subscales are: Attention, Orientation, Language, Memory, Visuoperception and Construction. In addition, there are brief assessments of social skills, praxis and responding to name. The first item in each subscale is typically one that would fall at the lower end of the scale of a standard test of the cognitive domain it purports to measure. Examples of the items in each subscale are as follows: Attention – digit span and counting auditory and visual stimuli; Orientation – name, date, city (spontaneously and multiple choice), time or day; Language – writing one's own name spontaneously, following simple verbal and written commands, naming shapes, naming photographs of objects and naming real objects; Memory – immediate and delayed recall of previously presented objects, colours and shapes, recalling a sentence and the examiner's name; Visuoperception – matching and identifying different colours and shapes; Construction – ability to draw shapes spontaneously, ability to copy and trace shapes. The total range of possible scores on the SIB is 0–100.

The SIB has been shown to be a valid assessment not only in the original English version (Schmitt *et al.*, 1997; Saxton *et al.*, 1990; Schmitt *et al.*, 1996; Wild *et al.*, 1993) but also in French (Boller *et al.*, 2002; Panisset *et al.*, 1994; Verny *et al.*, 1999), Italian (Pippi *et al.*, 1999) and Spanish

(Barbarotto *et al.*, 2000). In addition, the SIB has been shown to reliably document cognitive change over time in severely demented patients with AD (Schmitt *et al.*, 1997; Wild and Kaye, 1998) and has recently been shown to be useful in clinical trials (Feldman *et al.*, 2001; Gauthier *et al.*, 2002; Reisberg *et al.*, 2003; Tariot *et al.*, 2004; Schmitt *et al.*, 1996). A shortened version of the SIB is available that allows the assessment of more profoundly impaired patients and takes only 15 minutes to administer (Boller *et al.*, 2004).

The SCIP (Peavy *et al.*, 1996) is another performance-based assessment of cognition that has been shown to provide a reliable, valid measure of neuropsychological functioning in severely demented patients. It has the ability to avoid both floor and ceiling effects and to evaluate a wide range of cognitive abilities, i.e. overall behaviour, attention, language, memory, motor, conceptualisation, arithmetic and visuospatial functioning. The maximum score on the SCIP is 245 but it can be completed in approximately 30 minutes. The SCIP assesses some cognitive functions that the SIB does not, e.g. arithmetic and conceptualisation. The SCIP also provides an assessment of some of the behavioural aspects of severe dementia.

The Test for Severe Impairment (TSI) (Albert and Cohen, 1992) has the advantage that it is relatively brief, taking only 10 minutes to complete, and requires no specific stimulus materials, making it particularly useful for bedside testing (Harrell *et al.*, 2000). The TSI has six subsections assessing overlearned motor skills, language comprehension, language production, immediate and delayed memory, general knowledge and conceptualisation. The TSI has been shown to be a valid and reliable test (Foldi *et al.*, 1999) that is particularly useful for assessment of patients in the very impaired range, that is, individuals with MMSE scores of less than five (Jacobs *et al.*, 1999).

The Modified-Ordinal Scales of Psychological Development (M-OSPD) (Auer *et al.*, 1994) is an assessment tool based on the Piagetian developmental model of sensorimotor functions that has been shown to reliably assess cognition in patients with Global Deterioration Scale (GDS) (Reisberg *et al.*, 1982) scores at stages 6 and 7, indicating profound dementia (Auer and Reisberg, 1996). Patients with GDS scores in this range can also be reliably evaluated with the Severe Mini-Mental State Examination (SMMSE) (Harrell *et al.*, 2000). This scale was designed to retain the attributes of the original MMSE (Folstein *et al.*, 1975), that is, brevity and ease of administration, while extending the sensitivity of the MMSE at the lower end of the range to allow the reliable assessment of patients in the severely impaired range. Like the original, the SMMSE is a 30-point scale that briefly assesses a range of cognitive abilities; in the case of the SMMSE these include overlearned information, simple visuospatial functioning, executive skills and language abilities.

Discussion

The development of tests that allow the reliable documentation of both preserved and impaired cognitive abilities in severe dementia offered the opportunity to examine changes in cognitive functioning with several new treatments. Four medications have been the focus of investigation in recent years: donepezil hydrocholide (Aricept); rivastigmine (Exelon); galantamine (Reminyl) and memantine (known in the US as Namenda and in Europe as Axura and Ebixa) and the SIB has been used as one of a number of outcome measures in clinical trials involving severely demented AD patients (Feldman *et al.*, 2001; Gauthier *et al.*, 2001; Reisberg *et al.*, 2003; Tariot *et al.*, 2004).

There have been no studies of the natural history of the cognitive decline in severe AD or any other dementia and little is known about the range, rate or extent of cognitive deterioration in the last stages of the disease. For example, it is not known whether AD patients who initially present with significant language dysfunction continue to exhibit a disproportionate language deficit as the disease progresses into the last stages or whether the pattern of impairment across cognitive domains evens out over time. Similarly, we do not know whether the progression of cognitive impairment mirrors the pathological progression of AD. It has been suggested that the global rate of cognitive decline slows down as the disease progresses (Katzman *et al.*, 1988; Wild and

Kaye, 1998). However, it is likely that this assertion is related to earlier studies in which severely demented patients were assessed using traditional neuropsychological measures that resulted in significant floor effects. The annual rate of global decline as measured by the MMSE in patients across all stages of AD is around 3 points (Boller *et al.*, 1991; Han *et al.*, 2000). For patients in the severe range (i.e. MMSE scores of 10 or less) the annual rate of decline has been reported to be slightly higher, around 4.0 (Wild and Kaye, 1998) to 5.0 points (Jacobs *et al.*, 1991) suggesting that decline may actually speed up, rather than slow down.

The development of tests specifically designed to allow the assessment of cognitive deficits associated with severe dementia offers the opportunity to more fully investigate the nature of the cognitive decline in severe dementia. Because of the behavioural problems associated with severe dementia, and the limited attention span of some severely demented patients, most tests of late-stage AD are brief and do not offer the opportunity to assess a range of cognitive domains in any depth. The SIB was designed as a research tool and assesses nine separate cognitive domains. In a group of subjects with MMSE scores of 17 or less (Wild and Kaye, 1997), the annual percentage change in eight of the nine subtests ranged from 7% to 25%. Only one item showed no change over time and that was the ability of the patient to orient to the sound of his or her own name, a subtest that had a range of only 0–2 points. The mean annual rate of change on the SIB in this sample was calculated to be 17.1 points. This is consistent with the mean annual SIB decline of 15 points observed at the University of Pittsburgh Alzheimer's Disease Research Center in patients with MMSE scores of 10 or less (unpublished data, Saxton). In general, there is no difference in the rate of decline on the SIB for patients with initial MMSE scores in the severely demented range and for patients with MMSE scores in the moderately impaired range (Wild and Kaye, 1997). This finding suggests that, contrary to previous suggestions, the rate of decline does not slow down as the disease progresses.

In summary, the increased interest by the research community in severe dementia over the past decade undoubtedly resulted directly from the development of cognitive scales designed specifically to allow direct, performance-based assessment of cognition in these patients. The SIB, SCIP and the TSI have all shown that even significantly impaired patients are able to complete cognitive assessments if the scales are appropriate to the level of the patients' abilities and, furthermore, that the progression of cognitive decline, even in the severe stages, can be reliably documented over time. Even these scales, however, have floor effects and there remains the possibility that even far more profoundly impaired patients may be capable of completing some form of cognitive 'testing' if an appropriate scale could be developed.

References

Albert M, Cohen C (1992) The Test for Severe Impairment: an instrument for the assessment of patients with severe cognitive dysfunction. *Journal of the American Geriatric Society*, 40:449–453.

Auer S, Reisberg B (1996) Reliability of the Modified Ordinal Scales of Psychological Development: a cognitive assessment battery for severe dementia. *International Psychogeriatrics*, 8(2):225–231.

Auer S, Sclan S, Yaffee Y, Reisberg B (1994) The neglected half of Alzheimer disease: cognitive and functional concomitants of severe dementia. *Journal of the American Geriatric Society*, 42:1266–1272.

Barbarotto R, Cerri M, Acerbi C, Molinari S, Capitani E (2000) Is SIB or BNP better than MMSE in discriminating the cognitive performance of severely impaired elderly patients? *Archives of Clinical Neuropsychology*, 15(1):21–29.

Boller F, Holland A, Forbes M, Hood P, McGonigle-Gibson K, Becker JT, (1991) Predictors of decline in Alzheimer's disease. *Cortex*, 27:9–17.

Boller F, Verny M, Hugonot-Diener L, Saxton J (2002) Clinical features and assessment of severe dementia: a review. *European Journal of Neurology*, 9(2):125–136.

Boller F, Saxton J, Kastengo KB, *et al.* (2004) Short version of the severe impairment battery (SIB). *Neurology*, 62 Suppl 5:A131–132.

Dartigues J, Helmer C, Letenneur L (2002) Epidemiologie des demences, in Les Demences. Edited by Duychaerts C, Pasquier F. Paris: Douin, pp 5–13.

Feldman H, Gauthier S, Hecker J, Vellas B, Subbiah P, Whalen E (2001) A 24-week, randomized, double-blind study of donepezil in moderate to severe Alzheimer's disease. *Neurology*, 57(4):613–620.

Foldi NS, Majerovitz SD, Sheikh K, Rodriguez E (1999) The test for severe impairment: validity with the dementia rating scale and utility as a longitudinal measure. *Clinical Neuropsychologist*, 13(1):22–29.

Folstein MF, Folstein SE, McHugh PR (1975). 'Mini Mental State': a practical method for grading the cognitive state of patients for the clinician. *Journal of Psychiatric Research*, 12:189–198.

Fratiglioni L, Aguero-Torres H, Winblad B (1994) The impact of dementia on our societies and current possibilities of prevention. *International Journal of Geriatric Psychopharmacology*, 1:179–183.

Gauthier S, Feldman H, Hecker J, Vellas B, Emir B, Subbiah P (2002) Functional cognitive and behavioral effects of donepezil in patients with moderate Alzheimer's disease. *Current Medical Research and Design*, 18(6):347–354.

Han L, Cole M, Bellavance F, McCusker J, Primeau F, (2000) Tracking cognitive decline in Alzheimer's disease using the Mini Mental State Examination: a meta-analysis. *International Psychogeriatrics*, 12(2):231–247.

Harrell LE, Marson D, Chatterjee A, Parrish JA (2000) The Severe Mini-Mental State Examination: a new neuropsychologic instrument for the bedside assessment of severely impaired patients with Alzheimer disease. *Alzheimer Disease and Associated Disorders: An International Journal*, 14(3):168–175.

Hughes, C.B., Berg L, Danziger WL (1982) A new clinical scale for the staging of dementia. *British Journal of Psychiatry*, 140:566–572.

Jacobs D, Albert SM, Sano M, del Castillo-Castaneda C, Paik M, Marder K, Bell K, Brandt J, Albert MS, Stern Y (1999) Assessment of cognition in advanced AD: the test for severe impairment. *Neurology*. 52(8):1689–1691.

Katzman R, Brown T, Thal LJ, *et al.* (1988) Comparison of rate of annual change of mental status score in four independent studies of patients with Alzheimer's disease. *Annals of Neurology*, 24:384–389.

Mattis S (1988) Dementia rating scale (DRS). Odessa FL: Psychological Assessment Resources.

Panisett M, Roudier M, Saxton J, Boller F (1994) Severe Impairment Battery: a neuropsychological test for severely demented patients. *Archives of Neurology*, 51:41–45.

Peavy GM, Salmon DP, Rice VA, *et al.* (1996) Neuropsychological assessment of severely demented elderly: the severe cognitive impairment profile. *Archives of Neurology*, 53:367–372.

Pippi M, Mecocci P, Saxton J, Bartorelli L, Pettenati C, Bonaiuto S, Cucinotta D, Masaraki G, Neri M, Tammaro AE, Vergani C, Chionne F, Senin U (1999) Neuropsychological assessment of the severely impaired elderly patients: validation of the Italian short version of the Severe Impairment Battery (SIB). *Aging, Clinical and Experimental Research*, 11(4):221–226.

Reisberg B (1988) functional assessment staging (FAST). *Psychopharmacology Bulletin*, 653–659.

Reisberg B, Ferris SH, de Leon MJ, Crook T (1982) The global deterioration scale for assessment of primary degenerative dementia. *American Journal of Psychiatry*, 139:1136–1139.

Reisberg B, Sclan G, Franzsen E, Klugger A, Ferris S (1994) Dementia staging in chronic care populations. *Alzheimer disease and Related Disorders*, 8(Suppl 1):S188–S205.

Reisberg B, Doody R, Stoffler A, *et al.* (2003) Memantine in moderate-to-severe Alzheimer's disease. *The New England Journal of Medicine*, 348:1333–1341.

Roudier M, Marcie P, Grancher AS, Starkstein S, Boller F (1998) Discrimination of facial indentity and of emotions in Alzhiemer's disease. *Journal of Neurological Sciences*, 154:151–158.

Saxton J, Swihart AA (1989) Neuropsychological assessment of the severely impaired elderly patient. *Clinical Geriatric Medicine*, 5:531–543.

Saxton J, McGonigle-Gibson K, Swihart A, Miller M, Boller F (1990) Assessment of the severely impaired patient: description and validation of a new neuropsychological test battery. *Psychological Assessment*, 2:298–303.

Schmitt FA, Ashford JW, Ferris S, *et al.* (1996) Severe Impairment Battery: a potential measure for AD clinical trials, in Alzheimer Disease: From Molecular Biology to Therapy. Edited by Becker R, Giacobini E. Boston, Birkhauser, pp 419–423.

Schmitt FA, Ashford W, Ernesto C, Saxton J, *et al.* (1997) The Severe Impairment Battery: concurrent validity and the assessment of longitudinal change in Alzheimer's disease. *Alzheimer Disease and Associated Disorders*, 11:S51–S56.

Tariot PN, Farlow MR, Grossberg GT, *et al.* (2004) Memantine treatment in patients with moderate to severe Alzheimer disease already receiving donepezil. *The Journal of the American Medical Association*, 291, No.3:317–324.

Venneri A, Pentore R, Coticelli B, Della Salla S (1998) Unilateral spatial neglect in the late stage of Alzheimer's disease. *Cortex*, 34:743–752.

Verny M, Hugonot-Diener L, Saillon A, *et al.* (1999) Evaluation de la démence sévère: échelles cognitives et comportementales (groupe de travail du GRECO). *L'année Gérontologica Serdi*, 156–168.

Wild KV, Kaye JA (1997) The rate of progression of Alzheimer's disease in the later stages: Evidence from the severe impairment battery. *Journal of the International Neuropsychological Society*, 4:512–516.

Wild KV, Kaye JA (1998) Rate of progression in the later stages of Alzheimer disease: evidence from the severe impairment battery. *Clinical Neuropsychologist*, 12(2):281.

Wild KV, Howieson D, Lear J, Carrsyn C, Kay J (1993) Assessing the severely impaired dementia patient – functional correlates of the severe impairment battery. *Journal of Clinical and Experimental Neuropsychology*, 15(1):29.

5

Behavioural and Psychological Symptoms of Dementia – Agitation

E. Jane Byrne, Deborah Collins and Alistair Burns

Introduction

Behavioural and psychological symptoms of dementia (BPSD, Finkel and Burns, 2000) are a common feature of Alzheimer's disease (AD) and other dementias. These include agitation, anxiety, depression, apathy, delusions, sleep and appetite disturbance, elation, irritability, disinhibition and hallucinations. BPSD are as clinically significant as disorders of cognition, and a key element of the dementia syndrome but these symptoms are not reflected in current nosological systems (e.g. Byrne, 1997), and rely on the 'cognitive paradigm' (Berrios, 1987), i.e. that dementia can be defined by cognitive symptoms alone. With a disease time risk of up to 90% BPSD are responsible for the majority of distress that both sufferers and carers experience (Donaldson *et al.*, 1997; Tariot, 2002).

There is variability in the presentation and pattern of BPSD between individual patients, with symptoms rarely occurring in isolation. Associations have been made between the different symptoms and new evidence is emerging to suggest that clusters of symptoms within BPSD may be of clinical relevance (Robert *et al.*, in press; *vide infra*). As with individual symptoms these clusters differ by time, severity and diagnosis. In this chapter agitation will be used as an illustrative symptom of BPSD.

Behaviour does not occur in isolation, it is a dynamic process involving the sufferer, their environment and those who observe the behaviour and/or interact with the sufferer. This applies to agitation as to all other BPSD. Concepts of the aetiology of agitation will be discussed below but centre around the debate as to whether behaviour is part of the disease or is due to disease (Byrne and Arie, 1990; Bird, 2005). The instruments that are used to measure BPSD may also influence concepts of behaviour in dementia.

Frequency of BPSD

There is some variability between the reported prevalence rates of BPSD owing to heterogeneity in both patient populations and assessment methods. Many studies have had a cross-sectional design. Margallo-Lana *et al.* (2001) found an estimated prevalence amongst patients in residential care environments of 80%. The prevalence of patients experiencing one or more BPSD symptoms in the Cache County Study was found to be 69% (Steinberg *et al.*, 2003). European studies have recorded comparable prevalence rates in population-based studies. The European Alzheimer's Disease Consortium (EADC) recently described the prevalence of at least one feature in a sample of 194 patients as 96% (Byrne *et al.*, 2003, Petrovic *et al.*, 2005a, 2005b). In other population based studies, prevalence rates have been shown to be lower at 20% (Burns *et al.*, 1990, and Lyketsos *et al.*, 2000).

Severe Dementia. Edited by A. Burns and B. Winblad.
Copyright © 2006 John Wiley & Sons, Ltd.   ISBN 0-470-01054-1

Recent studies in Europe have investigated the longitudinal course of BPSD. A large, longitudinal French study found that patients experience increased behavioural disturbances as the disease progresses (Benoit *et al.*, 2003). Aalten *et al.*, (2005) proposed that different symptoms might have individual specific courses. Margallo-Lana *et al.*, (2001) found that in patients with mild dementia depression was the most common symptom, whereas in those with moderate dementia delusions were more common. Teri *et al.*, (1988) investigated 127 outpatients and divided the population by severity of illness, mild, moderate and severe dementia, based on the Mini Mental State Examination (MMSE, Folstein *et al.*, 1975). In severe dementia, agitation (24%) was amongst the most commonly noted behavioural disturbances. Agitation was found to be significantly associated with delusions and hallucinations (Petrovic *et al.*, 2005a, 2005b).

Agitation

'Agitation' is one of the commonest of the cluster of signs and symptoms that make up the constellation of BPSD and is associated with both the progression of dementia and distress in carers (Cohen-Mansfield *et al.*, 1995a, 1995b; Donaldson *et al.*, 1997; Tariot, 2002). The original report by Alzheimer (1906, 1907), on the first person (Auguste D) to be described as suffering from the disease that now bears his name had, amongst other symptoms, agitation as a prominent feature (Alzheimer, 1906; Burns *et al.*, 2002). Both agitation and aggression impact on the quality of life of both people with dementia and their families and the behaviours affect the quality of social interactions (Collins *et al.*, 2005).

Definitions of agitation

Cohen-Mansfield and Billig (1986) define agitation as: 'inappropriate verbal, vocal, or motor activity that is not judged by an outside observer to be an obvious outcome of the needs or confusion of the individual'. Cohen-Mansfield *et al.*, (1989) further characterised agitated behaviours into four key categories based on the Cohen-Mansfield Agitation Inventory (CMAI): (i) physically non-aggressive (restlessness, pacing, mannerisms, hiding things, dressing or undressing inappropriately); (ii) physically aggressive (hitting, pushing, scratching, biting, kicking and grabbing); (iii) verbally non-aggressive (negativism, repetitions, interruptions, constant requests for attention); and (iv) verbally aggressive (screaming, making strange noises, cursing and outbursts of temper). The International Psychogeriatric Association in their educational pack (IPA, 2003) subdivide 'verbal agitation' into two types: verbally non-aggressive behaviour (e.g. constant requests for attention) and verbally aggressive behaviour (e.g. screaming). The latter subdivision of verbal agitation is echoed in the Neuropsychiatric Inventory (NPI, Cummings *et al.*, 1994) and the initial formulation of Cohen-Mansfield and colleagues (1989). Examples of other definitions of agitation and aggression are listed in Table 1. Hurley *et al.*'s (1999) definition is similar to Cohen-Mansfield and Billig (1986) in including a consideration of both 'disease and dis-ease'. The definition of Bird (2005) is included as BPSD, especially agitation, are frequently seen as 'challenging'.

Tariot (2002), used a semi-operational definition of agitation. He suggested that it is possible to discover the meaning for disturbed behaviour by considering factors related to their dementia (dis-ease); others are specific to it (disease). Factors related to dementia include: side effects of medications, pain, physical problems (infections, sensory impairments), anxiety, depression and psychosis. Dementia-specific causes of agitation include the way that a sufferer interacts with their social and physical environment as a result of their cognitive dysfunction. Both dementia-related and dementia-specific causes of agitation should be viewed in the context of the individual and their life history. In many cases, examining the interaction of the patient within their environment will explain the agitation. However, agitation may occasionally be a primary feature of a dementia syndrome (*vide infra*).

Table 1. Definitions of agitation and aggression

Authors	Definition
Patel *et al.* (1992) – Aggression	'An overt act involving the delivery of noxious stimuli to (but not necessarily aimed at) another organism, object or self which is clearly not accidental.'
Mingas *et al.* (1989) – Agitation	'Overt behaviour that indicates restlessness, hyperactivity or subjective distress. Verbal or physical aggressive behaviour not directed at a specific target should be rated as agitation.'
Hurley *et al.* (1999) – Agitation	'Those observed patient behaviours which communicate to others that the patient is experiencing an unpleasant state of excitement and which remain after interventions to reduce internal and external stimuli by managing resistiveness, alleviating adverse physical signs and decreasing sources of accumulated stress have been carried out.'
Bird (2005) – Challenging behaviour	'Any behaviour associated with the dementing illness which causes distress or danger to the person with dementia or others, or is a manifestation of distress.'

Frequency of agitation

Reisberg and colleagues (Reisburg *et al.*, 1987) identified agitation and aggression in more than 40% of the 57 patients. Of these, violence was present in 30% and wandering in 3%. Significant aggression was found in 65% of 183 demented outpatients (Ryden, 1988). In a further study of outpatients with dementia, outbursts of anger were recorded in 51% and aggression in 21%. These authors noted that in this population the reported behaviours worsened as the dementia progressed (Swearer *et al.*, (1988). Burns *et al.*, (1990) found the overall prevalence rate of aggression (defined as behaviours resulting in violence) in 178 patients with AD to be 20%. They also found aggression to be positively associated with more severe illness and admission to hospital, wandering was found in 19%.

Recent cross-sectional European studies examining the frequency of agitation (as defined by the NPI) are shown in Table 2. It can be seen that agitated behaviours are amongst the commonest of BPSD, occurring in up to 45% of patients. Logsdon *et al.*, (1999) suggest that agitation may occur in between 70% and 90% of people with dementia at some point during the course of their illness. Other studies found agitated behaviours in more than half of demented patients during the course of the illness (Tariot and Blazina, 1993; Mega *et al.*, 1996; Devanand *et al.*, 1997; Marin *et al.*, 1997).

Associations of agitation

Agitation in dementia has been found to be correlated with depression (Olin *et al.*, 2002; Leroi and Lyketsos, 2005), psychosis (Levy *et al.*, 1996; Jeste and Finkel, 2000), severity of dementia (Levy *et al.*, 1996; Aalten *et al.*, 2005) and sleep disorders (Cohen-Mansfield and Marx, 1990; Allen *et al.*, 2003). One example of a correlation matrix between BPSD is shown in Table 3. This data is derived from the EADC/BPSD study (Byrne *et al.*, 2003; Petrovic *et al.*, 2005a, 2005b). In this study the assessment of BPSD included some items not found in the NPI (Cummings *et al.*, 1994). Agitation

Table 2.   Frequency of BPSD in European studies (as defined by the NPI)

Symptom	EADC/BPSD $N = 131$	Maasbed $N = 199$	REAL1 $N = 255$	REAL2 $N = 244$	Burns *et al.* (1990) $N = 178$
Delusions	26.0	19.4	24.7	10.2	16
Hallucinations	9.2	7.9	7.8	5.7	23
Agitation	**38.2**	**30.9**	**44.3**	**32.8**	—
Depression	58.0	45.3	42.7	36.9	43
Anxiety	44.3	33.8	46.3	44.3	—
Elation	9.2	7.0	9.8	4.5	3.5
Apathy	65.6	59.3	63.5	47.9	—
Disinhibition	21.4	12.6	13.3	10.2	—
Irritability	45.0	39.7	25	28.3	20 (aggression)
Motor	29.8	34.7	29.8	14.7	—
Sleep	25.2	18.1	12.9	13.5	—
Appetite	25.2	24.6	24.3	20.5	16

Key: EADC/BPSD, Byrne *et al.* (2003), Petrovic *et al.* (2005a, 2005b). Maasbed, Aalten *et al.* (2005). REAL 1 (MMSE = 11–20); REAL 2 (MMSE = 21–30), Benoit *et al.* (2003), Burns *et al.* (1990).

and psychosis (i.e. delusions and hallucinations) were significantly associated. Agitation was also significantly correlated with depression.

Cohen-Mansfield and Libin (2005) investigated the correlations of two major types of agitation: verbal agitation and physically non-aggressive agitation. Verbal agitation included; repetition of sentences or questions, screaming, constant demands for attention and complaining. Physically non-aggressive agitation included: pacing or wandering, inappropriate handling of objects, repetitive mannerisms, fidgeting and restlessness. The authors found verbally agitated behaviours to be correlated with female gender, impaired activities of daily living, impaired social functioning, and cognitive decline. Physically non-aggressive agitation was correlated with cognitive impairment and less concurrent medical illness.

There is a growing literature on the complex interrelationships amongst the symptoms of BPSD. The concept of 'clusters' of BPSD symptoms (Lyketsos *et al.*, 2001; Robert *et al.*, in press; Verhey *et al.*, 2005) has a clinical resonance and there exists a degree of concordance between recently published studies.

Frisoni *et al.*, (1999) found three factors in a study of 162 patients with Alzheimer's disease: a mood factor, a frontal lobe factor and a psychosis factor. Three factors were also identified in a study of 199 patients with mixed aetiologies of dementia (de Vugt *et al.*, 2003). These factors were a mood/apathy factor (80%), a psychosis factor (37%) and a hyperactivity factor (60%). Most recently, four factors have been identified in a study of 194 patients with different types of dementia to include: a psychosis factor, a psychomotor factor, a mood-lability factor and an instinctual factor (Petrovic *et al.*, 2005a, 2005b).

Many studies (such as those reviewed by Robert *et al.*, in press) have found the factors of psychosis and hyperactivity to include agitation. Lyketsos *et al.*, (2001) in a population-based study found that BPSD in Alzheimer's disease cluster into three categories: patients with none or only one, symptom; patients with mainly affective symptoms; and patients displaying a psychotic syndrome. Nevertheless, they did not find a predominately agitated group of patients and agitation was considered to be a non-specific symptom. de Vugt *et al.*, (2003) did report a group of agitated patients, interestingly within the 'hyperactivity' subsyndrome of the study not the psychosis factor

Table 3. Correlations between BPSD ($N = 194$)

	Per	Mir	Hoa	Sex	Cur	Mis	Sho	App	Slee	Mot	Irr	Dis	Apa	El	Anx	Dep	Ag	Hal
Del	.276**	.326**	.233**	.229**	.218**	.334**		.167*		.402**	.160*		.200**				.271**	.169*
Hall	.326**			.145*		.296**	.366**			.289**	.219**		.215**	.175*		.178*	.280**	
Ag	.385**			.181*	.290**	.183*	.242**			.295**	.513**	.174*				.247**		
Dep	.231**		.143*				.174*				.224**	.211**	.219**					
Anx							.207*	.157*			.224**							
El	.205**			.213**	.178*		.287**				.202**	.332**						
Apa						.269**	.246**	.171*	.219**	.289**	.259**	.175*						
Dis	.196**			.173*	.222**		.148*				.253*							
Irr				.225**	.348**		.281**		.217**	.156*								
Mot	.274**	.212**	.144*			.395**		.179*										
Slee	.266**				.185**	.252**												
App	.144*						.145*											
Sho	.247**				.395**	.285**												
Mis	.337**		.185**															
Cur	.379**																	
Sex																		

(Continued)

Table 3. *(Continued)*

	Per	Mir	Hoa	Sex	Cur	Mis	Sho	App	Slee	Mot	Irr	Dis	Apa	El	Anx	Dep	Ag	Hal
Hoa	.331**	.289**																
Mir	.188*																	

*indicates relationships significant at the 5% level ($p \leq 0.05$).
**indicates relationships significant at the 1% level ($p \leq 0.01$).
Key: Del, delusions; Hall, hallucinations; Ag, agitation; Dep, depression; Anx, anxiety; El, elation; Ap, apathy; Dis, disinhibition; Irr, irritability; Slee, sleep; App, appetite; Sho, shouting and screaming; Mis, misidentification; Cur, cursing; Sex, Sexual disinhibition; Hoa, hoarding; Mir, mirror sign; Mot, aberrant motor behaviour.
(Source: Byrne *et al.* (2003); Petrovic *et al.* (2005a, 2005b)

(explaining 29.54% of the variance). The psychosis factor of their study, although less prevalent, was associated with more severe total behavioural problems.

The REAL study (Benoit *et al.*, 2003) stratified their sample on the basis of severity of illness (as measured by the MMSE) into two groups: mild (MMSE score 21–30) and moderate/severe (MMSE score 11–20). They found that the components of the factors were influenced by severity. In the mild group the factor was delusions-agitation-irritability/mood/hallucinations; in the moderate/severe group the factor was mood/frontal/sensorimotor.

Most studies of clustering of BPSD have used the Neuropsychiatric Inventory (NPI, Cummings *et al.*, 1994) as the measure of BPSD. We have recently demonstrated in the EADC/BPSD study (Byrne *et al.*, 2003) that derived factors are influenced by this symptom measure (NPI) and by the inclusion of symptoms not included by the NPI. (Petrovic *et al.*, 2005a, 2005b)

Aetiology of agitation
Psychosocial
The concept that human behaviour (whether arising in dementia sufferers or in other people) is a dynamic construct between the observed, the observers and the context in which the behaviour arises is not new. In dementia care, the voice, or perspective, of the dementia sufferer has often been neglected (Byrne and Arie, 1990; Kitwood, 1988; Nolan *et al.*, 2004). The concept of 'person-centred' dementia care, which the late Tom Kitwood pioneered, reasserted that voice, and contributed to improvements in dementia care. Unfortunately, some have misinterpreted the concept of Kitwood at the expense of other components of the dynamics of behaviour in dementia (Nolan *et al.*, 2004; Bird; 2005). For example coping strategies employed by carers have been shown to increase the occurrence of delusions, aggressiveness or hyperactive behaviour (de Vugt *et al.*, 2004; Riello *et al.*, 2002; Hamel *et al.*, 1990).

Similarly the nature of the social interaction between care staff and their perception of behaviour in residents has been shown to contribute to whether a behaviour is problematic (reviewed by Bird (2005)). Whilst 'respect for personhood' is essential in dementia care (Nolan *et al.*, 2004), it is insufficient alone to completely understand behaviour as a dynamic process; the other components of the dynamic (the environment, other people) need also to be considered. Psychosocial approaches to dementia care take this view (Moniz-Cook *et al.*, 2000; Bird, 2002) and inform the assessment of BPSD.

Pathophysiology
Whilst there are differences in the pathology and neurochemistry of the major causes of the dementia syndrome, they all affect, to a greater or lesser degree, areas of the brain implicated in the genesis of BPSD. One of the first studies to investigate the pathophysiology of BPSD was conducted by Gusatafson and Hagberg (1975). They investigated the relationship between several psychiatric symptoms and cerebral blood flow (CBF) in 75 patients with dementia. Anxious and depressed patients were found to have an extensive reduction in CBF. For all severities of cognitive functioning, paranoid symptoms and liability of mood were recorded. Patients with severe dementia had low frontal blood flow and associated features of psychomotor overactivity and elation.

Karim and Burns (2003) have reviewed the pathophysiology of psychosis in dementia. The authors concluded that psychotic symptoms in AD were associated with: genetic predisposition (e.g. Presenilin 1, polymorphic variations in serotonin receptor genes, 5HT2A and 5HT2C); differing degrees of cell loss in CA1 and dorsal raphe neuclus when compared to non-psychotic AD patients; and differences in hemispheric size, blood flow and glucose metabolism (between people with psychosis in AD and those without).

Aggression is modulated principally by the hypothalamus (Ovsiew and Yudofsky, 1983), temporal lobe and limbic structures (Elliot, 1992), and the prefrontal cortex (Lishman, 1968; Luria, 1980). Altered (reduced) function of serotoninergic systems has also been shown to modulate aggressive behaviour in humans (Asberg *et al.*, 1976; Brown *et al.*, 1982).

The characteristics and aetiology of agitation were examined in 427 outpatients with dementia by Senanarong and colleagues (Senanarong *et al.*, 2004). They found AD patients had an increased prevalence of agitation (as measured by the NPI) with increasing dementia severity. They also found that behaviours mediated by the frontal lobes (such as irritability, delusions and disinhibition) explained most of the variance in agitation levels.

Biopsychosocial

A cursory glance at the literature on interventions for the management of BPSD might suggest that biological factors (disease) are antithetically opposed to psychosocial factors (dis-ease). We concur with the views of the International Psychogeriatric Association (IPA, 2003) in their BPSD educational publication. They concluded that 'the best model' to explain the aetiology of BPSD (and implicitly to assess and manage BPSD) was one which encompassed biological, psychological and social factors.

Assessment and measurement of BPSD

Implicit in the biopsychosocial model of BPSD is the requirement that each component of the behavioural dynamic (the person and their illness; their environment and social circumstances; and those around them) should be assessed. A detailed strategy for the biopsychosocial assessment of BPSD can be found in Alexopoulos *et al.*, (1998). This consensus guideline to the treatment of agitation in dementia is recommended as it is available (free of charge) on the Internet, provides a comprehensive review of the literature and includes a version for carers (in small or in large print).

This 'holistic' approach to the assessment of behaviour is found in the 'ABC' assessment of behaviour (Mahoney *et al.*, 2000) outlined in Table 4.

Individual symptoms of BPSD may be measured using either observational (e.g. the Agitated Behaviours Mapping Instrument (ABMI) Cohen-Mansfield *et al.*, 1989a) or informant measures (e.g. the Cohen-Mansfield Agitation Inventory CMAI Cohen-Mansfield *et al.*, 1989b). Direct observations assess specific patterns of behaviours/activities during a particular time frame. They are often time-consuming and thus costly. Direct observation requires training for observers, but inter-rater reliability is high, ranging from 85% to 90% (Cohen-Mansfield *et al.*, 1986). Informant measures are potentially subject to observer bias (Bird, 2005). With trained observers, however, the two methods may show an acceptable level of concordance (Cohen-Mansfield and Libin, 2004).

Table 4.   The 'ABC' approach to the assessment of behaviour in dementia

Domain	Observations
Antecedents	Events that occurred before the behaviour – in the person, in the environment, in other people
Behaviour	An exact description of the behaviour
Consequences	The effects of the behaviour on the person and on others

Source: Adapted from Mahoney *et al.* (2000).

There are numerous measures for BPSD both observational and informant. One of the most comprehensive descriptions of these measures is to be found in Burns *et al.*, (2004). Of the inform-ant measures of BPSD, probably the most widely used is the NPI (Cummings *et al.*, 1994) or the NPI-D, which incorporates a measure of carer distress (Kaufer *et al.*, 1998). For agitation the most widely used measure is that of Cohen-Mansfield's group; the informant measure (CMAI, Cohen-Mansfield *et al.*, 1989b).

Conclusion

BPSD are common and distressing to both the sufferer and to their carers. They are now the subject of good quality research. A 'holistic' approach to their understanding and assessment, the biopsy-chosocial model, offers hope for the alleviation of the suffering that they cause.

References

Aalten P, de Vugt, ME, Jaspers N, Jolles J, Verhey F (2005) The course of neuropsychiatric symptoms in demen-tia. Part 1: findings from the two-years longitudinal Maasbed study. *Int J Geriatr Psychiatry*, 20:523–30.

Alexopoulos GS, Silver JM, Kahn DA, Frances A, Carpenter D, eds (1998) The Expert Consensus Guideline Series: Agitation in Older Persons with Dementia. A Postgraduate Medicine Special Report, McGraw-Hill.

Alzheimer A. (1906) Über einen eigenartigen schweren Erkrankungsprozeß der Hirnrinde. *Neurologisches Centralblatt*, 23:1129–36.

Alzheimer A. (1907) Über eine eigenartige Erkrankung der Hirnrinde. *Allegmine Zeitschrift für Psychiatrie und Psychisch-Gerichtliche Medizin*, 64:146–8.

Asberg M, Thoren P, Traskman L, Bertilsson L, Ringberger V (1976) Serotonin depression – a biochemical subgroup within the affective disorders? *Science*, 191(4226):478–80.

Benoit M, Staccini P, Brocker P, Benhamidat T, Bertogliati C, Lechowski L, Tortrat D, Robert PH (2003) Be-havioral and psychologic symptoms in Alzheimer's disease: results of the REAL. *FR study Rev Med Interne*, 24 Suppl 3:319s-324s. In French.

Bird M, Llewellyn-Jones R, Smithers H, Korten A (2002) Psychosocial approaches to challenging behaviour in dementia. A controlled trial. Canberra, Commonwealth Dept of Health and Aging.

Brown G, Ebert M, Grayer P, *et al.* (1982) Aggression, suicide, and serotonin. *Am J Psychiatry*, 139:741–746.

Burns A, Jacoby R, Levy R (1990) Psychiatric phenomena in Alzheimer's disease, *Br J Psychiatry*, 157:72–93.

Burns A, Byrne EJ, Ballard C, Holmes C (2002) Sensory stimulation in dementia: an effective option for man-aging behavioural problems. *British Medical Journal*, 325:1312.

Byrne EJ (1997) Differential diagnosis of dementia. *International Psychogeriatrics*, 9:39–50.

Byrne EJ, Arie T (1990) Coping with dementia in the elderly. In: Current Medicine 2, ed. Lawson DH. Church-ill Livingstone, Edinburgh, 137–155.

Byrne EJ, Robert P, Hurt C (2003) BPSD in Europe:an EADC study of behavioural and psychological symp-toms of dementia(BPSD): a report of th EADC BPSD thematic group. *Int Psychogeriatr*, 15(suppl 2):96.

Cohen-Mansfield J (1995) Assessment of disruptive behavior/agitation in the elderly: function, methods and difficulties. *J Geriatr Psychiatry Neurol*, 8(1):52–60. Review.

Cohen-Mansfield J, Billig N (1986) Agitated behaviors in the elderly. I. A conceptual review. *Journal of the American Geriatrics Society*, 34:711–21.

Cohen-Mansfield J, Libin A (2004) Assessment of agitation in elderly patients with dementiacorrelations be-tween informant rating and direct observation. *Int J Geriatr Psychiatry*, 19:881–91.

Cohen-Mansfield J, Marx MS (1990) *Journal of Aging and Health*, 2(1):42–57.

Cohen-Mansfield J, Marx M, Rosenthal A (1989) A description of agitation in a nursing home. *Journal of Gerontology*, 44:M77–M84.

Cohen-Mansfield J, Culpepper W, Werner P (1995a) The relationship between cognitive function and agitation in senior day care participants. *Int J Geriatr Psychiatry*, 10:585–95.

Cohen-Mansfield J, Werner P, Watson V, Pasis S (1995b) Agitation among elderly persons at adult day-care centers: the experiences of relatives and staff members. *Int Pyschogeriatr*, 7(3):447–58.

Cummings JL, Mega M, Gray K *et al.* (1994) The Neuropsychiatric Inventory: comprehensive assessment of psychopathology in dementia. *Neurology*, 44:2308–14.

Devanand DP, Jacobs DM, Tang MX, Del Castillo-Castaneda C, Sano M, Marder K, Bell K, Bylsma FW, Brandt J, Albert M, Stern Y (1997) The course of psychopathologic features in mild to moderate Alzheimer disease. *Arch Gen Psychiatry*, 54(3):257–63.

de Vugt ME, Stevens F, Aalten P. Lousberg R, Jaspers N, Winkens I, Jolles J, Verhey Fr (2003) Behavioural disturbances in dementia patients and quality of the marital relationship. *Int J Geriatr Psychiatry*, 18:149–54.

de Vugt ME, Stevens F, Aalten P, Lousberg R, Jaspers N, Winkens I, Jolles J, Verhey FR (2004) Do caregiver management strategies influence patient behaviour in dementia? *Int J Geriatr Psychiatry*, 19(1):85–92.

Donaldson C, Tarrier N, Burns A (1997) The impact of the symptoms of dementia on caregivers. *British Journal of Psychiatry*, 170:62–8.

Elliot FA (1992) Violence: the neurological contribution: an overview. *Arch Neurol*, 49:595–603.

Folstein ME, Folstein SE, McHugh PR (1975) 'Mini-Mental State'. A practical method for grading the cognitive state of patients for the clinician. *Journal of Psychiatric Research,* 12:189–98.

Frisoni GB, Rozzini L, Gozzetti A, Binetti G, Zanetti O, Bianchetti A, Trabucchi M, Cummings JL (1999) Behavioral syndromes in Alzheimer's disease: description and correlates. *Dement Geriatr Cogn Disord*, 10(2):130–8.

Gustafson L, Hagberg B (1975) Emotional behaviour, personality changes and cognitive reduction in presenile dementia: related to regional cerebral blood flow. *Acta Psychiatr Scand Suppl*, 257:37–71.

Hamel M, Gold DP, Andres D, Reis M, Dastoor D, Grauer H, Bergman H (1990) Predictors and consequences of aggressive behavior by community-based dementia patients. *Gerontologist*, 30(2):206–11.

Hurley AC, Volicer L, Camberg, Ashley J *et al*. (1999) *Journal of Mental Health and Aging*, 5(2).

Jeste DV, Finkel SI (2000) Psychosis of Alzheimer's disease and related dementias. Diagnostic criteria for a distinct syndrome. *Am J Geriatr Psychiatry*, 8(1):29–34.

Karim S, Burns A (2003) The biology of psychosis in older people. *J Geriatr Psychiatry Neurol*, 16(4):207–12. Review.

Kaufer DI, Cummings JL, Christine D, Bray T, Castellon S, Masterman D, MacMillan A, Ketchel P, DeKosky ST (1998) Assessing the impact of neuropsychiatric symptoms in Alzheimer's disease: the Neuropsychiatric Inventory Caregiver Distress Scale. *J Am Geriatr Soc*, 46(2):210–15.

Kitwood T (1998) From free associations: a new radicalization of psychoanalysis. *Hist Human Sci*, 1(2):263–73.

Levy ML, Cummings JL, Fairbanks LA, Bravi D, Calvani M, Carta A (1996) Longitudinal assessment of symptoms of depression, agitation, and psychosis in 181 patients with Alzheimer's disease. *Am J Psychiatry*, 153(11):1438–43.

Lishman WA (1968) Brain damage in relation to psychiatric disability after head injury. *Br J Psychiatry*, 114(509):373–410.

Logsdon RG, Gibbons LE, McCurry SM, Teri L (1999) Quality of life in Alzheimer's disease: patient and caregiver reports. *Journal of Mental Health and Aging*, 5(1).

Luria MH (1980) Long-term survival after recovery from acute myocardial infarction. *Compr Ther*, 6(6):36–41.

Luria SM (1980) Target size and correction for empty-field myopia. *J Opt Soc Am*, 70(9):1153–4.

Lyketsos CG, Steinberg M, Tschanz, Norton MC, Steffens DC, Breitner JC (2000) Mental and behavioural disturbances in dementia, findings from cache County study on memory and Aging. *Am J Psychiatry*, 157:708–14.

Lyketsos CG, Sheppard JM, Steinberg M, Tschanz JA, Norton MC, Steffens DC, Breitner JC (2001) Neuropsychiatric disturbance in Alzheimer's disease clusters into three groups: the Cache County study. *Int J Geriatr Psychiatry*, 16:1043–53.

Mahoney E, Volicer L, Hurley A (2000) Challenging Behaviors in Dementia. Health Professions Press, Baltimore, MD.

Margallo-Lano M, Swann A, O'Brien J *et al*. (2001) Prevalence and pharmacological management of behavioural and psychological symptoms amongst dementia sufferers living in care environments. *Int J Geriatr Psychiatry*, 16(1):39–44.

Marin DB, Green CR, Schmeidler J, Harvey PD, Lawlor BA, Ryan TM, Aryan M, Davis KL, Mohs RC (1997) Noncognitive disturbances in Alzheimer's disease: frequency, longitudinal course, and relationship to cognitive symptoms. *J Am Geriatr Soc*, 45(11):1331–8.

Mega MS, Cummings JL, Fiorello T, Gornbein J (1996) The spectrum of behavioral changes in Alzheimer's disease. *Neurology*, 46(1):130–5.

Moniz-Cook E, Woods R, Gardiner E (2002) Staff factors associated with perception of behaviour as 'challenging' in residential and nursing homes. *Aging and Mental Health*, 4:48–55.

Nolan MR, Davies S, Brown J, Keady J, Nolan J (2004) Beyond 'person-centred' care: a new vision for gerontological nursing. *International Journal of Older People Nursing* in association with *Journal of Clinical Nursing*, 13(3a):45–53.

Olin JT, Katz IR, Meyers BS, Schneider LS, Lebowitz BD (2002) Provisional diagnostic criteria for depression of Alzheimer disease: rationale and background. *Am J Geriatr Psychiatry*, 10(2):125–8; 129–41. Review. Erratum in: *Am J Geriatr Psychiatry*, 10(3):264.

Ovsiew F, Yudofsky S (1983) Aggression: a neuropsychiatric perspective, in rage, power, and aggression. In *The Role of Affect in Motivation, Development and Adaptation*. Yale University Press, pp 213–30.

Petrovic M *et al.* Clustering of Behavioural and psychological symptoms in Dementia (BPSD) within and beyond the 12 items of Neuropsychiatric Inventory: a European Alzheimer's Disease (EADC) study. (Submitted.)

Reisberg B, Burns A (1997) Preface: Diagnosis of Alzheimer's Disease. *International Psychogeriatrics*, 9(Suppl 1):5–7.

Riello R, Geroldi C, Parrinello G, Frisoni GB (2002) The relationship between biological and environmental determinants of delusions in mild Alzheimer's disease patients. *Int J Geriatr Psychiatry*, 17(7):687–8.

Ryden M *et al.* (1988) Aggressive behaviour in persons with dementia who live in the community. *Alzheimer Disease and Associated Disorders*, 2(4):342–55.

Senanarong V, Cummings JL, Fairbanks L, Mega M, Masterman DM, O'Connor SM, Strickland TL (2004) Agitation in Alzheimer's disease is a manifestation of frontal lobe dysfunction. *Dement Geriatr Cogn Disord*, 17(1–2):14–20.

Steinberg M, Sheppard JM, Tschanz JT, Norton MC, Steffens DC, Breitner JC, Lyketsos CG (2003) The incidence of mental and behavioral disturbances in dementia: the Cache County study. *J Neuropsychiatry Clin Neurosci*, 15(3):340–5.

Swearer JM, O'Donnell BF, Kane KJ, Hoople NE, Lavoie M (1998) Delayed recall in dementia: sensitivity and specificity in patients with higher than average general intellectual abilities. *Neuropsychiatry Neuropsychol Behav Neurol*, 11(4):200–6.

Teri L, Larson EB, Reifler BV, Behavioural disturbance in dementia of the Alzheimer's type. *J Am Geriatr Soc*, 36:1–6.

Verhey FR, Ponds RW, Rozendaal N, Jolles J (1995) Depression, insight and personality changes in Alzheimer's disease and vascular dementia. *Journal of Geriatric Psychiatry and Neurology*, 8:23–27.

6

Depression in Severe Dementia

Kate Bielinski and Brian Lawlor

Introduction

Depression in dementia is a potentially treatable component of what is otherwise an irreversible disorder. While depression as a complication of the mild and moderate stages of dementia is increasingly well recognised and understood, less is known about depression complicating severe dementia. This chapter focuses on the aetiology, phenomenology and management of depression in severe dementia and addresses the key issues faced by clinicians in caring for these patients.

Diagnostic challenges

The diagnosis of depression in severe dementia poses challenges to the clinician for a number of reasons.

Severe cognitive impairment, particularly short-term memory deficits, as well as compromised comprehension and communication skills, may impair a patient's ability to recall and report recent depressive symptoms, thereby making the assessment process more difficult. The evaluation may be further complicated by anosognosia, whereby the patient is unable to recognise his or her own disability.

In Alzheimer's dementia (AD), depressive symptoms may fluctuate, being present for short periods of time but recurring frequently (Lee and Lyketsos, 2003; Marin *et al.*, 1997). Many symptoms of depression such as sleep and appetite disturbance, weight loss and psychomotor retardation overlap with the neuropsychiatric symptoms of dementia, and this overlap may make these symptoms less useful in detecting depression in patients with severe dementia. Apathy is a common neuropsychiatric symptom in dementia, affecting over 90% of patients in the later stages of dementia (Robert, 2002), and while distinguishing between the two can be difficult, depression can be distinguished from apathy on the basis of the presence of dysphoric symptoms of sadness, hopelessness and guilt, which are typically absent in apathy (Boyle and Malloy, 2004). This distinction is an important one, as apathy may not respond to antidepressant treatment.

A further potential challenge is the issue of depressive symptoms being seen as 'understandable' in the context of severe dementia, or the failure to recognise symptoms as part of a depressive disorder. Ageist attitudes, such as the belief that depressive symptoms are part of normal ageing, and the attitude that the treatment of depression in the patient with severe dementia is ultimately futile, may mean that, even where symptoms are identified and recognised, clinicians may see them as not being worth treating.

Provisional diagnostic criteria for the diagnosis of depression in AD have been developed (Olin *et al.*, 2002); see Table 1. While these criteria acknowledge and address some of the differences in the presentation of depression in the context of AD, their use may still be of limited value in patients with severe dementia, owing to some of the factors referred to above.

Severe Dementia. Edited by A. Burns and B. Winblad.
Copyright © 2006 John Wiley & Sons, Ltd.   ISBN 0-470-01054-1

Table 1.   Provisional diagnostic criteria for depression of AD

1. All criteria for dementia of Alzheimer type are met.
2. More than 3 symptoms of depression, rather than the five required for diagnosis of idiopathic depression:
   - depressed mood,
   - decreased positive affect or pleasure in response to social contact and usual activities,
   - social isolation or withdrawal,
   - disruption in appetite,
   - disruption in sleep,
   - psychomotor changes,
   - irritability,
   - fatigue or loss of energy,
   - feelings of worthlessness, hopelessness, guilt,
   - recurrent thoughts of death or suicide, or suicidal plan or attempt.
3. Items of social isolation/withdrawal and irritability were added.
4. Symptoms required to *occur* during the same two-week period but not required to *persist* over the two-week period.

Assessment of depression in severe dementia

The detection of depression or depressive symptoms should be based on a comprehensive assessment of the patient and their mental state, with supplementary information obtained from a suitable informant. Careful consideration must be given to the *nature* and *quality* of symptoms, and to whether there has been any *change* in symptom profile. Rating scales may also be used to assist in the assessment process and there are a number of informant-based objective rating scales that are appropriate for use in severe dementia.

Rating scales for use in detecting depression in severe dementia

The Geriatric Depression Scale (Yesavage *et al.*, 1983), which is used widely in Old Age Psychiatry, loses validity below a score of 15 on the Mini Mental State Examination (McGivney *et al.*, 1994) and is therefore less useful in detecting depression in severe dementia. Other scales have been designed to detect depression in patients with severe dementia and are briefly described:

- **Cornell Scale for Depression in Dementia** (Alexopoulos *et al.*, 1988) is a rating scale that uses a combination of observation and informant-based questions, focusing on signs and symptoms within the week prior to interview. Scores on the CSDD range between 0 and 38, with a higher score indicating more severe depression. A score of 8 or more suggests depressive symptoms that require monitoring, if not treatment. Scores over 12 suggest a significant depressive episode requiring treatment (Lyketsos and Lee, 2004).
- **Depressive Signs Scale** (Katona and Aldridge, 1985) aims to detect depressive signs in patients with severe dementia and has been validated against the dexamethasone suppression test. It is completed on the basis of an interview with the subject and separate interview with an informant.
- **Neuropsychiatric Interview** (Cummings *et al.*, 1994) was developed to gather data on the presence and nature of psychopathological symptoms in patients with cerebral pathologies, particularly patients with AD or dementias of other aetiologies. Utilising information from an

informant, it assesses 12 domains – delusions, hallucinations, agitation, depression, anxiety, euphoria, apathy, disinhibition, irritability, aberrant motor behaviour, nighttime behaviours and eating disorders – and is a useful instrument for recording the behavioural disorders that are frequent in severe dementia (Mirakhur *et al.*, 2004; Hart *et al.*, 2003; Menon *et al.*, 2001).
- The **Gestalt scale** is a five-item observational scale designed to detect depression among persons with severe dementia (Greenwald and Kramer, 1991). It has been shown to have a high concordance with DSM-III-R diagnosis. Items are rated as absent (0) or present (1), and scores range from 0 to 5 (most depressed). It is based on the presence of one of more of the following in a non-delirious patient:

—lack of environmental reactivity in previously interactive person
—affective anxiety
—beseeching quality to speech
—depressed appearance
—affect-laden psychomotor agitation

Phenomenology of depression in severe dementia

Somatic symptoms, such as sleep or appetite disturbance, psychomotor retardation, loss of interest and decreased social activity, are common in dementia, occurring in more than half of patients with dementia (Gruber-Baldini *et al.*, 2003) and increase with dementia severity. Therefore, symptoms with a predominantly affective quality such as guilt, hopelessness, helplessness, worthlessness, sadness or sad appearance, unhappiness and mood congruent delusions should be given more weighting in the assessment process. A 'knit-brow' facial appearance, characterised by the brows being slightly lowered and drawn together, might also be an index of dysphoria and sadness in elderly patients with severe dementia (Magai *et al.*, 2000). In severe dementia, behavioural disturbances, including verbal agitation and disturbed vocalisation (Gruber-Baldini *et al.*, 2003), physical aggression (Lyketsos *et al.*, 1999a; Menon *et al.*, 2001) and food refusal (Draper, 1999) may accompany depressive symptoms, are often the presenting problem and may be a depressive equivalent (Table 2).

Table 2. Phenomenology of depression in severe dementia

Guilty feelings
Hopelessness
Helplessness
Worthlessness
Sadness or sad appearance
Unhappiness
Mood congruent delusions
Behavioural disturbances
Verbal agitation
Disturbed vocalisation
Physical aggression
Food refusal
'Knit-brow' facial appearance

Epidemiology of depression in severe dementia

There is a wide variability of the estimated prevalence rates of depression and depressive symptoms across all stages of dementia. The variability of these prevalence rates may be accounted for by a number of factors, including the use of different patient populations, differing diagnostic criteria and differing assessment methods for depression. In severe dementia, an added factor contributing to the wide discrepancy are the difficulties in diagnosing depression accurately in the patient with severe dementia. A summary of the studies examining the prevalence of major depression and depressive symptoms in severe dementia are shown in Table 3.

The reported prevalence rate of depression and depressive symptoms in severe dementia ranges widely from 6% to 61%, with reported prevalence of major depression in severe AD varying between 6% and 27%.

Few studies have examined the longitudinal course and incidence of depression in severe dementia. Payne *et al.* (2002) reported that among residents of a specialist long-term care facility with dementia the prevalence rates of depression were highest on admission and declined at six-month and twelve-month follow-up.

Aetiology of depression in severe dementia

The prevalence of depression in dementia is higher than would be expected to occur by chance, and it is unlikely to simply reflect the co-occurrence of the two disorders (Ballard *et al.*, 2001), and the occurrence of depression in the late stages of dementia, beyond the point of the patient having insight into their condition, suggests that the genesis of depressive symptoms in dementia is not purely due to a reaction to the awareness of loss of cognitive function, and gives credence to the biological hypotheses about the aetiology of depression in dementia. In examining the evidence for the aetiology of depression in severe dementia, most of the literature refers to AD and very little refers to other forms of dementia or specifically to late-stage or severe dementia.

Environmental factors and life events

People with dementia, even those with severe dementia can develop depressive symptoms in response to stress and environmental change. Anthony *et al.* (1987) examined the effect on patients with dementia of an enforced move following the closure of a psychiatric hospital. A large proportion of patients with dementia demonstrated significant depressive behaviours following their transfer to another facility and these persisted for up to three months after the move. The implication of these findings is that admission to a nursing home or other care facility is inherently associated with a change of routine and environment and may therefore precipitate depression in patients with dementia. Furthermore, events which were associated with a high degree of threat to the person's wellbeing were strongly associated with depressive symptoms in patients with dementia (Orrell and Bebbington, 1995).

Overall, these studies highlight that people with dementia may be sensitive to distressing experiences and that life events can play a role in precipitating depression in this population.

Genetic factors

The development of depression in dementia may also be due in part to genetic factors. A family history of depression in first-degree relatives may be a risk factor for the development of depression in AD (Fahim *et al.*, 1998; Lyketsos *et al.*, 1996; Pearlson *et al.*, 1990), although some studies have not replicated this finding (Heun *et al.*, 2001). Furthermore, significant familial effects on mood state have been shown in a study of siblings with AD (Tunstall *et al.*, 2000). From a diagnostic point of view, the presence of a personal or family history of depression provides supporting evidence

Table 3. Prevalence studies of depression in severe dementia

Study (year)	Population	Number	Diagnosis of dementia	Severity of dementia	Diagnostic criteria for depression	Major depression	Minor depression/ depressive symptoms
Forstl *et al.* (1992)	AD patients	178	NINCDS-ADRDA criteria	Mean MMSE 5.8	DSM-III-R	27%	
Payne *et al.* (1998)	Outpatient clinic	AD VaD UN	NINCDS-ADRDA criteria NINCDS-AIREN criteria	MMSE <10 PGDRS score >6	CSDD >12		AD 19% VaD 42% UN 60%
Ballard *et al.* (1999)	Clinical cohort	AD 18 DLB 20	NINCDS-ADRDA	MMSE <10	DSM-III-R	AD 6% DLB 20%	
Lyketsos *et al.* (2000)	Community dwelling	105	NINCDS-ADRDA criteria NINCDS-AIREN criteria	CDR >3	NPI		Depression item present in 19%
Ballard *et al.* (2000)	Hospital dementia case register VaD AD	16 18	NINCDS-ADRDA criteria NINCDS-AIRENS criteria	MMSE <10	CSDD >10 DSM-III-R	VaD 19% AD 6%	
Evers *et al.* (2002)	Post-mortem retrospective chart review. Nursing home residents	185		CDR >3	DSM-III-R	23%	>3 depressive symptoms 14%
Watson *et al.* (2003)	Residents with dementia in assisted living facilities	144		MDS-Cogs score 9–10	CSDD score >7	20%	
Samuels *et al.* (2004)	Post mortem DLB AD	16 39	Neuropathological confirmation	CDR >3 in 6 months prior to death	16-item check list based on DSM-IV	AD 21% DLB 25%	AD 18% DLB 31%

AD, Alzheimer's disease. CDR, Clinical Dementia Rating (Hughes *et al.*, 1982; Morris, 1993). CSDD, Cornell Scale for Depression in Dementia. DLB, Dementia with Lewy bodies. MDS-Cogs, Minimum Data Set – Cognition Scale (Hartmaier *et al.*, 1994). MMSE, Mini Mental State Examination (Folstein *et al.*, 1975). NINCDS-ADRDA, National Institute of Neurological and Communicative Disorders and Stroke – Alzheimer's disease and related disorders. NINCDS-AIRENS, National Institute of Neurological and Communicative Disorders and Stroke – Association Internationale pour l'Enseignement en Neurosciences. NPI, Neuropsychiatric Inventory. PGDRS, Psychogeriatric Dependency Rating Scales (Wilkinson *et al.*, 1980). UN, Undifferentiated dementia – diagnostic group included Lewy body dementia, fronto-temporal dementia, dementia secondary to anoxia or dementia secondary to traumatic brain injury. VaD, Vascular dementia.

for the diagnosis of depression in a patient with dementia in whom depression in suspected but not certain (Greenwald, 1995).

A number of susceptibility genes have been studied with respect to depression in AD. Polymorphisms of the 5-HT receptor and transporter genes have been positively associated with depression in AD (Holmes *et al.*, 2002a; Zil *et al.*, 2000); however, ApoE4 allele does not appear to be a risk factor for depression in dementia (Scarmeas *et al.*, 2002; Schmand *et al.*, 1998; Lyketsos *et al.*, 1997; Zubenko *et al.*, 1996). These studies, taken together suggest that certain genetic factors may increase the risk of depression being 'uncovered' by the Alzheimer disease process.

Neurobiological factors

Post-mortem studies, examining neurotransmitter systems in patients with dementia who were depressed in life compared to those who were not depressed, provide some support for the role of neurochemical systems in the aetiology of depression in dementia. Potential methodological weaknesses of these studies include the inclusion of small numbers, the use of retrospective chart review to diagnose depression and the time lapse between depressive symptoms being documented or recorded and the post-mortem examination. A summary of post-mortem neurochemical studies in severe dementia is shown in Table 4. All of the studies cited included dementia patients who were severely affected.

Structural and functional brain changes are also implicated as aetiological factors of depression in dementia particularly changes in frontal lobe function in patients who are depressed. White matter hyperintensities in the frontal lobes on magnetic resonance imaging have been associated with higher depression scores in patients with AD, dementia with Lewy bodies and vascular dementia of moderate severity (Barber *et al.*, 1999). Glucose metabolism has been shown to be impaired in the superior frontal lobes bilaterally and in the left anterior cingulate cortex in patients with AD who were depressed compared to non-depressed Alzheimer's subjects (Hirano *et al.*, 1998).

Other putative risk factors for the development of depression in vascular dementia include the degree of morbidity and disability associated with cerebrovascular insults and comorbid cardiovascular disease and the potential depressogenic effects of some centrally acting cardiovascular medications (Greenwald, 1995).

Treatment strategies

An important goal of treatment of people with severe dementia is the use of strategies to improve quality of life and enhance mood and behaviour. Treatment of depression is important because of the impact of depression on function, behaviour and cognition even in severe dementia. Severe dementia complicated by depression is associated with increased cognitive and functional impairment of patients (Rovner *et al.*, 1989), as well as greater behavioural disturbances such as aggression (Lyketsos *et al.*, 1999a), and increased utilisation of health care resources (Bartels *et al.*, 2003; Kales *et al.*, 1999).

Identification of a depressive episode in a patient with severe dementia should trigger the initiation of a comprehensive management plan that is tailored to the individual physical and psychological needs of the patient and which may, depending on the severity and persistence of symptoms, include non-pharmacological and pharmacological interventions.

Non-pharmacological treatments for depression in severe dementia

Non-pharmacological treatment strategies may be used as an adjunct to biological treatments, or may be used on their own in the management of milder forms of depression in severe dementia and may be directed towards both the patient and the caregiver. A regular routine and a schedule of

Table 4. Post-mortem neurochemical studies in severe dementia

Study	Population studied	Dementia severity	Diagnostic criteria for depression	Findings
Zweig et al. (1988)	Pathologically confirmed AD Depressed n = 8 Non-depressed n = 13	MMSE <10 in all except one patient	Retrospective chart review Structured retrospective interviews with family members DSM-III-R	Significantly fewer neurons in locus coeruleus and rostral central raphe nucleus in AD patients with depression compared to non-depressed
Forstl et al. (1992)	Neuropathologically confirmed cases of AD Depressed n = 14 Non-depressed n = 38	Mean MMSE 5.8 Depressed 7.4 Non-depressed 4.2	GMSS DSM-III-R Patients examined within 12 months before death	Depressed AD cases had significantly greater loss of neurons in LC. Higher neuronal counts in nucleus of Meynert in depressed AD cases (not statistically significant)
Forstl et al. (1994)	Neuropathologically confirmed AD Non-depressed n = 30 History of depression n = 12	Mean MMSE 5.8	GMSS DSM-III-R	Depressed cases had significantly lower neuron numbers in LC. Depressed cases had slightly higher neuronal counts in basal nucleus of Meynert and substantia nigra
Chen et al. (1996)	Post-mortem study AD n = 20 Controls n = 16	Mean MMSE 7.1	Present behaviour examination	Significantly fewer serotonin uptake sites in temporal and frontal cortex in AD patients with history of persistent depressive symptoms compared to non-depressed AD subjects
Hoogendijk et al. (1999)	AD n = 18 6 depressed 6 transiently depressed 6 non-depressed Controls n = 8	GDS at death Mean 6.43 FAST score within 6 months of death 6–7f	HDRS CSDD DSM-III-R Mean interval between last assessment and death, 4.3 months	Loss of neurons in LC in AD patients confirmed. No correlation between loss of neurons and depression
Ballard et al. (2002a)	21 prospectively assessed patients with DLB 7 depressed 14 not depressed	Mean MMSE 10.3 Mean MMSE at death 6.6	DSM-III-R	DLB patients with major depression had relative preservation of 5-HT transporter reuptake sites compared to those without depression

FAST, Functional Assessment Staging (Reisberg, 1988). GDS, Global Deterioration Scale (Reisberg et al., 1982). GMSS, Geriatric Mental State Schedule (Copeland et al., 1976; Gurland et al., 1976). HDRS, Hamilton Depression Rating Scale (Hamilton, 1960). LC, Locus coeruleus. 5-HT, 5-hydroxytryptamine.

pleasurable activities for the patient, as well as on-going education of the caregiver about dementia and depression provide a platform to which other treatment strategies may be added. One of the key determinants of the likely success of an intervention is that it is tailored to the individual patient's needs and preferences. Non-pharmacologic interventions for depression in severe dementia should identify and address any underlying environmental or psychosocial stressors and unmet patient needs, and reduce the use of pharmacological interventions where possible, thus minimising the risk of adverse side effects and drug interactions (Cohen-Mansfield, 2001).

Non-pharmacologic strategies that have been investigated in severe dementia include the behavioural and mood effects of Snoezelen therapy (van Weert et al., 2005; Baillon et al., 2004), the use of Simulated Presence (a personalised, interactive audiotape containing one side of a live telephone conversation with a family member or surrogate, which is rich in selected memories and positive emotions) and its effect on wellbeing in persons with AD (Camberg et al., 1999), the effect of bright-light therapy on agitation (Lyketsos et al., 1999b; Ancoli-Israel et al., 2003), and the effect of massage and aromatherapy on agitation (Ballard et al., 2002b; Holmes et al., 2002b; Smallwood et al., 2001). While these have been demonstrated to have positive effects on agitation and quality of life measures, as well as having a high degree of patient acceptability, there have been few studies specifically investigating the effects of these treatments on depression in severe dementia. Van Weert et al. (2005) demonstrated that, in patients with moderate to severe dementia, the integration of Snoezelen into 24-hour dementia care was associated with a significant improvement in behaviour, agitation and mood measures, compared to a control group of patients who received standard care. A study by Camberg et al. (1999) investigated the effect of Simulated Presence on observations of facial expressions, withdrawn behaviour and interest in patients with severe dementia. Simulated Presence was equivalent to standard care and superior to placebo in producing happy facial expressions, and was superior to both standard care and placebo in observations of 'interest'.

Biological treatment strategies
Antidepressants in the treatment of depression in severe dementia
There are few systematic treatment trials for depression in dementia, and the studies that have been carried out have been with small numbers, of limited duration of treatment and have investigated the efficacy of antidepressant medication in community-dwelling patients with depression in the context of mild to moderate dementia. There are very few studies investigating the use of selective serotonin reuptake inhibitors (SSRIs) in patients with depression with severe dementia. A small ($n = 10$) open-label study investigating the use of sertraline in depressed patients with severe AD found that sertraline improved affect in eight patients and decreased food refusal in five out of six patients with eating difficulties (Volicer et al., 1994). An eight-week, randomised control trial, examining the effect of sertraline in 31 nursing home residents with late stage AD and a diagnosis of DSM-IV major or minor depression found that the treatment group improved on all measures over eight weeks, although there was no significant difference between treatment and placebo groups (Magai et al., 2000).

In general, SSRIs should be first-line agents in treating syndromal depression in dementia. The recommended duration of treatment is uncertain; the limited naturalistic studies suggest that depressive symptoms can fluctuate but the natural history of major depression in dementia is largely unknown. Treatment should usually be for six months for a single episode of major depression with longer-term maintenance if there is a relapse on discontinuation.

Acetylcholinesterase inhibitors in the treatment of depression in severe dementia
The cholinergic deficit in AD has been linked to neuropsychiatric disturbances including depression and there is increasing interest in the use of cholinesterase inhibitors in the management of the

non-cognitive symptoms of dementia (Holmes *et al.*, 2004). Treatment with cholinomimetic agents may improve non-cognitive symptoms of dementia, such as depression, as well as the cognitive symptoms (Cummings, 2000). A large, multi-centre study investigating the use of donepezil in patients with moderate to severe AD demonstrated a significant improvement on the Neuropsychiatric Inventory in the treatment group compared to placebo, particularly in the domains of apathy, depression and anxiety (Feldman *et al.*, 2001). However, there is no evidence for a benefit from cholinesterase inhibitors on syndromal depression in AD.

Electroconvulsive treatment in severe dementia
Evidence on the use of ECT in depression in severe dementia is sparse, there is no randomised evidence and existing evidence is from case reports, small case series and retrospective reviews (Van der Wurff *et al.*, 2003). A chart review study (Rao and Lyketsos, 2000) of 31 patients with a primary dementia and depression who were treated with ECT, concluded that ECT is an effective treatment for depression in dementia, with delirium being the most common adverse event (49%). Of the three patients in the case series with severe dementia, one developed a transient delirium and none had serious cardiac or neurological complications and all patients with severe dementia were reported as improved on the global outcome score. Weintraub and Lippmann (2001) also reported a positive outcome in a case report of a woman with advanced AD complicated by depression. The use of electroconvulsive therapy may be considered in patients suffering from severe depression, particularly with psychosis.

Addressing the needs of caregivers
Caring for a person with illness has been recognised as a risk factor for mental and physical health problems in the caregiver (Vitaliano *et al.*, 1997; Schulz *et al.*, 1990), and this risk may be higher when caring for a person with dementia (Hooker *et al.*, 1998; Schulz *et al.*, 1995). The presence of neuropsychiatric symptoms in a person with dementia can result in a lower quality of life for the patient as well as for their carers (Finkel *et al.*, 1998) and the research indicates that neuropsychiatric symptoms of dementia have a greater negative impact than cognitive impairments on the mental health of caregivers (Hooker *et al.*, 2002). The management plan of a person with severe dementia should therefore recognise and aim to address the potential needs of caregivers.

Summary
Depression is a common complication of severe dementia but can be difficult to detect and diagnose. Atypical features such as agitation, disturbed vocalisation and food refusal, together with withdrawal, irritability and more typical features of guilt, worthlessness and hopelessness point to the presence of depression. The cause of depression in severe dementia may be multifactorial and it is important to remember that people with severe dementia can develop depressive reactions in response to negative life events and can respond negatively to environmental change. Depression in severe dementia is associated with increased cognitive and functional impairment and can be linked to aggression and for these reasons warrants detection and treatment. While there is a limited evidence base to work from, behavioural and pharmacological treatments can be effective.

References

Alexopoulos GS, Abrams RC, Young RC *et al.* (1988) Cornell Scale for Depression in Dementia. *Biological Psychiatry*, 23:271–284.

American Psychiatric Association (1987) Diagnostic and Statistical Manual of Mental Disorders, 3rd edition, revised. American Psychiatric Association, Washington, DC.

American Psychiatric Association (1994) Diagnostic and Statistical Manual of Mental Disorders, 4th edition. American Psychiatric Association, Washington, DC.

Ancoli-Israel S, Martin JL, Gehrman P *et al.* (2003) Effect of light on agitation in institutionalized patients with severe AD. *Am J Geriatr Psychiatry*, 11:194–203.

Anthony K, Proctor AW, Silverman AM *et al.* (1987) Mood and behaviour problems following the relocation of elderly patients with mental illness. *Age and Ageing*, 16:355–365.

Baillon S, van Diepen E, Prettyman R *et al.* (2004) A comparison of the effects of Snoezelen and reminiscence therapy on the agitated behaviour of patients with dementia. *Int J Geriatr Psychiatry*, 19:1047–1052.

Ballard C, Holmes C, McKeith I *et al.* (1999) Psychiatric morbidity in dementia with Lewy bodies: a prospective clinical and neuropathological comparative study with Alzheimer's disease. *Am J Psychiatry*, 156:1039–1045.

Ballard C, Neill D, O'Brien J *et al.* (2000) Anxiety, depression and psychosis in vascular dementia: prevalence and associations. *Journal of Affective Disorders*, 59:97–106.

Ballard C, O'Brien J, James I, Swann A (2001) Dementia: management of behavioural and psychological symptoms. Oxford University Press.

Ballard C, Johnson M, Piggott M *et al.* (2002a) A positive association between 5HT re-uptake binding sites and depression in dementia with Lewy bodies. *Journal of Affective Disorders*, 69:219–223.

Ballard CG, O'Brien, Reichelt K *et al.* (2002b) Aromatherapy as a safe and effective treatment for the management of agitation in severe dementia: the results of a double blind, placebo controlled trial. *J Clin Psychiatr*, 63:553–558.

Barber R, Scheltens P, Gholkar A *et al.* (1999) White matter lesions on magnetic resonance imaging in dementia with Lewy bodies, Alzheimer's disease, vascular dementia, and normal aging. *J Neurol Neurosurg Psychiatry*, 67:66–72.

Bartels SJ, Horn SD, Smout RJ *et al.* (2003) Agitation and depression in frail nursing home elderly patients with dementia. Treatment characteristics and service use. *Am J Geriatr Psychiatry*, 11:231–238.

Boyle PA, Malloy PF (2004) Treating apathy in Alzheimer's disease. *Dement Geriatr Cogn Disord*, 17:91–99.

Camberg L, Woods, Ooi WL *et al.* (1999) Evaluation of simulated presence: a personalized approach to enhance well-being in persons with Alzheimer's disease. *JAGS*, 7:446–452.

Chen CP, Alder JT, Bowen DM *et al.* (1996) Presynaptic serotonergic markers in community acquired cases of Alzheimer's disease: correlations with depression and neuroleptic medication. *Journal of Neurochemistry*, 66:1592–1598.

Cohen-Mansfield J (2001) Nonpharmacologic Interventions for Inappropriate Behaviours in Dementia. A review, summary and critique. *Am J Geriatr Psychiatry*, 9:361–381.

Copeland JRM, Kelleher MJ, Kellett JM *et al.* (1976) A semi-structured clinical interview for the assessment of diagnosis of mental state in the elderly: the Geriatric Mental State Schedule. I. Development and reliability. *Psychological Medicine*, 6:439–449.

Cummings JL (2000) Cholinesterase inhibitors: a new class of psychotropic compounds. *Am J Psychiatry* 157:4–15.

Cummings JL, Mega M, Gray K *et al.* (1994) The Neuropsychiatric Inventory: comprehensive assessment of psychopathology in dementia. *Neurology*, 44:2308–2314.

Draper B (1999) Practical geriatrics: the diagnosis and treatment of depression in dementia. *Psychiatr Serv*, 50:1151–1153.

Evers MM, Samuels SC, Lantz M *et al.* (2002) The prevalence, diagnosis and treatment of depression in dementia patients in chronic care facilities in the last six months of life. *Int J Geriatr Psychiatry*, 17:464–472.

Fahim S, van Duijn CM, Baker FM *et al.* (1998) A study of familial aggregation of depression, dementia and Parkinson's disease. *Eur J Epidemiol*, 14:233–238.

Feldman H, Gauthier S, Hecker J *et al.* (2001) A 24-week, randomized, double-blind study of donepezil in moderate to severe Alzheimer's disease. *Neurology*, 57:613–620.

Finkel SI, Silva JCE, Cohen GD *et al.* (1998) Behavioural and psychological symptoms of dementia: a consensus statement on current knowledge and implications for research and treatment. *Am J Geriatr Psychiatry*, 6:97–100.

Folstein MF, Folstein SE, McHugh PR (1975) 'Mini Mental State'. A practical method for grading the cognitive state of patients for the clinician. *J Psychiatr Res*, 12:189–192.

Forstl H, Burns A, Luthert P (1992) Clinical and neuropathological correlates of depression in Alzheimer's disease. *Psychol Med*, 22:877–884.

Forstl H, Levy R, Burns A *et al.* (1994) Disproportionate loss of noradrenergic and cholinergic neurons as cause of depression in Alzheimer's disease – a hypothesis. *Pharmacopsychiatry*, 27:11–15.

Greenwald BS, Kramer E (1991) Major depression in severe dementia, in New Research Program and Abstracts: American Psychiatric Association 144th Annual Meeting, New Orleans, LA, May 11–16, p 170.

Greenwald BS (1995) Depression in Alzheimer's disease and related dementias, in Behavioural Complications in Alzheimer's Disease (Ed B Lawlor), American Psychiatric Press, Washington, DC, pp 19–53.

Gruber-Baldini AL, Zimmerman S, Watson L *et al.* (2003) Recognition and treatment of depressive symptoms among residents with dementia in assisted living. Symposium 117. Presented at the 56th Annual Scientific Meeting of The Gerontological Society of America, San Diego, Nov 22.

Gurland BJ, Fleiss JL, Goldberg K *et al.* (1976) A semi-structured clinical interview for the assessment of diagnosis of mental state in the elderly: the Geriatric Mental State Schedule. II. A factor analysis. *Psychological Medicine*, 6:451–459.

Hamilton M (1960) A rating scale for depression. *Journal of Neurology, Neurosurgery and Psychiatry*, 23:56–62.

Hart DJ, Craig D, Compton SA *et al.* (2003) A retrospective study of the behavioural and psychological symptoms of mid and late phase Alzheimer's disease. *Int J Geriatr Psychiatry*, 18:1037–1042.

Hartmaier SL, Sloane PD, Guess HA *et al.* (1994) The MDS Cognition Scale: a valid instrument for identifying and staging nursing home residents with dementia using the minimum data set. *JAGS*, 42:1173–1179.

Heun R, Papassotiropoulos A, Jessen F *et al.* (2001) A family study of Alzheimer's disease and early and late-onset depression in elderly patients. *Arch Gen Psychiatry*, 58:190–196.

Hirano N, Mori E, Ishii K *et al.* (1998) Frontal lobe hypometabolism and depression in Alzheimer's disease. *Neurology*, 50:380–383.

Holmes C, Arranz M, Collier D *et al.* (2002a) Depression in Alzheimer's disease: the effect of serotonin receptor gene variation. Abstracts from the 8th Int Congress on Alzheimer's Disease and Related Disorders, Stockholm.

Holmes C, Hopkins V, Hensford C *et al.* (2000b) Lavender oil as a treatment for agitated behaviour in severe dementia: a placebo controlled study. *Int J Geriatr Psychiatry*, 17:305–308.

Holmes C, Wilkinson D, Dean C *et al.* (2004) The efficacy of donepezil in the treatment of neuropsychiatric symptoms in Alzheimer's disease. *Neurology*, 63:214–219.

Hoogendijk WJ, Sommer IE, Pool CW *et al.* (1999) Lack of association between depression and loss of neurons in the locus coeruleus in Alzheimer disease. *Archives of General Psychiatry*, 56:45–51.

Hooker K, Monahan DJ, Bowman SR *et al.* (1998) Personality counts for a lot: predictors of mental and physical health of spouse caregivers in two disease groups. *Journal of Gerontology: Psychological Sciences*, 53B:73–85.

Hooker K, Bowman SR, Padgett Coehlo D *et al.* (2002) Behavioural change in persons with dementia: relationship with mental and physical health of caregivers. *Journal of Gerontology: Psychological Sciences*, 57B:453–460.

Hughes CP, Berg L, Danziger WL *et al.* (1982) A new clinical scale for the staging of dementia. *Br J Psychiatry*, 140:566–572.

Kales HC, Blow FC, Copeland LA *et al.* (1999) Health care utilization by older patients with coexisting dementia and depression. *Am J Psychiatry*, 156:550–556.

Katona CLE, Aldridge CR (1985) The dexamethasone suppression test and depressive signs in dementia. *Journal of Affective Disorders*, 8:83–9.

Lee HB, Lyketsos CG (2003) Depression in Alzheimer's disease: heterogeneity and related issues. *Biol Psychiatry*, 54:353–362.

Lyketsos CG, Lee HB (2004) Diagnosis and treatment of depression in Alzheimer's disease. A practical update for the clinician. *Dement Geriatr Cogn Disord*, 17:55–64.

Lyketsos CG, Tune LE, Pearlson G *et al.* (1996) Major depression in Alzheimer's disease: an interaction between gender and family history. *Psychosomatics*, 37:380–389.

Lyketsos CG, Baker L, Warren A *et al.* (1997) Depression, delusions and hallucinations in Alzheimer's disease: no relationship to apolipoprotein E genotype. *J Neuropsychiatry Clin Neurosci*, 9:64–77.

Lyketsos CG, Steele C, Galik E *et al.* (1999a) Physical aggression in dementia patients and its relationship to depression. *Am J Psychiatry*, 156:66–71.

Lyketsos CG, Veiel LL, Baker *et al.* (1999b) A randomized controlled trial of bright light therapy for agitated behaviours in dementia patients residing in long-term care. *Int J Geriatr Psychiatry*, 14:520–525.

Lyketsos CG, Steinberg M, Tschanz JT *et al.* (2000) Mental and behavioural disturbances in dementia: findings from the Cache County Study on Memory in Aging. *Am J Psychiatry*, 157:708–714.

Magai C, Kennedy G, Cohen CI, Gomberg D (2000) A controlled clinical trial of sertraline in the treatment of depression in nursing home patients with late-stage Alzheimer's disease. *Am J Geriatr Psychiatry*, 8:66–74.

Marin DB, Green CR, Schmeidler J *et al.* (1997) Noncognitive disturbances in Alzheimer's disease: frequency, longitudinal course, and relationship to cognitive symptoms. *JAGS*, 45:1331–1338.

McGivney SA, Mulvihill M, Taylor B (1994) Validating the GDS depression screen in the nursing home. *JAGS*, 42:490–492.

Menon AD, Gruber-Baldini AL, Hebel JR *et al.* (2001) Relationship between aggressive behaviours and depression among nursing home residents with dementia. *Int J Geriatr Psychiatry*, 16:139–146.

Mirakhur A, Craig D, Hart DJ *et al.* (2004) Behavioural and psychological syndromes in Alzheimer's disease. *Int J Geriatr Psychiatry*, 19:1035–1039.

Morris J: The CDR (1993) current version and scoring rules. *Neurology*, 43:2412–2413.

Olin JT, Katz IR, Meyers BS *et al.* (2002) Provisional diagnostic criteria for depression of Alzheimer disease. Rationale and background. *Am J Geriatr Psychiatry*, 10:129–141.

Orrell M, Bebbington P (1995) Life events and senile dementia. Affective symptoms. *Br J Psychiatry*, 166: 613–620.

Payne JL, Lyketsos CG, Steele C *et al.* (1998) Relationship of cognitive and functional impairment to depressive features in Alzheimer's disease and other dementias. *J Neuropsychiatry Clin Neurosci*, 10:440–447.

Payne JL, Sheppard J-ME, Steinberg M *et al.* (2002) Incidence, prevalence and outcomes of depression in residents of a long-term care facility with dementia. *Int J Geriatr Psychiatry*, 17:247–253.

Pearlson GD, Ross CA, Lohr WD *et al.* (1990) Association between family history of affective disorder and the depressive syndrome of Alzheimer's disease. *Am J Psychiatry*, 147:454–456.

Rao V, Lyketsos CG (2000) The benefits and risks of ECT for patients with primary dementia who also suffer from depression. *Int J Geriatr Psychiatry*, 15:729–735.

Reisberg B (1988) Functional assessment staging (FAST). *Psychopharm Bull*, 24:653–659.

Reisberg B, Ferris SH, de Leon MJ *et al.* (1982) The Global Deterioration Scale (GDS) for assessment of primary degenerative dementia. *Am J Psychiatry*, 139:1136–1139.

Robert P (2002) Understanding and managing behavioural symptoms in Alzheimer's disease and related dementias: focus on rivastigmine. *Curr Med Res Opin*, 18:156–171.

Rovner BW, Broadhead J, Spencer M *et al.* (1989) Depression and Alzheimer's disease. *Am J Psychiatry*, 146:350–353.

Samuels SC, Brickman AM, Burd JA *et al.* (2004) Depression in autopsy confirmed dementia with Lewy bodies and Alzheimer's disease. *The Mount Sinai Journal of Medicine*, 71:55–62.

Scarmeas N, Brandt J, Albert M *et al.* (2002) Association between the APOE genotype and psychopathologic symptoms in Alzheimer's disease. *Neurology*, 58:1182–1188.

Schmand B, Hooijer C, Jonker C *et al.* (1998) Apolipoprotein E phenotype is not related to late-life depression in a population based sample. *Soc Psychiatry Psychiatr Epidemiol*, 33:21–26.

Schulz R, Visintainer P, Williamson G (1990) Psychiatric and physical morbidity effects of caregiving. *Journal of Gerontology: Psychological Sciences*, 45:181–191.

Schulz R, O'Brien A, Bookwala J *et al.* (1995) Psychiatric and physical morbidity effects of dementia caregiving: prevalence, correlates and causes. *The Gerontologist*, 35:771–791.

Smallwood J, Brown R, Coulter F *et al.* (2001) Aromatherapy and behaviour disturbances in dementia: a randomized controlled trial. *Int J Geriatr Psychiatry*, 16:1010–1013.

Tunstall N, Fraser L, Lovestone S *et al.* (2000) Familial influence on variation in age of onset and behavioural phenotype in Alzheimer's disease. *Br J Psychiatry*, 176:156–159.

Van der Wurff FB, Stek ML, Hoogendijk WJG *et al.* (2003) The efficacy and safety of ECT in depressed older adults: a literature review. *Int J Geriatr Psychiatry*, 18:894–904.

Van Weert JC, van Dulmen AM, Spreeuwenberg PM *et al.* (2005) Behavioural and mood effects of Snoezelen integrated into 24-hour dementia care. *JAGS*, 53:24–33.

Vitaliano P, Schulz R, Kiecolt-Glaser J *et al.* (1997) Research on psychological and physical concomitants of caregiving: Where do we go from here? *Annals of Behavioural Medicine*, 19:117–123.

Volicer L, Rheaume Y, Cyr MS (1994) Treatment of depression in advanced Alzheimer's disease using sertraline. *J Geriatr Psychiatry Neurol*, 7:227–229.

Watson LC, Garrett JM, Sloane PD *et al.* (2003) Depression in assisted living. Results from a four-state study. *Am J Geriatr Psychiatry*, 11:534–542.

Weintraub D, Lippmann SB (2001) ECT for major depression and mania with advanced dementia. *J ECT*, 17:65–7.

Wilkinson IM, Graham-White J (1980) Psychogeriatric Dependency Rating Scales (PGDRS). A method of assessment for use by nurses. *Br J Psychiatry*, 137:558–565.

Yesavage JA, Brink TL, Rose TL *et al.* (1983) Development and validation of a geriatric depression screening scale: a preliminary report. *Journal of Psychiatric Research*, 17:37–49.

Zil P, Padberg F, de Jonge S *et al.* (2000) Serotonin transporter (5-HT) polymorphism in psychogeriatric patients. *Neurosci Let*, 84:113–115.

Zubenko GS, Moossy J (1988) Major depression in primary dementia. Clinical and neuropathological correlates. *Archives of Neurology*, 45:1182–1186.

Zubenko GS, Henderson R, Stiffler S *et al.* (1996) Association of the APOE d4 allele with clinical subtypes of late life depression. *Biol Psychiatry*, 40:1008–1016.

Zweig RM, Ross CA, Hedreen JC *et al.* (1988) The neuropathology of aminergic nuclei in Alzheimer's disease. *Annals of Neurology*, 24:233–242.

Physical Aspects of Severe Alzheimer's Disease

Bruno Vellas

Introduction

Severe dementia is characterised by a significant cognitive, behavioural and functional decline towards a severe dependence, as well as, social troubles caused by an increase of caregiver burden, which requires greater resources utilisation, both medical and non-medical, representing a major health public problem.

Alzheimer's disease is characterised clinically by cognitive impairment, dominated by memory complaints, which may or may not be associated with a syndrome of aphasia, apraxia and agnosia. All these lead to disorders of instrumental function, executive function and judgement. The clinical presentation and the course of the disease may be extremely varied. The clinical disorders observed often differ widely from one subject to another, depending on factors such as age at onset, rapidity of progression and the diversity of cognitive and behavioural disturbances. Later, the disease progresses and gradually affects other cognitive domains (language, attention, arithmetic, orientation to time and place) as well as more complex functions such as executive functions which allow planning and performance of successive, organised tasks. The course of the disease is also marked by major disturbances of judgement and reasoning which may result in behavioural problems. These problems have a progressive impact on the activities of daily living and on independence which is initially revealed in certain domestic activities, and then in essential activities of daily living, and the patient becomes dependent. Problems of sphincter control, alteration of nutritional status, and disturbances of balance and gait accelerate the process of dependence.

The evolution of Alzheimer's disease

Alzheimer's is a chronic disease. Various complications can cause the subject to lose his or her independence and eventually even become permanently bedridden. Such a state is always accompanied by its own complications: pressure sores, infections, undernutrition, and therefore by high morbidity, loss of quality of life, and suffering, all of which also result in high medical costs.

One of the essential aims of medical follow-up of Alzheimer's patients is to preserve satisfactory physical independence and in consequence a better quality of life. It is possible to maintain patients' independence for the activities of daily living even at very advanced stages of the disease. There is in fact no correlation between the histopathological lesions and the quality of life or independence of the patients.

The natural history of Alzheimer's disease is today better known, through some long-term or retrospective studies which have recently been published. Alzheimer's disease is one of the most frequent causes of death, even if this has long been disregarded. Study of the causes of death in

Severe Dementia. Edited by A. Burns and B. Winblad.

1995 in the United States reveals that 7.1% of all deaths can be attributed to this disease, which is the third leading cause of death (Ewbank, 1999). A prospective study recently carried out in the state of Washington found concordant results, and revealed that certain factors decreased the duration of the patients' life, and in particular rapid decline of cognitive function, loss of independence, and falls were factors of poor prognosis. Identification and follow-up of these factors may help the patient and his or her family to better plan their future (Larson *et al.*, 2004). Median survival also appears to depend on age at the time of diagnosis (Brookmeyer *et al.*, 2002). The mean time elapsing between the onset of symptoms and the clinical diagnosis of the disease was 32.1 months (±37.9) and time elapsing between clinical diagnosis and institutionalisation was 23.9 months (±33.6). Institutionalisation therefore occurred at a mean of 56.5 months after the onset of the first symptoms. The mean duration of the disease after the onset of the first symptoms to the death of the patient was 101.3 months, or nearly 8.5 years. The longest duration of the disease was 252.1 months, or nearly 21 years, for one of these patients. In typical Alzheimer's disease, the diagnosis was made at the age of 75 years, or 32 months after the onset of the first signs. Admission to a retirement home took place on average 25 months after diagnosis, or 57 months (4.5 years) after the onset of the first signs of the disease at 71 years. The subject then spent about 44 months in the retirement home before decease (Grossberg *et al.*).

The main physical symptoms of the disease

Three signs should attract the attention of the physician caring for a patient with severe Alzheimer's disease:

- weight loss
- disturbances of balance and posture with risk of falls, and loss of mobility
- infections, mostly pneumonia

These are the basic essentials of non-cognitive follow-up of these patients.

Weight loss and Alzheimer's disease

When he first described the disease in 1906, Alois Alzheimer emphasised the occurrence of weight loss in his patient. However, this weight loss has long been mistakenly considered as occurring at the late stages of the disease. We now know than it can occur as soon as the first symptoms of the disease appear.

The sooner a management strategy is set up, the more effective it will be. Otherwise, we may rapidly find ourselves confronted with undernourished, anorexic subjects, where there is very little room for manoeuvre between doing nothing (often seen as abandonment of treatment) or setting up enteral nutrition (which is then seen as artificial prolongation of life), whereas early on, especially in subjects who live alone at home, a visit from a home help will often be sufficient to assist these patients in doing their shopping and preparing their meals. It therefore appears to be essential to assess the nutritional status of each Alzheimer's patient, particularly if he or she lives alone or has little family support.

The pathophysiological mechanisms of weight loss are complex and have only partially been elucidated. Alteration of nutritional status may be secondary to the development of inability to perform the activities of everyday living or to disturbances of eating behaviour. However, numerous studies have shown that weight loss is observed in the course of the disease even when the subjects still have a satisfactory energy intake. Certain authors suggest that atrophy of the internal temporal cortex or the effect of the e4 allele may play a role in weight regulation (Grundman *et al.*, 1996; Vanhanen *et al.*, 2001). Clinical practice shows that weight loss is accompanied by a variety of complications (decreased immunity, muscle atrophy, falls and fractures) which affect the state of health and increase the risk of institutionalisation and mortality. In the severe stages of the disease, behavioural disturbances and food disorders, e.g. refusal to eat, agitation, are some of the most difficult compications of the disease for health practitioners. Studies have shown that in the eight years after the onset of Alzheimer's disease, approximately 50% of patients require artificial nutrition or assistance in feeding; moreover, weight loss has been frequently observed in AD patients before and after institutionalisation. Poor nutritonal status can be responsible for alterations in immune response, infections, anorexia and pressure sores. Involuntary loss of muscle mass with aging, termed sarcopaenia, is a widespread condition in AD patients, associated with a reduction in muscle strength and function which gradually leads to impairment in the activities of daily living, increased risk of falls and fall-related fractures.

The nutritional status of the elderly person with AD can be quickly and easily evaluated with the MNA (Mini Nutrition Assessment). The MNA is the most validated tool to assess nutritional status in the elderly? It is also useful in Alzheimer's patients. The MNA is able to differentiate individuals with good nutritional status (>23.5), with poor nutritional status (<17) or at risk of malnutrition (between 17 and 23.5).

Among 595 patients living at home and followed in our Alzheimer centre in Toulouse, 166 (27.9%) presented moderately severe to severe AD defined by a MMS score below 16. Their MMS score mean was 11.4 ± 3.5. When we follow these patients for a one-year period, patients with moderate to severe dementia worsen their nutritional status with a statiscally significant decrease on the MNA score ($p = 0.0029$). A clinically signifant weight loss is also observed in nearly 40% of Alzheimer patients. When weight loss is more than 4% of total body weight it is related to a significant increase in morbidity and mortality.

It is very important to assess weight regularly, every six months, in AD patients, as well as assessing their nutritional status with the MNA at least once a year. If the patients have some life events it is important to assess again weight and nutrition status. If the MNA is less than 23.5 it is necessary to look carefully at each MNA item to determine where the patient loses points to as to be able to correct the risk factors. If the MNA score is less than 17 the patient is more likely already to present protein-caloric undernutrition and it is necessary to measure plasma albumin and CRP and to discuss more extensive refeeding. We have demonstrated in some previous studies that with caregiver education and/or with oral supplementation it is possible to increase weight, MNA score and muscle mass in Alzheimer's patients. It is really important to improve nutritional intake as soon as possible in the earliest stage of malnutrition so as to be able to avoid tube-feeding. Complications related to tube-feeding are clearly more important than the benefit in the severely demented patients.

Mobility problems, falls and risk of accidents

In patients with Alzheimer's disease, posture rapidly becomes incorrect as a consequence of ageing (arthritis, impaired vision, muscle wasting etc.) but this may also be directly related to Alzheimer's disease (Kluger *et al.*, 1997; Franssen *et al.*, 1999) or to medication. Disturbances of equilibrium can lead to numerous falls and fractures, or to abusive use of restraint. Accidents generally occur in patients in whom Alzheimer's disease has not been diagnosed: drug-related accidents, accidents in the street or in the home. Balance and mobility problems have major psychological consequences leading to anxiety and a feeling of insecurity. They can result in decreased physical activity and loss of social contacts.

Alzheimer's disease is one of the causes of epilepsy in the elderly subject. Numerous patients develop extrapyramidal symptoms. Resting tremor is rarer than in idiopathic Parkinson's disease or in drug-induced striatal syndromes. On the other hand, rigidity and bradykinesia or a 'parkinsonian' gait are more frequent (Mitchell, 1999). An underlying brain disorder, in this instance Alzheimer's disease, is a risk factor for confusion in the elderly. Sphincter problems generally develop in advanced forms.

At a late stage of Alzheimer's disease muscle and joint contractures may develop, leading to a permanently bedridden state and to death because of the complications of decubitus. The value of walking and passive mobilisation of the joints to prevent such contractures must be stressed.

Infections
Weight loss, difficulty in walking, falls and behaviour disorders, will develop in almost all Alzheimer's subjects at one time or another in the course of the disease. They sometimes occur simultaneously. Undernutrition increases the likelihood of muscle wasting and falls. Falls often lead staff to use restraint during the day, resulting in agitation at night. All these factors rapidly end in the patient becoming permanently bedridden. Bedridden severely demented elderly patients are more likely to develop infections. Urinary infections are common in those patients with urinary incontinence. But major problems are related to pneumonia. Pneumonia in these patients with severe dementia are common and a frequent cause of death. Protein-calorie undernutrition will decrease immunity function capacity; moreover swallowing disorders are frequent and could be responsible for pneumonia aspiration. In very severe dementia and bedridden patients, palliative care must be discussed.

Medical follow-up
Once the diagnosis has been established, patients can be followed by standardised gerontological evaluation (Rubenstein *et al.*, 1984). One of the principal aims of management is to postpone the period of loss of independence which precedes death. It is very important to provide therapeutic management for these patients and their families. This need is felt by the family, and if it is not met they will turn to alternative medicine. Standardised evaluation allows rapid and objective exploration of several facets of the elderly patient: dependence (ADL, IADL), memory deficit and the syndrome of aphasia/apraxia/agnosia (MMS), the risk of pressure sores (Norton's scale), nutritional status with the MNA (Mini Nutritional Assessment), and study of walking and balance (Tinetti's test). Two other tools may also be useful: the Neuropsychiatric Inventory (NPI), which explores the psychiatric complications of the disease, and the Zarit scale (Zarit *et al.*, 1980) which assesses caregiver burden. The Zarit scale, by exploring caregiver burden, makes it possible to adapt the services proposed or helps to pose the indication of admission to a retirement home when this seems necessary.

It is in fact preferable to decide on a move to a retirement home in advance and under good conditions, rather than wait until the last minute and then have to resort to emergency admission under poor conditions for all those concerned: the patient, the family and those close to them.

Clinical examination
Complete clinical examination of the patient must be carried out initially and then every three months. This examination must be repeated if a new incident occurs (agitation, fever etc.). In particular, bladder distension should be sought (in women and in men), as well as pollakiuria and altered general status. It should include examination of vision and hearing, and of the teeth and mouth to seek for poor dental condition or fungal infections. Signs of depression or anxiety and mobility problems should be sought. It is also important to look for a faecaloma, constipation, gastric or abdominal pain in these patients who cannot adequately express their complaints. The same is true of rheumatological pain, which may be the cause of unexplained refusal to walk.

Interview
The interview should yield information on the living arrangements of the patient, the quality of support from his or her family and relatives and the impact of the disease on the couple.

Radiological examination and biological tests

Among the radiological examinations and biological tests, a chest X-ray is advisable (this is particularly useful for patients who attend a day centre or who live in an institution, if a resident with whom the patient may have been in contact develops tuberculosis or a lung infection). It will serve as a reference.

Study of the cardiac silhouette can show associated heart failure. Plain abdominal X-ray can exclude a high faecaloma which could not be found by digital rectal examination. Lastly, a basic ECG is useful, as well as a battery of laboratory tests which should include a complete blood count, hydroelectrolyte and liver tests, and urine culture.

Gerontological evaluation

The standardised gerontological evaluation should be carried out in all patients at the time of diagnosis and then every six months or when a change in circumstances occurs, either social (death of a family member or relative, change of living arrangements, institutionalisation, hospitalisation), or at the onset of an intercurrent disease.

Social evaluation should look at the living arrangements of the patient (alone, with family, in institution), and the characteristics of family and relatives (availability, state of health, age etc.).

The family must also be fully informed about the services available and the possibilities of legal protection when this is necessary, bearing in mind that it is better to anticipate and prevent problems than have to suffer them. Similarly, when admission to an institution becomes necessary, it is preferable it should take place under good conditions a little early, rather than wait until the last minute and have to resort to emergency admission under unsatisfactory conditions. On the other hand, when the family has not made up their mind to institutionalise the patient, it is better to make a last attempt to keep the patient at home rather than leave the family with feelings of remorse.

Specific treatment for Alzheimer's disease can only be contemplated as part of a care plan which includes treatment of behavioural problems, nutritional problems and mood, appropriate social management (services delivered to relieve the informal caregiver) and psychological support.

Management structures

The concern of the clinician at the present time must be to identify patients as early as possible in order to rapidly set up a medical and non-medical intervention strategy, with the aim of maintaining as long as possible satisfactory independence for the patient and his or her family and friends.

Management at home with increased support

Pharmacological and non-pharmacological management of the patient and support and assistance to family and relatives remain the decisive factors in postponing admission to an institution. The majority of patients with dementia live at home, and they are often cared for by the family alone, without any help from professionals.

However, intermediate solutions between care at home by the family and institutionalisation have been developed in recent years: care at home with increased support, respite families, day care centres or temporary care centres are possibilities which offer specific and appropriate management to persons with Alzheimer's disease. But families are still too often insufficiently informed, the facilities available differ widely depending on location, and the financial cost of the services proposed or of the accommodation are still an obstacle to appropriate management of the elderly person with dementia.

Management at home with increased support calls upon external professional help, working as a team with a common objective, and usually coordinated by the general practitioner. Various professionals and services intervene, which are adapted and modulated according to the needs of the patient and his or her family. The following assistance can be provided:

- *nursing care* for toileting, prevention of decubitus ulcers and distribution of medication; this is provided by a nurse in private practice or by a care association
- *physiotherapy*
- *the help of an occupational therapist* with if necessary *conversion of the accommodation* to reduce the risk of accidents in the home (increased security, prevention of the risk of falls, locking of doors and potentially dangerous places etc.)
- *the services of a home nurse or a helper* – the latter is trained in the physical and psychological management of dependent persons
- *a home help* for the daily activities the person can no longer carry out (shopping, housework, meal preparation etc.); visits may be daily except for weekends and public holidays; these services are organised by the local councils and the hourly cost depends on the beneficiary's financial resources; similar assistance may be provided by an independent home help
- some town councils run a *meal delivery service*, which is subject to the same conditions as domestic help
- *provision of a tele-alarm* – this type of device is indicated in mild to moderate dementia without marked temporospatial disorientation and above all without major behavioural disturbance.

Relatives and family also require support if maintenance at home is to be prolonged. Numerous studies have shown that the decisive factor in institutionalisation of patients was less the severity of the disease than the stamina of the caregiver, usually the spouse. The family need information and assistance if they are to react and adjust well to the disease. This information and support can be provided by the family doctor, the staff of specialised centres (day care centre, day hospital, memory clinic etc.) aided by the various associations.

Hospitalisation at home and hospitalisation in medium- or long-stay units

The physician plays an essential role in detecting disorders or complications of the disease. He may make it possible to avoid hospitalisation by preventing or treating factors of aggravation such as urinary, bronchial or skin infections, foot care problems, constipation, dehydratation, sensory deficits, etc.

Hospitalisation at home, always planned for a limited period, is often a more beneficial alternative than hospitalisation in a medium-stay unit or admission to a convalescent home. It comprises the intervention in the home of a genuine medical team with a doctor, nurse and nursing auxiliary.

But admission to hospital may become necessary to manage an acute psychiatric or medical problem or to give the family some respite. The following structures all have as primary aim the rehabilitation of the subject and discharge to his or her own home:

- *departments of medicine* (*geriatrics, neurology, internal medicine or psychiatry*) offer specialised management of the problem which motivated the admission to hospital; but sometimes these facilities are not adapted to aged, demented patients (for example, in internal medicine departments the premises are not suited to management of a behavioural problem, while in psychiatry departments it may be difficult to give a physical complication the specialised medical management required).
- *the acute care unit* can take in Alzheimer's patients whatever the stage of the disease and whatever the intercurrent or associated diseases for a stay lasting a few days; there are very few of these facilities

Community residences, respite families and short-stay centres

Between the home and long-stay facilities (private retirement home or long-stay unit in a hospital) community residences offer patients some independence, with the possibility of access to catering services (restaurant, room service).

Retirement homes and long-stay units

Admission to a long-stay unit may become unavoidable when management at home becomes too heavy a burden for the family. Many innovative experiments are being carried out in the hospital setting. They all try to improve the quality of life and management of these patients. Specialised units are being developed; these may be either day care units, sheltered units, or true units for diagnosis and rehabilitation. Unfortunately, such initiatives are still very rare and there are many difficulties in the way of their creation, owing to lack of funding.

The general practitioner accompanies Alzheimer's patients for perhaps 10 years, and copes, with the help of a specialised centre, with all the complications which develop throughout the course of the disease. Some can be managed at home, others will require hospitalisation. Hospitalisation is known to be in itself a factor aggravating the problems of the elderly person in general (frequent episodes of confusion), and these are all the more likely when the care facility is not adapted to behavioural disturbances. This raises the problem of how these hospital facilities can be converted to meet the specific needs of this very particular population.

Conclusion

The variety and frequency of complications are factors which increase the risk of hospitalisation and admission to an institution in severely demented patients. Development of a care plan within a coherent, effective multidisciplinary partnership will allow patients, as well as their families, to be better prepared to live with the disease.

References

Brickman AM, Riba A, Bell K *et al.* (2002) Longitudinal assessment of patient dependence in Alzheimer disease. *Arch Neurol*, 59:1304–1308.

Brookmeyer R, Corrada MM, Curriero FC *et al.* (2002) Survival following a diagnosis of Alzheimer disease. *Arch Neurol*, 59:1764–1767.

Cummings JL, Mega M, Gray K *et al.* (1994) The Neuropsychiatric Inventory: comprehensive assessment of psychopathology in dementia. *Neurology*, 44:2308–2314.

Ewbank DC (1999) Deaths attributable to Alzheimer's disease in the United States. *Am J Public Health*, 89:90–92.

Folstein M, Folstein S, McHugh PR (1975) 'Mini-mental State'. A practical method for grading the cognitive state patients for the clinicien. *J Psychiatr Res*, 12:189–198.

Franssen EH, Souren LE, Torossian CL *et al.* (1999) Equilibrium and limb coordination in mild cognitive impairment and mild Alzheimer's disease. *J Am Geriatr Soc*, 47:463–469.

Freels S, Cohen D, Eisdorfer C *et al.* (1992) Functional status and clinical findings in patients with Alzheimer's disease. *J Gerontol A Biol Sci Med Sci*, 47A:M177–M182.

Grundman M, Corey-Bloom J, Jernigan T *et al.* (1996) Low body weight in Alzheimer's disease is associated with mesial temporal cortex atrophy. *Neurology*, 46:1585–1591.

Hughes CP, Berg L, Danziger WL *et al.* (1982) A new clinical scale for the staging of dementia. *Br J Psychiatry*, 140:566–572.

Katz S, Downs TD, Cash HR *et al.* (1970) Progress in development of the index of ADL. *Gerontologist*, 10:20–30.

Knopman D, Donohue JA, Gutterman EM (2000) Patterns of care in the early stages of AD: impediments to timely diagnosis. *J Am Geriatr Soc*, 48:300–304.

Larson EB, Shadlen MF, Wang L *et al.* (2004) Survival after initial diagnosis of Alzheimer disease. *Ann Intern Med*, 140:501–509.

Lawton MP, Brody EM (1969) Assessment of older people: self-maintaining and instrumental activities of daily living. *Gerontologist*, 9:179–186.

Mitchell SL (1999) Extrapyramidal features in Alzheimer's disease. *Age Ageing*, 28:401–409.

Rubenstein LZ, Josephson KR, Wieland GD *et al.* (1984) Effectiveness of a geriatric evaluation unit. A randomised clinical trial. *N Engl J Med*, 311:1664–1670.

Vanhanen M, Kivipelto M, Koivisto K *et al.* (2001) ApoE-epsilon4 is associated with weight loss in women with AD: a population-based study. *Neurology*, 56:655–659.

Vellas B, Guigoz Y, Garry PJ *et al.* (1999) The Mini Nutritional Assessment (MNA) and its use in grading the nutritional state in elderly patients. *Nutrition*, 15:116–122.

Weiner MF, Doody RS, Sairam R *et al.* (2002) Prevalence and incidence of major depressive disorder in Alzheimer's disease: findings from two databases. *Dement Geriatr Cogn Disord*, 13:8–12.

Zarit SH, Reever KE, Bach-Peterson J (1980) Relatives of the impaired elderly: correlates of feelings of burden. *Gerontologist*, 20:649–655.

8

Clinical Features of Severe Dementia: Staging

Barry Reisberg, Jerzy Wegiel, Emile Franssen, Sridhar Kadiyala,
Stefanie Auer, Liduïn Souren, Marwan Sabbagh and James Golomb

Definition of Severe Dementia

From a clinical perspective the phase of Severe Dementia can be defined as, 'the portion of the dementia disease process in which cognitive deficits are of sufficient magnitude as to compromise an otherwise healthy person's capacities to independently perform basic activities of daily life, such as dressing, bathing, and toileting'. From this clinical perspective, the phase of Severe Dementia is enormously important since this is clearly the portion of the disease in which both caregivers, individually, and society, more generally, are most burdened. Equally importantly, the Severe Dementia phase is the portion of dementia in which patients may suffer to the greatest extent. It is also a portion of dementia in which interventions can be most meaningful in alleviating distress and suffering for patients. For the most part, such interventions require an understanding of the clinical process of the Severe Dementia phase.

In the context of Alzheimer's disease (AD), Global Deterioration Scale (GDS) (Reisberg *et al.*, 1982) stage 5 has been termed Moderate AD, GDS stage 6 has been termed Moderately Severe AD, and GDS stage 7 has been termed Severe AD (e.g. see Reisberg and Saeed, 2004). The Severe Dementia phase includes GDS stage 6 and GDS stage 7, Moderately Severe and Severe AD.

The definition of the Severe Dementia phase provided above is consistent with the GDS stage definitions for the AD stages. It is also consistent with the definitions used for currently approved treatments for AD. In terms of pharmacologic treatment approvals, memantine has been approved in the United States for the treatment of moderate to severe AD. This severity range for the memantine approval corresponds to GDS stages of 5 and 6 and Mini Mental State Examination (MMSE) (Folstein *et al.*, 1975) scores of ≤ 14 to ≥ 3 in two of the three pivotal trials (Reisberg *et al.*, 2003; Tariot *et al.*, 2004). The severity range in the third trial (Winblad and Poritis, 1999) cited in the approval product labelling (Namenda™ tablets, Thompson PDR, 2005), is GDS stages of 5 to 7 and MMSE scores of <10. These approval ranges are consistent with definitions for the GDS stages in AD which have been applied. Similarly, at the upper end of the severity spectrum, the cholinesterase inhibitors have been approved for the treatment of mild to moderate AD in the United States and elsewhere, using definitions which are consistent with the definition of the Severe Dementia phase proposed in this chapter (i.e. Moderate AD is less severe than the Severe Dementia phase range provided herein).

However, the terminology which has been employed in the Clinical Dementia Rating (CDR) (Hughes *et al.*, 1982; Berg, 1988; Morris, 1993), is not consistent with the definitions proposed in this chapter. Specifically, the CDR 2 stage, termed 'Moderate Dementia', in the CDR scale publications, is a stage in which patients 'require ... assistance in dressing, hygiene, keeping of personal effects'. Clearly, the CDR 2 stage, as well as the subsequent CDR 3 stage, fits the definition of Severe Dementia proposed herein. Therefore, these CDR 2 and CDR 3 stages will be discussed in the context of severe dementia in this chapter.

Time course and stages of Severe Dementia

A schema of the time course of the Severe Dementia phase in Alzheimer's disease (AD), the major aetiopathogenic dementia entity, and the relationship of the course of Severe Dementia to the clinical process of AD from its earliest clinical manifestations, is shown in Figure 1.

From the standpoint of time course, the Severe Dementia phase, encompassing both the Moderately Severe AD and Severe AD stages, is the major portion of AD. The clinically observed potential duration of the Severe Dementia phase in AD in patients who survive into the final substage of the disease is potentially ~10 years, and some AD patients will survive for even longer periods in this phase of the disease. If the current usual time of demise in AD is used in calculating the typical time course of the Severe Dementia phase in AD, patients on average survive for approximately 5 to 6 years in the Severe phase of AD. By comparison, the total duration of Mild to Moderate AD combined is approximately 3.5 years. Figure 1 also illustrates the temporal course of the pre-dementia stages in AD progression, namely the Subjective Cognitive Impairment (SCI) and Mild Cognitive Impairment (MCI) stages, in comparison with the temporal duration of the phase of Severe Dementia.

An understanding of the nature of the Severe Dementia phase must necessarily begin with the stages of the condition. Stages of the Severe Dementia phase have been elaborated for AD. However, it is increasingly apparent that common aetiopathogenic processes pertain in many non-AD dementias, particularly the other tauopathies, as well as AD, and produce similar clinical stages. Hence, the stages of AD are more or less applicable for other degenerative dementias as well. Two different staging systems for AD have been developed. These are: (1) the Clinical Dementia Rating (CDR), and (2) the Global Deterioration Scale (GDS) and Functional Assessment Staging (FAST) system (GDS/FAST). As illustrated in Figure 1, the CDR (Hughes *et al.*, 1982; Berg, 1988; Morris, 1993) stages 2 and 3 fall within the Severe Dementia phase range. These stages are as follows:

	CDR Stage 2	CDR Stage 3
Memory	Severe memory loss; only highly learned material retained; new material rapidly lost	Severe memory loss; only fragments remain
Orientation	Usually disoriented in time; often to place	Orientation to person only
Judgement and problem solving	Severely impaired in handling problems, similarities, differences; social judgement usually impaired	Unable to make judgements or solve problems
Community affairs	No pretence of independent function outside house	
Home and hobbies	Only simple chores preserved; very restricted interests, poorly sustained	No significant function in home outside of own room
Personal care	Requires assistance in dressing, hygiene, keeping of personal effects	Requires much help with personal care, often incontinent

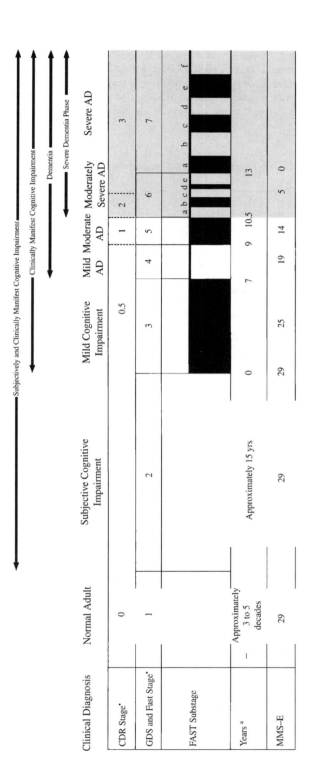

Figure 1. Typical time course of normal brain ageing, mild cognitive impairment and Alzheimer's disease.

Source: Adapted from: Reisberg, et al., *Alzheimer's Disease and Associated Disorders*, 1994; 8 (Suppl.): S 1884–205

AD, Alzheimer's disease; CDR, Clinical Dementia Rating; GDS, Global Deterioration Scale; FAST, Functional Assessment Staging; MMSE, Mini-Mental State Examination.

*Stage range comparisons shown between the CDR and GDS/FAST stages are based upon published functioning and self –care descriptors.

[a] "Numerical values represent time from the earliest clinically manifest symptoms of mild cognitive impairment associated with subsequently manifest Alzheimer's disease (i.e., the beginning of GDS and FAST stage 3). For GDS and GDS/FAST stages are based upon published functioning symptoms. for GDS and FAST stages 3 and above, the values are subsequent to the onset of mild cognitive impairment symptoms. All temporal estimates were initially published in Reisberg, 1986, and have been supported by subsequent clinical and pathological cross-sectional and longitudinal investigations (e.g., Reisberg, et al., 1996; Robinski, et al., 1995, 1997; Kluger, et al., 1999).

[b] FAST stages 1 and 2, the temporal values are prior to onset of mild cognitive impairment symptoms, for GDS and FAST stages 3 and above, the values are subsequent to the onset of mild cognitive impairment symptoms. All temporal estimates were initially published in Reisberg, 1986, and have been supported by subsequent clinical and pathological cross-sectional and longitudinal investigations (e.g., Reisberg, et al., 1996; Robinski, et al., 1995, 1997; Kluger, et al., 1999).

Collectively, the GDS/FAST staging system provides a much more detailed description of the nature and course of the Severe Dementia phase. The GDS itself provides global descriptions of two clinical stages in the Severe Dementia phase. For an optimal appreciation of the stages of the Severe Dementia phase, Table 1 shows the preceding stage of Moderate AD (sometimes referred to as the stage of Moderate Dementia), as well as the stages of Moderately Severe and Severe AD

Table 1. Global Deterioration Scale (GDS) for age-associated cognitive decline and Alzheimer's disease*

GDS stage	Clinical characteristics	Diagnosis	Phase
5	Patient can no longer survive without some assistance. Patient is unable during interview to recall a major relevant aspect of their current life, e.g., (a) their address or telephone number of many years. (b) the names of close members of their family (such as grandchildren). (c) the name of the high school or college from which they graduated. Frequently some disorientation to time (date, day of the week, season, etc.) or to place. An educated person may have difficulty counting back from 40 by 4s or from 20 by 2s. Persons at this stage retain knowledge of many major facts regarding themselves and others. They invariably know their own names and generally know their spouse's and children's names. They require no assistance with toileting or eating, but may have difficulty choosing the proper clothing to wear.	Moderate Alzheimer's Disease	Moderate Dementia Phase
6	May occasionally forget the name of the spouse upon whom they are entirely dependent for survival. Will be largely unaware of all recent events and experiences in their lives. Retain some knowledge of their surroundings: the year, the season, etc. May have difficulty counting by 1s from 10, both backward and sometimes forward. Will require some assistance with activities of daily living. (a) may become incontinent. (b) will require travel assistance but occasionally will be able to travel to familiar locations. Diurnal rhythm frequently disturbed. Almost always recall their own name.	Moderately Severe Alzheimer's Disease	Severe Dementia Phase

Table 1. (*Continued*)

GDS stage	Clinical characteristics	Diagnosis	Phase
	Frequently continue to be able to distinguish familiar from unfamiliar persons in their environment. Personality and emotional changes occur. These are quite variable and include: (a) delusional behavior, e.g., patients may accuse their spouse of being an imposter; may talk to imaginary figures in the environment, or to their own reflection in the mirror. (b) obsessive symptoms, e.g., person may continually repeat simple cleaning activities. (c) anxiety symptoms, agitation, and even previously non-existent violent behavior may occur. (d) cognitive abulia, e.g., loss of willpower because an individual cannot carry a thought long enough to determine a purposeful course of action.		
7	All verbal abilities are lost over the course of this stage. Early in this stage words and phrases are spoken but speech is very circumscribed Later there is no speech at all—only babbling. Incontinent of urine; requires assistance toileting and feeding. Basic psychomotor skills (e.g. ability to walk) are lost with the progression of this stage. The brain appears to no longer be able to tell the body what to do. Generalized and cortical neurologic signs and symptoms are frequently present.	Severe Alzheimer's Disease	

Source: Reisberg *et al.* (1982). Copyright © 1983 by Barry Reisberg, MD. Reproduced with permission.
*GDS stages 6 and 7, encompassed within the Severe Dementia phase, are shaded.

(sometimes referred to as the Moderately Severe Dementia stage and the Severe Dementia stage, respectively).

The Severe Dementia phase of AD is marked by a succession of dramatic and characteristic losses in functional abilities. These losses occur in a characteristic pattern in the dementia of AD. The FAST staging procedure describes this characteristic pattern of functional losses in AD (Reisberg, 1986; Reisberg, 1988; Sclan and Reisberg, 1992). The FAST stages have been enumerated to be optimally concordant with the corresponding GDS stages in AD (hence the GDS/FAST staging system). There is a strong correlation between the FAST stages and the GDS stages in AD patients who are free of non-AD related physical or mental disabilities (*r* values ~ 0.9, Reisberg *et al.*, 1985a). Despite this very strong relationship between the GDS and the FAST, there remains some variability, even in subjects with uncomplicated probable AD. To provide a full context of the progression of functional losses in AD described with the FAST, Table 2 provides an enumeration

Table 2. Functional Assessment Stages (FAST) and time course of functional loss in normal ageing and Alzheimer's disease[*]

Fast stage	Clinical characteristics	Clinical diagnosis	Estimated duration in AD[a]	Mean MMSE[b]	Clinical phase[c]
1	No decrement	Normal Adult		29–30	Normal
2	Subjective deficit in word finding or recalling location of objects	Subjective Cognitive Impairment	15 years	29	Normal Aging
3	Deficits noted in demanding employment settings	Mild Cognitive Impairment	7 years	25	MCI
4	Requires assistance in complex tasks, e.g., handling finances, planning dinner party	Mild AD	2 years	19–20	Mild Dementia
5	Requires assistance in choosing proper attire	Moderate AD	18 months	15	Moderate Dementia
6a	Requires assistance in dressing	Moderately Severe AD	5 months	9	Severe Dementia Phase
b	Requires assistance in bathing properly		5 months	8	
c	Requires assistance with mechanics of toileting (such as flushing, wiping)		5 months	5	
d	Urinary incontinence		4 months	3	
e	Fecal incontinence		10 months	1	
7a	Speech ability limited to about a half-dozen words	Severe AD	12 months	0	
b	Intelligible vocabulary limited to a single word		18 months	0	
c	Ambulatory ability lost		12 months	0	
d	Ability to sit up lost		12 months	0	
e	Ability to smile lost		18 months	0	
f	Ability to hold head up lost		12 months or longer	0	

Adapted from Reisberg (1986). Copyright ©1984 by Barry Reisberg, MD. Reproduced with permission.

[a] In subjects without other complicating illnesses who survive and progress to the subsequent deterioration stage.

[b] MMSE = Mini Mental State Examination score (Folstein *et al.*, 1975). Estimates based in part on published data summarised in Reisberg, Ferris, de Leon *et al.* (1989) and obtained in Reisberg, Ferris, Torossian *et al.* (1992), These MMSE score estimates apply for subjects who are free of non-AD-related physical and mental morbidities or conditions.

[c] The clinical phase applies for subjects who are free of non-AD-related physical and mental comorbidities or conditions.

[*] The stages and phases within the dementia range are shaded. The Severe Dementia phase is shaded more darkly.

of the FAST stages from normal ageing to most severe AD. This comprehensive description is particularly appropriate, even in this chapter focusing on the Severe Dementia phase of AD, since it will be noted from Table 2 that of the 16 FAST stages and substages, 11 substages fall within the Severe Dementia phase range. The 11 FAST substages of the Severe Dementia phase can be grouped into five categories: I. Deficient Activities of Daily Life [ADLs], FAST stages 6a to 6c; II. Incipient Incontinence, FAST stages 6d and 6e; III. Incipient Nonverbal, FAST stages 7a and 7b; IV. Incipient Nonambulatory, FAST stage 7c; and V. Immobile, FAST stages 7d, 7e and 7f (Auer *et al.*, 1994). These categories of the Severe Dementia phase are illustrated in Table 3. Table 2 also shows approximate mean MMSE scores for the FAST stages and substages, from published data in subjects with AD (Reisberg *et al.*, 1989a; Reisberg *et al.*, 1992). Additionally, Table 2 shows approximate mean temporal course estimates of the duration of the FAST stages and substages in AD. These temporal estimates have been supported for the Severe Dementia phase both through longitudinal study (Reisberg *et al.*, 1996), and through direct neuropathologic observations (Bobinski *et al.*, 1995; Bobinski *et al.*, 1997). Table 4 describes the precise characteristics of the very important 11 FAST substages of the Severe Dementia phase in greater detail. For comparison, Table 4 also contains a description of the preceding Moderate AD stage. Table 5 summarises some of the extensive validity data for the FAST staging procedure in charting the course of AD, and especially the Severe Dementia phase of AD. The FAST stages of Moderate AD and the stages of the Severe Dementia phase of AD are illustrated in Figures 2 to 8.

Some of the validity data regarding the FAST staging of AD will be described later in this chapter in relation to clinical aspects of AD. However, since the severe phase of AD is characterised by

Table 3. Severe Dementia Phase: categories of functional loss and corresponding Functional Assessment Stages (FAST stages) in Alzheimer's disease

Clinical phase	Categories of functional loss	FAST stages	Clinical diagnosis
Severe Dementia Phase	I. Deficient activities of daily life [ADLs]	6a. Requires assistance in dressing	Moderately Severe Alzheimer's Disease
		6b. Requires assistance in bathing properly	
		6c. Requires assistance with mechanics of toileting	
	II. Incipient Incontinence	6d. Urinary incontinence	
		6e. Fecal incontinence	
	III. Incipient Nonverbal	7a. Speech ability limited to about a half-dozen words	Severe Alzheimer's Disease
		7b. Intelligible vocabulary limited to a single word	
	IV. Incipient Nonambulatory	7c. Ambulatory ability lost	
	V. Immobile	7d. Ability to sit up lost	
		7e. Ability to smile lost	
		7f. Ability to hold head up lost	

Table 4. Sequence of functional loss in the moderate and severe dementia phases of Alzheimer's disease (functional assessment staging with annotations)*†

FAST stage	Characteristics	Clinical diagnosis	Category of functional loss
5	*Deficient performance in choosing proper attire, and assistance is required for independent community functioning* – the spouse or other caregiver frequently must help the individual choose the appropriate clothing for the occasion and/or season (e.g., the individual will wear incongruous clothing unless appropriate counseling is provided); over the course of this stage some patients may also begin to forget to bathe regularly (unless reminded) and automobile driving capabilities becomes compromised (e.g., carelessness in driving an automobile and violations of driving rules).	Moderate AD	Incipient deficit in activities of daily life [ADLs]
6a	*Requires actual physical assistance or active direction in putting on clothing properly* – the caregiver must provide increasing assistance with the actual mechanics of helping the individual clothe himself properly (e.g., putting on clothing in proper sequence, tying shoelaces, putting shoes on proper feet, buttoning and/or zipping clothing, putting on blouse, shirt, pants, skirt, etc., correctly).	Moderately Severe AD	Deficient in activities of daily life [ADLs]
6b	*Requires assistance bathing properly* – the patient's ability to adjust bathwater temperature diminishes; the patient may have difficulty entering and leaving the bath; there may be problems with washing properly and completely drying oneself.	Moderately Severe AD	Deficient in activities of daily life [ADLs]
6c	*Requires assistance with mechanics of toileting* – patients at this stage may forget to flush the toilet and may begin to wipe themselves improperly or less fastidiously when toileting.	Moderately Severe AD	Deficient in activities of daily life [ADLs]
6d	*Urinary incontinence* – this occurs in the absence of infection or other genitourinary tract pathology; the patient has episodes of urinary incontinence. Frequency of toileting may mitigate the occurrence of incontinence somewhat.	Moderately Severe AD	Incipient Incontinence
6e	*Fecal incontinence* – in the absence of gastrointestinal pathology, the patient has episodes of fecal incontinence. Frequency of toileting may mitigate the occurrence of incontinence somewhat.	Moderately Severe AD	Incipient Incontinence

7a	*Speech limited to about 6 words in the course of an average day* – during the course of an average day the patient's speech is restricted to single words (e.g., 'Yes,' 'No,' 'Please') or short phrases (e.g., 'please don't hurt me'; 'get away'; 'get out of here'; 'I like you').	Severe AD	Incipient Nonverbal
7b	*Intelligible vocabulary limited to generally a single intelligible word or less in the course of an average day* – as the illness progresses, the ability to utter even short phrases on a regular basis is lost so that the spoken vocabulary becomes limited to generally 1 or 2 single final intelligible words as an indicator for all things and needs (e.g., 'Yes,' 'No,' 'O.K.' for all verbalization – provoking phenomena). Alternatively, there may be no remaining intelligible words in an average day.	Severe AD	Incipient Nonverbal
7c	*Ambulatory ability lost* – patients gradually lose the ability to ambulate independently; in the early part of this substage they may require actual support (e.g., being physically supported by a caregiver) and physical assistance to walk, but as the substage progresses, the ability to ambulate even with assistance is lost; the onset is somewhat varied with some patients simply taking progressively smaller and slower steps – other patients begin to tilt forwards, backwards or laterally when ambulating; twisted gaits have also been noted as antecedents of ambulatory loss.	Severe AD	Incipient Nonambulatory
7d	*Ability to sit up lost* – the patients lose the ability to sit up without assistance (e.g., they need some form of physical brace – an arm rest, a belt, or other brace or other special devices to keep them from sliding down in the chair).	Severe AD	Immobile
7e	*Ability to smile lost* – patients are no longer observed to smile, although they do manifest other facial movements and sometimes grimace.	Severe AD	Immobile
7f	Ability to hold head up lost – patients can no longer hold up their head unless the head is supported. Alternatively, the head may become immobile because of contractures.	Severe AD	Immobile

*Adapted from Reisberg (1986). Copyright © 1984 by Barry Reisberg, MD. Reproduced with permission.
†The FAST stage is the highest ordinally enumerated score (i.e. the highest consecutive score).

Table 5. The FAST staging procedure in charting the characteristic clinical course of Alzheimer's disease (AD): validity and unique utility, particularly in the Severe Dementia phase

I. Criterion validity

A. Longitudinal course of AD

Progression of AD on the FAST accounted for about twice the variance in temporal course of AD (change in measure vs. time elapsed) as that accounted for by the MMSE in a five-year prospective study of course of patients with probable AD (Reisberg *et al.*, 1996).

B. Neuropathologic investigations of AD

1. Relationships between neuropathologically assessed volumes of hippocampal formation subdivisions and FAST stage 7 substages (N.B. in FAST stage 7 MMSE scores are virtually uniformly zero [bottom]) (Bobinski *et al.*, 1995).

   Cornu ammonis $r = 0.70$ $(p \leq 0.05)$
   Subiculum complex $r = 0.79$ $(p \leq 0.001)$
   Entorhinal cortex $r = 0.62$ $(p \leq 0.05)$

2. Correlations between total number of neurons in hippocampal formation subdivisions and FAST stage 7 substages (Bobinski *et al.*, 1997).

   Cornu ammonis $r = 0.90$ $(p \leq 0.01)$
   CA1 $r = 0.88$ $(p \leq 0.01)$
   Subiculum $r = 0.79$ $(p \leq 0.001)$

3. Percentages of remaining neurons in hippocampal brain regions with neurofibrillary changes (Bobinski *et al.*, 1997).

	Control	FAST 7a to 7c	FAST 7e to 7f
Cornu ammonis			
CA 1	5.5%	43.2%	71.0%
CA 2	5.2%	22.4%	32.7%
CA 3	0.6%	9.5%	26.4%
CA 4	0.8%	10.3%	27.8%
Subiculum	2.3%	21.4%	52.4%

C. Pharmacologic treatment of AD

The FAST staging has demonstrated sensitivity to pharmacologic treatment of AD in AD patients in the Moderately Severe FAST staging range. Specifically, in a 32-site multi-center trial conducted throughout the USA, subjects treated with memantine showed significantly less deterioration over the course of the 28-week double-blind, randomized, controlled trial (Reisberg *et al.*, 2003). Last observation carried forward analysis, $p < 0.05$, Observed cases analysis, $p < 0.01$

II. Concurrent validity

A. Neurologic reflexes and release signs

Correlations with a summary measure of neurologic reflexes and release signs (Franssen *et al.*, 1991, 1993; Franssen and Reisberg, 1997).

1. In 480 subjects at all severity levels (Franssen and Reisberg, 1997).

	Correlation	% variance
MMSE	$r = 0.74$	55%
FAST	$r = 0.80$	64%

2. In 37 subjects with MMSE scores of zero (Franssen and Reisberg, 1997).

Table 5.   (*Continued*)

	Correlation	% variance
FAST	$r = 0.80$	64%

B. Cognitive change	Correlations with cognitive change assessments (Reisberg *et al.*, 1983, 1984, 1985b, 1992; Shimada *et al.*, 2003; Auer *et al.*, 1994).

	FAST correlations
Concentration	0.88
Recent memory	0.90
Remote memory	0.83
Orientation	0.94
MMSE	0.83
Binet scale (stages 5 to 7)	0.85
M-OSPD (stages 6 and 7)	0.77

III. Utility

A. Identification of major physical disabilities in AD, which could not be charted with traditional assessments	Contractures occur in approximately a million AD patients in the US alone: 95% of AD patients with contractures have MMSE scores of zero. FAST correlation with contracture occurrence in AD is 0.70 (Souren *et al.*, 1995).
B. Identification of a physical, neurologic marker of AD course	Neurologic reflexes distinguished early stage 6 AD patients (FAST 6a to 6c) from early stage 7 AD patients (FAST 7a to 7b), with a specificity, sensitivity and overall accuracy of > 85% (Franssen *et al.*, 1997). This differentiation corresponds to the point of emergence of incontinence in AD.

FAST = Functional Assessment Staging; MMSE = Mini Mental State Examination; M-OSPD = Modified-Ordinal Scales of Psychological Development

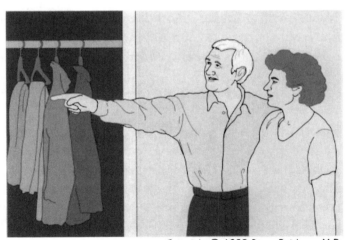

Copyright © 1999 Barry Reisberg, M.D.

Figure 2.   FAST Stage 5: Moderate Alzheimer's disease. Incipient deficits in activities of daily life. Decreased ability to choose proper clothing to wear. © 1999 Barry Reisberg, M.D. Reproduced with permission.

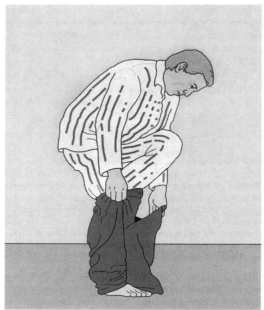

Figure 3. FAST Stage 6a: Moderately Severe Alzheimer's disease. ADL Deficient: decreased ability to put on clothing properly without assistance. © 1999 Barry Reisberg, M.D. Reproduced with permission.

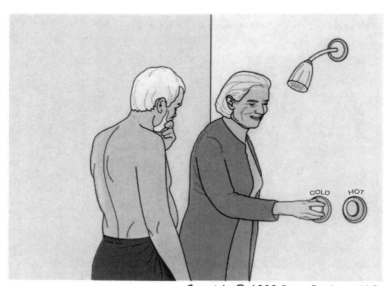

Figure 4. FAST Stage 6b: Moderately Severe Alzheimer's disease. ADL Deficient: requires assistance bathing independently. © 1999 Barry Reisberg, M.D. Reproduced with permission.

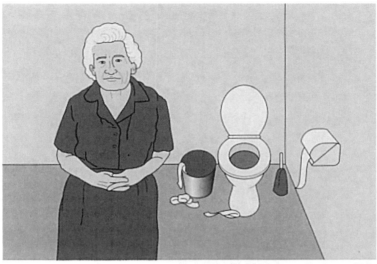

Copyright © 1999 Barry Reisberg, M.D.

Figure 5. FAST Stage 6c: Moderately Severe Alzheimer's disease. ADL Deficient: requires assistance with cleanliness in toileting. © 1999 Barry Reisberg, M.D. Reproduced with permission.

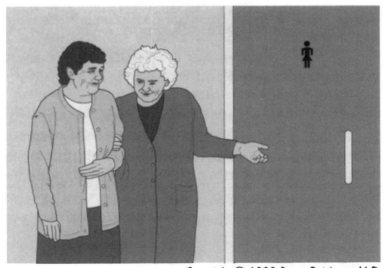

Copyright © 1999 Barry Reisberg, M.D.

Figure 6. FAST Stages 6d and 6e: Moderately Severe Alzheimer's disease. Incipient Incontinence: requires assistance to maintain continence. © 1999 Barry Reisberg, M.D. Reproduced with permission.

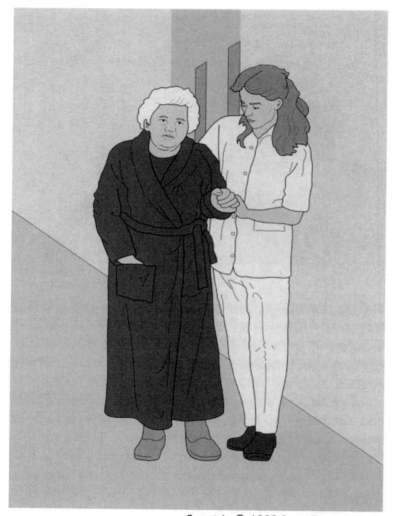

Copyright © 1999 Barry Reisberg, M.D.

Figure 7.   FAST Stages 7a to 7c: Severe Alzheimer's disease. Incipient Nonverbal: Speech ability is limited to a few words (7a), then serviceable speech is lost (7b). Incipient Nonambulatory: subsequently, patient requires assistance in walking (7c). © 1999 Barry Reisberg, M.D. Reproduced with permission.

a GDS/FAST stage 6 in which MMSE scores begin to have floor effects, and a final seventh stage in which the MMSE is generally zero, it is clear that conventional measures and procedures cannot be used for the detailed concurrent validity assessment of the FAST in the Severe Dementia phase of AD. Longitudinal, neuropathologic and pharmacologic criterion validity investigations have been necessary for the detailed and presently extensive establishment of criterion validity of the FAST staging procedure for the Severe Dementia phase of AD (Table 5).

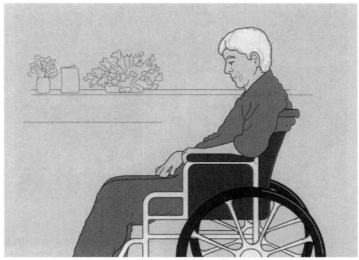

Copyright © 1999 Barry Reisberg, M.D.

Figure 8. FAST Stage 7d: Severe Alzheimer's disease. Immobile: without armrests on the chair, the patient would fall over (7d). Subsequently, patients lose the ability to smile (7e) and to hold up or move their head independently (7f). © 1999 Barry Reisberg, M.D. Reproduced with permission.

One example of criterion validity data with respect to the FAST staging has been the longitudinal study of the course of AD. In a five-year prospective study which examined the correlation between change in measures versus change in time in a cohort of AD patients who were community residing at baseline, the change in FAST score measures accounted for twice the variance in temporal change as the MMSE score change (see Table 5) (Reisberg *et al.*, 1996).

Another form of criterion validity investigation of the FAST staging measure has been the relationship to change in neuropathologic measures of AD. The hippocampus is considered to be the brain region most affected in AD. Therefore, a series of studies of the relationship between neuropathologic changes in the hippocampus and the FAST stage at the time of demise have been conducted. The patients in these neuropathologic studies were all in GDS stage 7 and in various substages of FAST stage 7 at the time of demise. Therefore, they were all at a point in AD when MMSE scores are generally zero. As summarised below, these studies show very interesting continuous linear changes in neuropathologic manifestations of AD over the approximately seven-year potential course of this final, frequently neglected, Severe stage of AD.

Changes in hippocampal volume correlated very robustly with FAST stages at the time of death in the post-mortem studies (Bobinski *et al.*, 1995). The strongest volumetric relationship was observed between volume of the subiculum complex of the hippocampus and the FAST stage ($r = 0.8$, $p \leq 0.001$) (see Table 5 and Figure 9).

In another neuropathologic investigation, the relationship between cell loss in the subdivisions of the hippocampus and the FAST stage at the time of demise has been examined (Bobinski *et al.*, 1997). The correlation between the number of remaining neurons in the Ammons horn and the FAST stage was 0.9 ($p \leq 0.01$) and the correlation between the number of remaining neurons in the subiculum and the FAST stage at demise was 0.8 ($p \leq 0.001$) (Table 5).

These robust relationships between neuropathologically assessed hippocampal volumes and neuronal numbers are some of the strongest relationships reported in the literature between any

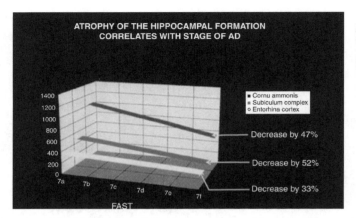

Figure 9. Atrophy of the hippocampal formation correlates with stage of Severe AD. Relationships between volumes of hippocampal formation subdivisions and Functional Assessment Staging (FAST) stages at the time of death in patients with clinically diagnosed and neuropathologically verified Alzheimer's disease are shown. Atrophic correlations were significant (cornu ammonis, $p < 0.05$; subiculum complex, $p \leq 0.001$; entorhinal cortex, $p \leq 0.05$). Data were derived from studies of 13 AD patients at the following FAST stages at the time of death: 7a, $n = 4$; 7b, $n = 3$; 7c, $n = 2$; 7e, $n = 3$; 7f, $n = 1$. Data and figure are from Bobinski *et al.*, (1995), © Sage Publications 1995. Reproduced by permission of Sage Publications, Thousand Oaks, London and New Delhi. www.sagepub.co.uk

neuropathologic changes and any clinical measures in AD, at any stage in the illness process. They are even more impressive in that these relationships were observed in the brains of patients all of whom were at various FAST stage 7 substages. Therefore, as noted, all of these patients probably would have scored zero on the MMSE at the time of their demise.

Another interesting study has examined the relationship of neurofibrillary changes in hippocampal brain regions to the FAST stage at the time of demise in Severe (FAST stage 7) AD (Bobinski *et al.*, 1997). The results are shown in Table 5 and Figure 10. These show the percentage of remaining neurons with neurofibrillary changes in the hippocampal brain regions. As might be anticipated, these percentages increase dramatically in the FAST stage 7a to 7c subject group (i.e. subjects who are incipient nonverbal or incipient nonambulatory in the earlier part of the Severe AD stage), in comparison with controls. However, importantly, the percentages also increase in the FAST stage 7e and 7f subject group (i.e. subjects who are immobile in the latter part of the Severe AD stage), in comparison with the FAST stage 7a to 7c subject group. With the exception of the dentate gyrus, which is relatively spared even in Severe AD, the changes in neurofibrillary burden in remaining hippocampal neurons are marked in early stage 7 and increase further, clearly and dramatically, in late stage 7.

These neuropathologic studies of the utility and validity of the FAST staging procedure for severe AD were all conducted in FAST stage 7 subjects. These are a particularly interesting subject group since these subjects are at various severity levels in the years after the MMSE is zero, and are frequently not staged or studied. Even when stage 7 severity level subjects are included in investigations, they are generally not differentiated and they are grouped together as having MMSE scores of zero or as being 'untestable'. Hence, the longest portion of the AD severity range is generally neglected.

Another criterion validity study has examined the FAST in the earlier stage of the Severe Dementia phase, stage 6. This study, with entry criteria of a GDS stage of 5 or 6 and a FAST stage ≥ 6a, found that patients treated with memantine for a 28-week period in a randomised controlled trial

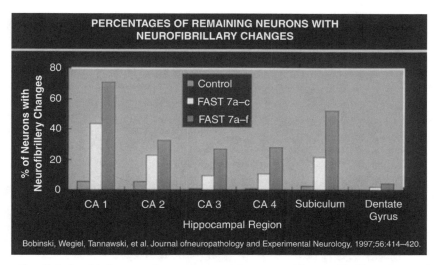

PERCENTAGES OF REMAINING NEURONS WITH NEUROFIBRILLARY CHANGES

Bobinski, Wegiel, Tannawski, et al. Journal ofneuropathology and Experimental Neurology, 1997;56:414–420.

Figure 10. Relationship between the percentages of neurons with neurofibrillary changes in hippocampal brain regions and Functional Assessment Staging (FAST) stages in Severe Alzheimer's disease. Data are derived from neuropathologic studies of 16 subjects with Severe Alzheimer's disease (AD) and five normal elderly controls. The AD subjects were divided into two groups. Group 1, Incipient Nonverbal and Incipient Nonambulatory, FAST stages 7a to 7c ($n = 9$) and group 2, Immobile, FAST stages 7e and 7f ($n = 4$). From Bobinski *et al.* (1997) Relationships between regional neuronal loss and neurofibrillary changes in the hippocampal formation and duration and severity of Alzheimer disease. Journal of Neuropathology and Experimental Neurology, 56:414–420. Copyright, Lippincott, Williams and Wilkins.

showed significantly less change on the FAST than placebo-treated patients (last observation carried forward analysis, $p < 0.05$, observed cases analysis, $p < 0.01$) (Reisberg *et al.*, 2003).

Hence, the FAST staging procedure clinical stages are: (1) superior to standard measures, such as the MMSE, in relating to the course of AD over time; (2) relate very strongly to known neuropathologic changes which occur over the course of AD, such as hippocampal atrophy, hippocampal neuronal cell loss, and increments in neurofibrillary degeneration; and (3) are sensitive to pharmacologic treatment effects. All of these aspects of the validity of the FAST staging procedure are particularly applicable to the Severe Dementia phase. In other studies, the construct validity (Sclan and Reisberg, 1992), and the concurrent validity of the FAST stages and substages throughout the severity spectrum have been demonstrated (Table 5). Some of these additional aspects will be discussed in greater detail later in this chapter in conjunction with the description of the clinical features of the Severe Dementia phase.

There are other aspects of the GDS/FAST staging system which are also applicable to the staging of Severe Dementia, namely the Brief Cognitive Rating Scale (BCRS) axes. The BCRS axes describe various elements of the dementia process. Each of these elements are described and enumerated ordinally so as to be optimally concordant with the corresponding GDS and FAST stages. As previously noted, the GDS and FAST stages per se, have also been enumerated and weighted for optimal concordance. In the context of cognitive changes in progressive normal ageing, MCI, and AD, this optimal concordance for the BCRS axes with each other, with the FAST, and with the GDS has been demonstrated (Reisberg and Ferris, 1988; Reisberg *et al.*, 1992; Reisberg *et al.*, 1993) (see Figure 11).

BCRS axes 1 to 4 have been widely used throughout the world, for example in the context of worldwide pharmacologic trials. More specifically, these axes are incorporated in the New York

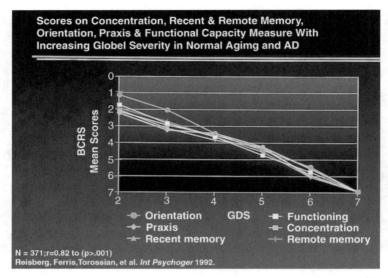

Figure 11. Scores on Brief Cognitive Rating Scale (BCRS) measures of concentration, recent memory, remote memory, orientation, praxis, and functional capacity with increasing global severity in normal ageing and AD. An identical subject sample ($N = 371$) was studied on each of the variables. This sample consisted of 241 women and 130 men, mean age $= 72.7 \pm 8.7$ years. Global Deterioration Scale (GDS) scores were as follows: GDS $= 2$, $n = 75$; GDS $= 3$, $n = 48$; GDS $= 4$, $n = 77$; GDS $= 5$, $n = 75$; GDS $= 6$, $n = 58$; GDS $= 7$, $n = 38$. All subjects were free of medical, psychiatric, neurologic, or neuroradiologic conditions that might interfere with cognition apart from normal ageing or probable AD (McKhann *et al.*, 1984). Assessments of BCRS Axis 1, concentration; BCRS Axis 2, recent memory; BCRS Axis 3, remote memory; BCRS Axis 4, orientation; and BCRS Axis 5, which is the FAST staging, without substages; and BCRS Axis 9, praxis, were obtained on the respective axes of the BCRS (Reisberg *et al.*, 1985b; Reisberg and Ferris, 1988). This figure was initially published in Reisberg *et al.* (1992), reproduced by permission of Cambridge University Press.

University – Clinician's Interview Based Assessment of Change Plus Informant interview (NYU-CIBIC-Plus) assessment. The NYU-CIBIC-Plus has been used in the worldwide approvals of both current classes of pharmacologic treatment for AD. Specifically, the NYU-CIBIC-Plus has been employed in the pivotal studies of the cholinesterase inhibitor, rivastigmine, and the NMDA receptor antagonist, memantine. The portions of these BCRS axes of greatest relevance for the assessment of the Severe Dementia phase of AD, as well as, the preceding, Mild and Moderate Dementia phases, are illustrated in Table 6.

Advantages of utilising the elements of the GDS/FAST staging system collectively, as well as independently, in the assessment of AD patients at all points in the illness process, including the Severe Dementia phase, have been demonstrated. One such syncretic benefit of the GDS/FAST staging which has been described is in the context of tracking the course of AD.

For example, in the five-year prospective longitudinal study of the course of AD (Reisberg *et al.*, 1996), the MMSE score correlation with time elapsed in the 65 AD patients' followed was 0.32 ($p < 0.05$), accounting for 10% of the temporal variance (see Table 5 and Figure 12). The BCRS Axis I to IV score correlation with elapsed time in these AD patients was 0.36 ($p < 0.01$), accounting for 13% of the temporal variance. The FAST score change correlated at 0.45 ($p < 0.001$), accounting for 20% of the variance in time elapsed. Finally, the GDS stage change correlation was

Table 6. Brief cognitive rating scale axes I–IV: abstracted stages optimally concordant with mild, moderate, moderately severe, and severe AD

	Axis 1: Concentration	Axis 2: Recent memory	Axis 3: Past memory	Axis 4: Orientation
Level 4	Definite concentration deficit for persons of their background (e.g., marked deficit on serial 7s, frequent deficit in subtraction of serial 4s from 40).	Cannot recall major events of previous weekend or week. Scanty knowledge (not detailed) of current events, favorite TV shows, etc. May not know telephone number and/or telephone area code and/or postal (zip) code.	Clear-cut deficit. The spouse recalls more of the patient's past than the patient. Cannot recall childhood friends and/or teachers but knows the names of schools attended. Confuses chronology in reciting personal history.	Mistakes day of the month by 10 days or more, and/or confuses month of the year by 1 month or more.
Level 5	Marked concentration deficit (e.g., giving months backwards or serial 2s from 20).	Unsure of weather, and/or may not know current president and/or current address.	Major past events sometimes not recalled (e.g., names of schools attended). Characteristically, at this stage patients recall some schools attended, but not others.	Unsure of month and/or year and/or season, unsure of locale.
Level 6	Forgets the concentration task. Frequently begins to count forward when asked to count backwards from 10 by 1s.	Occasional knowledge of some recent events. Little or no idea of current address, weather, etc. Given the current president's first name, may recall their last name.	Some residual memory of past (e.g., may recall country of birth or former occupation, may or may not recall mother's name, may or may not recall father's name). Generally, patients do not recall any of the schools which they attended.	No idea of date. Identifies spouse but may not recall name. Knows own name.
Level 7	Marked difficulty counting forward to 10 by 1s.	No knowledge of any recent events.	No memory of past (cannot recall country, state, or town of origin, cannot recall names of parents, etc.)	Cannot identify spouse. May be unsure of personal identity.

Adapted from Reisberg and Ferris (1988). Copyright © 1984 by Barry Reisberg, M.D. Reproduced with permission.
Level 4 is optimally concordant with mild AD, Level 5 with moderate AD, Level 6 with moderately severe AD, and Level 7 with severe AD.

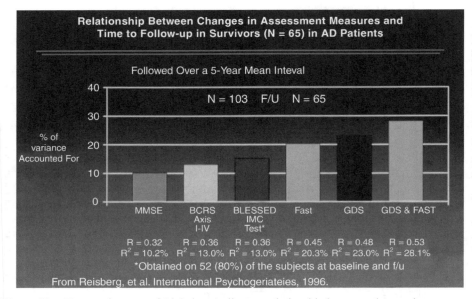

Figure 12. Temporal course of Alzheimer's disease: relationship between changes in assessment measures and time to follow-up in survivors ($N = 65$) followed over a five year mean interval. As a criterion for entry, all subjects had probable AD (McKhann *et al.*, 1984) and were at GDS and FAST stages $\geq$ 4. At baseline, survivors had a mean ($\pm$SD) MMSE score of 15.7$\pm$5.6. FAST stage distribution at baseline, was as follows: FAST stage 4, $n = 34$; FAST stage 5, $n = 22$; FAST stage 6, $n = 8$; FAST stage 7, $n = 1$. At follow-up, mean ($\pm$ SD) MMSE scores were 5.1$\pm$6.9. Approximately half, 33 of 65 subjects, had an MMSE score of 0 at follow-up. FAST stage distribution at follow-up was: FAST stage 4, $n = 2$; FAST stage 5, $n = 7$; FAST stage 6, $n = 27$; FAST stage 7, $n = 29$. Changes in FAST scores were calculated using ordinally enumerated FAST scores with stages 4 to 7f enumerated from 4 to 16. AD denotes Alzheimer's disease; BCRS, Brief Cognitive Rating Scale; FAST, Functioning Assessment Staging; GDS, Global Deterioration Scale; MMSE, Mini Mental State Examination; Blessed IMC, Information, Memory and Concentration Test of Blessed *et al.* (1968). Data from Reisberg *et al.* (1996), reproduced by permission of Cambridge University Press.

0.48 ($p < 0.001$), accounting for 23% of the temporal variance. Importantly, the GDS and FAST together explained the greatest proportion of the temporal variance. Specifically, the GDS and the FAST together correlated at 0.53 (multiple r) with the time elapsed in the 65 AD patients followed over the five year interval, explaining 28% of the variance in temporal change, almost three times that accounted for by MMSE score change. Furthermore, all of the variance in MMSE score change was subsumed within the GDS/FAST changes.

Another example of the utility of the GDS/FAST staging system measures when employed in combination comes from studies using the NYU-CIBIC-Plus assessment. This assessment incorporates a cognitive component which is guided by BCRS Axis I to IV assessments, a functional component which is guided by the FAST staging, and, additionally, behavioural components. In the range of the Severe Dementia phase, the NYU-CIBIC-Plus has been sensitive to pharmacologic treatment with memantine in comparison with placebo-treated patients in a 32-site, multi-centre, pivotal trial (Reisberg *et al.*, 2003). Although the NYU-CIBIC-Plus incorporates elements apart from the GDS/FAST staging system, these findings would seem to support the synergistic value of using multiple components of the system in combination.

Clinical features of Severe Dementia

Clinically the Severe Dementia phase includes marked changes in cognition, behaviour, functioning, neurologic reflexes and physical capacities and movement.

Cognition

Patients throughout the Severe Dementia phase continue to demonstrate cognitive capacities. However, assessments designed for the measurement of cognitive capacity at earlier points in the dementia process become increasingly less useful in measuring and/or demonstrating residual cognitive capacities as this phase progresses.

In Moderately Severe AD (GDS/FAST stage 6), patients generally still score on the MMSE. The MMSE range is approximately from 12 to 1 (or, sometimes, zero), as this Moderately Severe stage of AD evolves (see Table 2). However, more specialised measures designed for the assessment of cognition in severe patients, are necessary for the sensitive assessment of cognition in this Moderately Severe AD stage.

The Severe Impairment Battery (SIB) (Panisset *et al.*, 1994) is a measure which is similar to the MMSE in terms of construction and the kinds of items which are assessed. However, the SIB was specifically designed to be sensitive for cognitive assessment in the Severe Dementia phase. It has, in fact, demonstrated sensitivity to pharmacologic interventions in the Moderately Severe AD range (e.g. Reisberg *et al.*, 2003). In the early portion of the Severe AD stage (early GDS/FAST stage 7), the SIB also appears to be subject to floor effects.

Traditional psychologic tests designed for adults are not useful in the assessment of patients in the Severe Dementia phase. However, assessments designed for young children and/or infants have proven very useful in eliciting and measuring residual cognitive capacities even in Severe AD, until FAST stage 7f (i.e. the final FAST substage).

For example, the well-known Binet intelligence test measure has been shown to be very useful in demonstrating residual intellectual capacity especially in the Moderately Severe AD range (GDS/FAST stage 6). Specifically, using a Japanese adaptation of the Binet test, the Tanaka–Binet Intelligence Scale (Tanaka Institute for Education, 1987), the basic age correlation with the FAST in subjects with Moderate to Severe AD (FAST stages 5 to 7) was found to be 0.85 (Shimada *et al.*, 2003). However, in FAST stage 7, this adaptation of the Binet intelligence scale showed uniform floor effects.

The Modified–Ordinal Scales of Psychological Development (M-OSPD) is a test measure which has been adapted for dementia assessment from a test measure originally applied to the assessment of cognitive abilities in infants and small children (Auer *et al.*, 1994). This assessment is very useful in demonstrating residual cognitive capacities in Moderately Severe AD and, especially, in Severe AD. As shown in Figure 13, patients in the final stage of Severe AD, who all had MMSE scores of zero (bottom), and who also had bottom scores on the Information, Memory and Concentration test of Blessed *et al.* (1968), continued to achieve scores on M-OSPD. Overall, the correlation between the M-OSPD test and the 11 FAST substages in FAST stage 6 and 7 in these AD patients was 0.77 ($p < 0.001$) (Auer *et al.*, 1994).

The importance of the findings regarding cognitive assessment in Moderately Severe and Severe AD is that thinking abilities can still be measured and that AD patients continue to think and display intelligence even after they can no longer speak. The cognitive abilities of Severe AD patients appear to be comparable to those of infants. Even before infants can speak, they can think, and they display intellectual capacities. The same appears to be true of AD patients with Severe, stage 7, AD.

Behavioural disturbances

Most studies of behavioural disturbances in AD have ignored the stage of Severe AD. Since many behavioural and psychological symptoms of dementia (BPSD) peak in the stage of Moderately

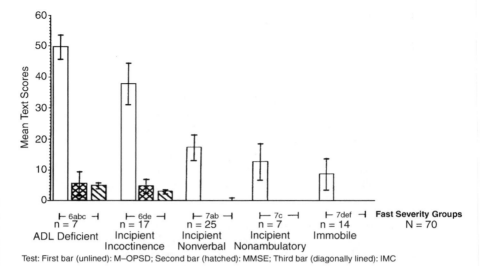

Test: First bar (unlined): M–OPSD; Second bar (hatched): MMSE; Third bar (diagonally lined): IMC

Figure 13. Functioning and cognition in the Severe Dementia phase of Alzheimer's disease. Comparative performance of five Functioning Assessment Staging (FAST) severity categories of AD patients in the Severe Dementia phase on cognitive assessments. The five FAST severity categories are labelled as follows: 6a, b, c (Deficient Activities of Daily Life [ADLs]), 6d, e (Incipient Incontinence), 7a, b (Incipient Nonverbal), 7c (Incipient Nonambulatory), and 7d, e, f (Immobile). M-OSPD: Modified–Ordinal Scales of Psychological Development scores; MMSE: Mini Mental State Examination scores; IMC: Information, Memory and Concentration Test scores (Blessed *et al.*, 1968). Using the M-OSPD, all comparisons between nonadjacent FAST severity groups are significant ($p_s < 0.001$). Significant differences between adjacent groups were found between 6d, e (Incipient Incontinence) and 7a, b (Incipient Nonverbal) FAST groups. Bars indicate 95% confidence limits above and below mean scores. From Auer *et al.* (1994) The neglected half of Alzheimer disease: cognitive and functional concomitants of severe dementia. Journal of the American Geriatrics Society, 42:1266–1272. Copyright, Blackwell Publishing Ltd.

Severe AD, these studies have concluded that many behavioural disturbances increase in magnitude throughout the course of AD. However, this clearly is not true. All behavioural disturbances decrease in magnitude in the final stage of Severe AD.

Figure 14 shows the incidence of BPSD in subjects with Moderate AD, Moderately Severe AD, and Severe AD. It will be noted that paranoid and delusional ideation appears to be more common in Moderate AD than in Moderately Severe AD. Similarly, sleep disturbances, primarily manifested as fragmented sleep, also appear to peak in Moderate AD. Activity disturbances and aggressivity, collectively referred to as agitation, are prominent in both Moderate AD and Moderately Severe AD stages.

It should be noted that the occurrence of BPSD symptoms such as those shown in Figure 14, is very much dependent on the environment (Reisberg *et al.*, 1998). If the patient has a means of productively channelling their energies, then activity disturbances will decrease or not be manifest. Similarly, if a patient is secure in their environment and experiences that their needs are being attended to, and believes that their verbalisations are appropriately addressed, then there will be little or no aggressivity.

The so-called delusions of AD have been observed to be similar in many ways to fantasies in children (Reisberg *et al.*, 1998). Unlike delusions in schizophrenia, which tend to be fixed false beliefs, the delusions in AD are not firmly held and not fixed, just as childhood fantasies are not

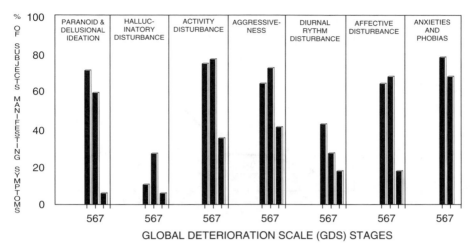

Figure 14. Incidence of behavioural and psychological symptoms of dementia (BPSD) in the stages of Moderate, Moderately Severe, and Severe AD. Subjects studied were initial or follow-up participants in an outpatient-based study at the New York University School of Medicine Aging and Dementia Research Center. Follow-up was sometimes conducted in residential home and nursing home settings as well as in the Research Center clinic setting. All dementia subjects fulfilled criteria for a diagnosis of probable AD (McKhann *et al.*, 1984), prior to evaluation. The aged subjects in the Moderate or the Severe Dementia phases had the following severity distribution; GDS stage 5, *n* = 28; GDS stage 6, *n* = 22; GDS stage 7, *n* = 17. For further details regarding these subjects and methods, see Reisberg *et al.* (1989b).

firmly held and not fixed. Just as a child from a more stressful environment will retreat into fantasy, an AD patient in a more stressful environment is more likely to be delusional.

Sleep disturbances, affective disturbances, anxiety and fears in the AD patient all vary markedly depending upon the kinds of activities, emotional support and basic level of security provided to the AD patient. These latter factors become increasingly important in the patient with Moderately Severe AD who can no longer survive independently and who clearly can no longer organise their own activities or environment.

Neurophysiologic changes

Various neurophysiologic changes occur in the Severe Dementia phase. These include progressive increments in rigidity, and the emergence of reflexes, such as the so-called infantile reflexes (also referred to as primitive reflexes, or alternatively termed frontal release signs, or, synonymously termed, developmental reflexes).

Figure 15 shows the emergence of the dominant form of rigidity in the AD patient, which is termed 'paratonic rigidity'. This is an involuntary resistance to passive motion of joints, most commonly extremities, such as the elbow. As can be seen from Figure 15, this rigidity begins to increase in the Moderate stage of AD. In Moderately Severe and Severe AD (GDS stages 6 and 7, respectively), this rigidity increases dramatically. The rigidity is probably related to decreased patient activities in a feedback loop whereby, for example, increased rigidity produces decreased activity. Decreased activity in turn eventuates in increased rigidity.

Other results of the increased rigidity in the AD patient in the Severe phase are probable relationships to decreased ambulation and the frequent development of contractures in the final stage of Severe AD.

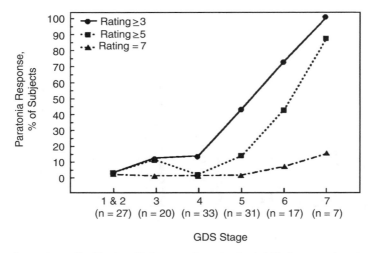

GDS Stage

Figure 15. Percentage of subjects with increased paratonic rigidity in normal ageing and AD of progressively increasing severity. The graph depicts the percentages of subjects showing paratonia as a function of the Global Deterioration Scale (GDS) stage, using three different ratings of activity. Paratonic rigidity, defined as stiffening of a limb in response to contact with the examiner's hand and an involuntary resistance to passive force necessary to elicit it. A rating of 1 denoted an absence of paratonic rigidity, whereas a rating of 7 indicated minimal passive force is required for elicitation of the sequence. Further detail regarding the scoring procedure can be found in Franssen (1993). Paratonic rigidity begins to emerge in Moderate AD patients. However, it becomes increasingly marked in Moderately Severe and Severe AD patients. From Franssen et al. (1991) Cognition-independent neurologic symptoms in normal aging and probable Alzheimer's disease. Archives of Neurology, 48:148–154. Copyright, the American Medical Association.

Developmental reflexes emerge in the Severe Dementia phase of AD. These include the sucking reflex, the hand and foot grasp reflexes, the rooting reflex, and the Babinski reflex. None of these reflexes are generally manifest either in normal aged adults, or in patients with Mild or Moderate AD. However, in GDS stage 6, approximately 40% of patients manifest one or more prehensile release signs to at least a mild extent, and about half of AD patients manifest a mild Babinski reflex (Figure 16) (Franssen et al., 1991). In GDS stage 7, the Severe stage of AD, nearly all patients manifest one or more mildly present prehensile reflexes and about 75% show a mild Babinski response.

These reflexes can impact on the care of the AD patient, particularly in the stage of Severe AD (GDS/FAST stage 7). For example, a stage 7 AD patient's grasp reflex may be so firm as to hurt the patient's caregiver. Also, an untrained caregiver may not know how to get the patient to relieve their grasp. Pulling away only serves to increase the force of the patient's hold. Gently stroking the back of the hand from distal to proximal will release the patient's painful or unpleasant hold (Souren et al., 1997).

The emergence of these developmental reflexes appears to relate strongly to fundamental physiologic functional changes which occur in the AD patient. For example, work of Franssen et al. (1997) has demonstrated that the emergence of incontinence in AD is associated with the emergence of developmental reflexes. Specifically, using the scale of Franssen (Franssen et al., 1991, 1993; Franssen, 1993), the prominent emergence of either a tactile sucking reflex, palmar or plantar grasp reflex, or a plantar extensor (Babinski) reflex is strongly associated with the emergence of incontinence in AD. In a study of nearly 800 subjects, less than 1% of normal elderly or MCI subjects manifested any of these reflexes. Less than 5% of Mild or Moderate AD subjects manifested

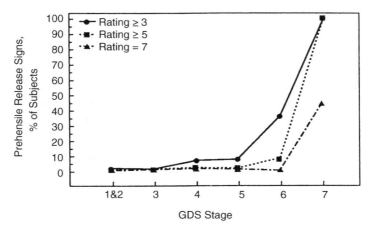

Figure 16. Percentages of subjects with presence of prehensile release signs (developmental reflexes) in normal ageing and AD of progressively increasing severity. The graph depicts the percentage of subjects showing prehensile release signs as a function of the Global Deterioration Scale (GDS) stage. The following prehensile release signs are represented: sucking reflex (tactile and visual), hand grasp, foot grasp, and the rooting reflex. The graph depicts the percentages of subjects with the presence of one or more of these reflexes to at least a mild degree according to the criteria of Franssen (1993). Presence on either right or left was credited for bilaterally tested reflexes (i.e. hand and foot grasp). It will be noted that these reflexes emerge in the Moderately Severe and Severe AD stages. Data and figure are adapted from Franssen *et al.* (1991).

any of these reflexes. In early stage 6, in patients with Deficient ADLs (FAST stages 6a to 6c), less than 15% of AD patients manifested any of these reflexes. In marked contrast, more than 85% of Incipient Nonverbal (FAST stage 7a and 7b) patients manifested one or more of these reflexes. The sensitivity, specificity and overall accuracy of these three developmental (infantile) reflexes in differentiating ADL Deficient but continent AD patients (FAST stage 6a to 6c) from Incipient Nonverbal AD patients (FAST stage 7a or 7b), were each found to be greater than 85% (Figure 17). Interestingly, if one translates the FAST stages into their developmental equivalents, these developmental reflexes appear to be just as robust markers of the transition from the Moderately Severe stage to the Severe stage of AD, as they are markers of the emergence from infancy to early childhood in normal development (Reisberg *et al.*, 1999). This phenomenon wherein degenerative mechanisms reverse the order of acquisition in normal development has been termed retrogenesis (Reisberg *et al.*, 1999).

The developmental reflexes in AD also appear to relate very strongly to other basic capacities in addition to continence. For example, a strong foot grasp reflex may be incompatible with ambulatory ability in the AD patient. This physiologic linkage also appears to be mirrored in normal development. Hand and foot grasp reflexes have disappeared at the end of the first year of life, at which time the infant begins to walk and simultaneously achieves increasing dexterity (Souren *et al.*, 1997; Peiper, 1963; Capute *et al.*, 1982).

Motor changes

Changes in balance, coordination and motor capacities occur even in MCI and Mild AD (Franssen *et al.*, 1999; Kluger *et al.*, 1997). These changes become increasingly overwhelming as the Severe Dementia phase of AD advances.

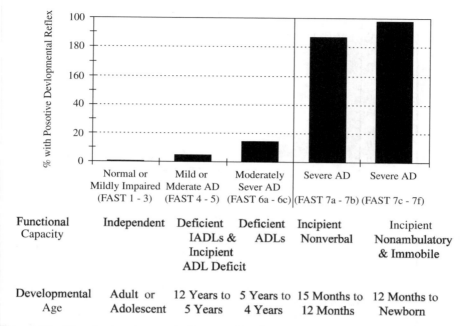

Figure 17. Neurologic retrogenesis. Percentages of patients with one or more of the following developmental reflexes (also known as primitive reflexes or frontal release signs) are shown: the tactile sucking reflex, the palmar grasp (hand grasp) reflex, the plantar grasp (foot grasp) reflex, and the plantar extensor (Babinski) reflex. All reflexes were elicited according to standard procedures and were assessed as being present when they were prominent and persistent, defined by a rating of ≥ 5 on the scale of Franssen (Franssen *et al.*, 1991, 1993; Franssen, 1993). For the three reflexes which were assessed bilaterally, specifically, the palmar grasp reflex, the plantar grasp reflex, and the plantar extensor reflex, a positive response on either side was assessed as positive. Subject samples were as follows: Deficient ADLs (FAST stages 6a to 6c), $n = 113$; Incipient Nonverbal (FAST stages 7a to 7b), $n = 29$; Incipient Nonambulatory and Immobile (FAST stages 7c to 7f), $n = 32$. IADLs are instrumental (complex) activities of daily life; ADLs are basic activities of daily life. Data and figure are adapted from Franssen *et al.* (1997).

In the Moderately Severe AD stage (GDS/FAST stage 6), patients tend to develop a small-stepped gait. AD patients in late stage 6 and early stage 7 are at increased risk for loss of ambulatory capacity. A brief period of immobilization will hasten this loss, as will excess physical disability. The development of rigidity, including paratonia, also contributes to decrements in ambulatory abilities. The closer a patient is to FAST stage 7c, at which point independent ambulating ability is invariably lost with the progression of AD, the more susceptible the AD patient is to 'premature' loss of ambulation.

Apart from loss of ambulatory ability, perhaps the most dramatic and debilitating physical changes which occur in the Severe Dementia phase are the development of contractures. A contracture can be defined as 'a permanent loss of joint mobility, measured through the determination of the passive range of motion of a joint' (Souren *et al.*, 1995). In perhaps the only systematic study of contracture occurrence in AD, that of Souren *et al.* (1995), contracture occurrence was defined as a limitation of 50%, or greater, of the passive range of motion of the joint. Using this definition, the prevalence of contractures in AD patients is illustrated in Figure 18. As can be seen from Figure 18, contractures

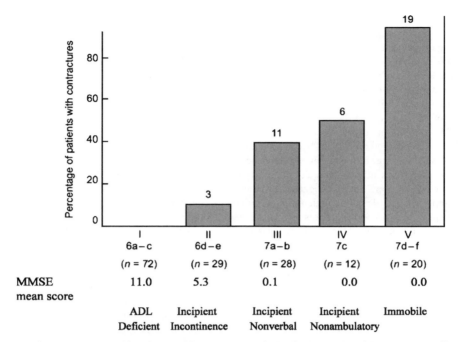

Figure 18. Percentages of patients with contractures in FAST Stage 6 and Stage 7 AD. All subjects fulfilled criteria for probable AD. FAST (Functional Assessment Staging (Reisberg, 1988)) categories are as follows: I. ADL (activities of daily life) Deficient, 6a, b, and c; II. Incipient Incontinence, 6d and e; III. Incipient Nonverbal, 7a and b; IV. Incipient Nonambulatory, 7c; and V. Immobile, 7d, e, and f. The numbers in parenthesis indicate the number of patients studied in the functional categories. The number on top of the bars indicates the numbers of subjects studied with presence of contractures. The significance of change in the prevalence of contractures from the preceding functional categories is as follows: between functional categories I and II: $p < 0.01$; between functional categories II and III: $p < 0.05$; between functional categories III and IV: not significant; and between functional categories IV and V: $p < 0.01$. Across the five functional categories, there are significant differences in the proportions of patients with contractures ($\chi^2 = 88.4$, df $= 4, p < 0.001$). The prevalence of contractures was highly correlated with FAST staging levels ($r = 0.70, p < 0.001$). Data and figure are adapted from Souren *et al.* (1995).

rarely occur before the point of development of incipient incontinence in AD (FAST stages 6d and 6e). In these FAST stages of incipient incontinence (the latter part of the Moderately Severe AD stage), 10% of AD patients manifested contracture occurrence. In the final stage of Severe AD, contractures are common, and increasingly prevalent as the stage progresses. In incipient averbal AD patients (FAST stages 7a and 7b), approximately 40% of AD patients manifested contractures. In incipient nonambulatory AD patients (FAST stage 7c), half of patients manifested contractures. In immobile AD patients (FAST stages 7d, 7e and 7f), contractures occurred in 95% of AD patients.

Although the statistics regarding contracture occurrence just reviewed should be of great concern, the magnitude of this problem is actually considerably greater. In 98% of the AD patients with contractures, more than one extremity was involved. Furthermore, more than two-thirds of patients who had contractures manifested these disabilities in all four extremities.

As might be anticipated from the severity range of contracture occurrence, 95% of the patients with contractures had MMSE scores of zero (bottom). The neglect of patients beyond the MMSE scoring range has contributed to the neglect of the study of contractures occurrence apart from the study of Souren *et al.*, 1995. Interestingly, the correlation noted between contracture occurrence and the FAST stage in the Souren *et al.* study was moderately strong, specifically, 0.70 (Table 5).

Another reason for the relative neglect of the study of contractures in AD patients is that these disabilities generally occur in nursing home or other institutionalized patients. In the Souren *et al.* study of AD patients in the Severe Dementia phase of AD (FAST ≥6a), only 7% of community residing patients manifested contractures (the mean FAST substage of the community residing patients was 6c). In contrast, 54% of AD patients in nursing homes manifested contractures (the mean FAST substage of the nursing home residing patients was 7b). Patients in nursing homes with dementia are frequently neglected to the extent that they do not receive specific diagnoses, such as AD, because they are not investigated as to the specific aetiopathogenesis of their condition. They are simply termed 'dementia patients'. Under these circumstances, contracture-related deformities are frequently attributed to strokes, arthritis or non-specific causes.

Contractures are important for many reasons. One reason is that contractures add considerably to the patient's level of disability and make care more difficult. Moving a patient with contractures is frequently painful for the patient. Therefore, these patients get even less movement and this in turn predisposes to additional contracture occurrence. Decubiti and resultant infections become more difficult to prevent in the presence of contractures. Additionally, patient physical deformity makes care psychologically less pleasing and less fulfilling for the caregiver.

One reason this discussion of contracture occurrence is so important is that these disabilities can probably be postponed if proper care is provided. The contractures appear to be, in part, the end result of the increasing rigidity which occurs in the AD patient. Additionally, the Severe Dementia phase AD patient becomes increasingly subject to contractures from periods of immobilization. The increasing rigidity appears to be treatable with proper exercises including strength, range of motion and maintenance of skills exercises. Immobilization can be guarded against and prevented with proper vigilance. Anecdotal evidence indicates that these procedures are effective in preventing rigidity and contractures even in the immobile, late stage 7, AD patient.

Utility of staging in dementias other than Alzheimer's disease

Detailed procedures for the staging of the Severe Dementia phase and the validity and utility of these staging procedures in AD have been reviewed in detail in the previous sections of this chapter. The occurrence of common aetiopathogenic mechanisms in many dementias not generally associated with AD has also been noted. How well does staging work in these other dementias? Two studies, which have addressed these issues in some detail, will be reviewed.

Normal pressure hydrocephalus

Normal pressure hydrocephalus (NPH) is a well-characterised clinical entity marked by: (1) ventricular dilatation out of proportion to the magnitude of cerebral cortical atrophy, (2) impairment of gait, (3) urinary incontinence, and (4) dementia. Golomb *et al.* (2000), investigated the nature and import of dementia in a consecutive series of 56 cognitively impaired patients undergoing shunt surgery for idiopathic NPH. In all cases, cognitive dysfunction either followed or evolved simultaneously with the onset of a gait disorder. Biopsies were obtained during shunt surgery consisting of a 5×7 mm wedge of tissue in the cortex adjacent to the shunt penetration site. The prevalence of cases exhibiting a positive biopsy for neuritic plaques increased in parallel with the GDS stage. Prevalence of a positive biopsy was 18% in MCI (GDS stage 3), and 75% for patients in the Severe Dementia phase (GDS stages 6 and 7) (see Figure 19). More specifically, 67% of the NPH patients

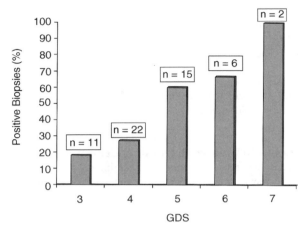

Figure 19. Percentages of biopsies of normal pressure hydrocephalus (NPH) patients evidencing neuritic plaques as a function of GDS (Global Deterioration Scale) score. A GDS score of 3 indicates Mild Cognitive Impairment while scores of 4 through 7 indicate progressively severe levels of dementia. The numbers on the top of the bars indicate the number of subjects in each GDS stage severity category. Data and figure are adapted from Golomb *et al.* (2000).

in GDS stage 6 had positive biopsies for neuritic plaques and both GDS stage 7 patients (100%) had positive biopsies. Hence, the magnitude of dementia assessed with the GDS procedure correlated with neuritic plaque burden in NPH patients with MCI or dementia including subjects in the Severe Dementia phase. Specifically, the Spearman rank correlation between GDS stage and the presence of neuritic plaques in the biopsy tissue sample in the NPH patients was 0.41 ($p = 0.0008$; one-sided).

Parkinson's disease

Parkinson's disease (PD) is a common condition, particularly in older persons, marked by progressive motoric changes. Cardinal clinical features include tremor, a slowing of movements (bradykinesia) and rigidity. Dementia is a common concomitant of PD. Prevalence estimates of dementia in PD range from approximately a quarter to more than three-quarters of all PD patients (Levy *et al.*, 2002; Giladi *et al.*, 2000; Aarsland *et al.*, 2003; Cummings, 1988).

Sabbagh *et al.* (2005), investigated the relationship between AD staging assessments and PD. The 75 PD patients had a mean age of 76 years and ranged from normal cognition (GDS stages 1 and 2, $n = 38$) to severe dementia (GDS stages 6 and 7, $n = 7$). The GDS and FAST staging procedures both correlated strongly both with the magnitude of cognitive change in this PD patient population and with the magnitude of motor disability in the PD patients.

Specifically, the correlation between cognitive capacity assessed with the MMSE and the GDS stage in the PD patients was $\rho = -0.65$ ($p < 0.001$) (the nonparametric Spearman rho [ρ] statistic was used for all of the correlations in this study). The correlation between the FAST and the MMSE in these PD patients was $\rho = -0.68$ ($p < 0.001$).

Perhaps the most interesting finding was in terms of the relationship between the standard Parkinson's disease motor assessment measure, the motor portion of the Unified Parkinson's Disease Rating Scale (UPDRS) (Hoehn and Yahr, 1967) and the dementia staging and MMSE assessments. The motor UPDRS scale includes the following items: speech; facial expression; tremor; rigidity;

finger tapping; hand movements; rapid alternating hand movements; leg agility; arising from a chair; posture; gait; postural stability; and body bradykinesia and hypokinesia. The motor UPDRS correlated with the MMSE in this PD subject population, with and without cognitive impairment ($\rho = -0.48$, $p < 0.001$). The correlation between the motor UPDRS and the staging assessments was somewhat more robust. Specifically, the motor UPDRS and the GDS correlation was $\rho = 0.58$, $p < 0.001$). The motor UPDRS correlation with the FAST stage in the PD patients was $\rho = 0.68$ ($p < 0.001$). Hence, the FAST staging procedure and the GDS, respectively, showed the most robust relationships to the current 'gold standard' measure of motor pathology in PD.

Utility of staging in the differential diagnosis of dementia

Although, as described in the preceding section, the staging procedures can be very useful in the assessment of non-AD dementias, the specific nature of the FAST staging procedure and the very salient functions assessed, nevertheless make the FAST, in particular, very useful in the identification of non-AD dementias. For example, fronto-temporal dementia (FTD) may present with a functional impairment out of proportion to the overall magnitude of cognitive change. Non-AD dementias, such as prion-associated sporadic Creutzfeldt–Jacob disease (CJD), commonly present with a more rapid course than AD. This more rapid course can readily be traced with the FAST staging procedure. Dementias associated with space occupying brain lesions, such as lesions from infarcts, tumours, etc., can produce 'premature' loss of ambulatory capacity, or premature incontinence, in comparison with the characteristic FAST ordinal progression in AD (Reisberg, 1986; Sclan and Reisberg, 1992).

Utility of staging in the identification of excess medical disability

The specific ordinal nature of the progression of dementia, particularly, but not exclusively, the dementia of AD outlined with the FAST staging procedure, permits the identification of non-dementia-related disabilities (Reisberg, 1986; Reisberg and Saeed, 2004). For example, premature occurrence of urinary incontinence can be identified, which may be associated with diuretic usage or other conditions. Similarly, premature compromise of ambulation associated with, for example, arthritis or sedating medication, can be identified using the FAST staging procedure. A rapid progression of disability along the ordinal pathway of the FAST can also occur secondary to diverse metabolic and central nervous system insults. This rapid progression can be readily identified by reference to the characteristic FAST time course of progression in AD. The source of this excess disability can be identified and, frequently, remediated.

Conclusion

The evolution of Severe Dementia can be described in great detail using staging procedures. The FAST staging procedure in particular is very useful in that it can provide clinicians and investigators with a detailed map of the progression of the Severe Dementia phase. Specifically, as this phase evolves, particularly in the dementia of AD, patients go through 11 FAST substages, which are grouped, into five broad functional categories. These 11 FAST substages, essential for on an understanding of the Severe Dementia phase are: (6a) decreased ability to put on clothing without assistance; (6b) decreased ability to handle the mechanics of bathing; (6c) decreased ability to handle the mechanics of toileting; (6d) incipient incontinence of urine; (6e) incipient incontinence of faeces; (7a) speech ability limited to approximately a half-a-dozen intelligible words in a seemingly average day; (7b) speech ability limited to, at most, a single intelligible word in a seemingly average day; (7c) loss of ability to ambulate independently; (7d) loss of ability to sit up independently; (7e) loss of ability to smile; (7f) loss of ability to hold up or, alternatively, to otherwise move one's head.

These characteristic FAST stages in the evolution of the Severe Dementia phase in AD have been extensively validated against AD related neuropathology, including hippocampal volume and cellular losses, and hippocampal neurofibrillary pathologic changes. The characteristic FAST stages of Severe AD have also been validated against concurrent cognitive and neurologic/neurophysiologic changes in the Severe Dementia phase AD patient.

Both research and patient care can potentially benefit substantially from more widespread application of staging procedures for the Severe Dementia phase.

In research, a neglected, final, major portion of dementia course can be described in detail instead of simply using the word 'severe' as is often done. Current research has demonstrated that extensive accurate staging is possible, through interviews with caregivers, post-mortem, even in patients for whom ante-mortem clinical data is not available (Rockwood *et al.*, 1998).

For patient care, excess disability can be identified and patient care can be optimised through an understanding of both patient capacities and disabilities. Extensive procedures for translating the insights achieved through the detailed staging of Severe Dementia phase patients into improved patient care have begun to be published and applied (Reisberg *et al.*, 2002). These care insights need to be applied in conjunction with staging towards the goals of optimising patient capacities and minimising patient distress.

Acknowledgements

Supported in part by US Department of Health and Human Services (DHHS) grants AG 03051, AG 08051, AG 019610, AG 09127, and AG 11505, from the National Institute on Aging of the US National Institutes of Health; by grants 90AZ 2791, 90AM 2552, and 90AR 2160 from the US DHHS Administration on Aging; by grant NCRR MO1 RR00096 from the General Clinical Research Center Program of the National Center for Disease Research Resources of the US National Institutes of Health; by the Fisher Center for Alzheimer's Disease Research Foundation; and by grants from Mr William Silberstein and Mr Leonard Litwin. The authors wish to thank Wei Zhu, PhD, from the statistical core of the NYU Alzheimer's Disease Center for assistance with analyses in this chapter.

References

Aarsland D, Andersen K, Larsen JP, Lolk A, Kragh-Sorensen P (2003) Prevalence and characteristics of dementia in Parkinson's disease. *Archives of Neurology*, 60:387–392.

Auer SR, Sclan SG, Yaffee RA, Reisberg B (1994) The neglected half of Alzheimer disease: cognitive and functional concomitants of severe dementia. *Journal of the American Geriatrics Society*, 42:1266–1272.

Berg L (1988) Clinical dementia rating (CDR). *Psychopharmacology Bulletin*, 24:637–639.

Blessed G, Tomlinson BE, Roth M (1968) The association between quantitative measures of dementia and senile change in the cerebral gray matter of elderly subjects. *British Journal of Psychiatry*, 114:797–811.

Bobinski M, Wegiel J, Wisniewski HM, Tarnawski M, Reisberg B, Mlodzik B, de Leon MJ, Miller DC (1995) Atrophy of hippocampal formation subdivisions correlates with stage and duration of Alzheimer disease. *Dementia*, 6:205–210.

Bobinski M, Wegiel J, Tarnawski M, Reisberg B, de Leon MJ, Miller DC, Wisniewski HM (1997) Relationships between regional neuronal loss and neurofibrillary changes in the hippocampal formation and duration and severity of Alzheimer disease. *Journal of Neuropathology and Experimental Neurology*, 56:414–420.

Capute AJ, Shapiro BK, Accardo PJ, Wachtel RL, Ross A, Palmer FB (1982) Motor functions: associated primitive reflex profiles. *Developmental Medicine and Child Neurology*, 24:662–669.

Cummings JL (1988) The dementias of Parkinson's disease: prevalence, characteristics, neurobiology, and comparison with dementia of the Alzheimer's type. *European Journal of Neurology*, 28:15–23.

Folstein MF, Folstein SE, McHugh PR (1975) Mini-mental state: a practical method for grading the cognitive state of patients for the clinician. *Journal of Psychiatric Research*, 12:189–198.

Franssen EH (1993) Neurologic signs in ageing and dementia, In: Burns, A. and Levy, R., eds., Aging and Dementia, A Methodological Approach. London: Edward Arnold, 144–174.

Franssen EH, Reisberg B (1997) Neurologic markers of the progression of Alzheimer disease. *International Psychogeriatrics*, 9:297–306.

Franssen EH, Reisberg B, Kluger A, Sinaiko E, Boja C (1991) Cognition-independent neurologic symptoms in normal aging and probable Alzheimer's disease. *Archives of Neurology*, 48:148–154.

Franssen EH, Kluger A, Torossian CL, Reisberg B (1993) The neurologic syndrome of severe Alzheimer's disease: relationship to functional decline. *Archives of Neurology*, 50:1029–1039.

Franssen EH, Souren LEM, Torossian CL, Reisberg B (1997) Utility of developmental reflexes in the differential diagnosis and prognosis of incontinence in Alzheimer disease. *Journal of Geriatric Psychiatry and Neurology*, 10:22–28.

Franssen EH, Souren LEM, Torossian CL, Reisberg B (1999) Equilibrium and limb coordination in mild cognitive impairment and mild Alzheimer's disease. *Journal of the American Geriatrics Society*, 47:463–499.

Giladi N, Treves TA, Paleacu D, Shabtai H, Orlov Y, Kandinov B, Simon ES, Korczyn AD (2000) Risk factors for dementia, depression and psychosis in long-standing Parkinson's disease. *Journal of Neural Transmission*, 107:59–71.

Golomb J, Wisoff J, Miller DC, Kluger A, Weiner H, Salton J, Graves W (2000) Alzheimer's disease comorbidity in normal pressure hydrocephalus: prevalence and shunt response. *Journal of Neurology, Neurosurgery, and Psychiatry*, 68:778–781.

Hoehn MM, Yahr MD (1997) Unified Parkinson's disease rating scale [UPDRS]: modified Hoehn and Yahr staging (1967), In: Herndon, R.M., ed., Handbook of Clinical Neurologic Scales. New York: Dernos Vermande, 81–91.

Hughes CP, Berg L, Danziger WL, Coben LA, Martin RL (1982) A new clinical scale for the staging of dementia. *British Journal of Psychiatry*, 140:566–572.

Kluger A, Gianutsos JG, Golomb J, Ferris SH, George AE, Franssen EH, Reisberg B (1997) Patterns of motor impairment in normal aging, mild cognitive decline, and early Alzheimer's disease. *Journal of Gerontology: Psychological Sciences*, 52B:P28–P39.

Kluger A, Ferris SH, Golomb J, Mittelman MS, Reisberg B (1999) Neuropsychological prediction of decline to dementia in nondemented elderly. *Journal of Geriatric Psychiatry and Neurology*, 12:168–179.

Levy G, Schupf N, Ming-Xin T, Cote LJ, Louis ED, Mejia H, Stern Y, Marder K (2002) Combined effect of age and severity on the risk of dementia in Parkinson's disease. *Annals of Neurology*, 51:722–729.

McKhann G, Drachman D, Folstein M, Katzman R, Price D, Stadlan EM (1984) Clinical diagnosis of Alzheimer's disease: report of the NINCDS-ADRDA work group under the auspices of Department of Health & Human Services Task Force on Alzheimer's disease. *Neurology*, 34:939–944.

Morris JC (1993) The Clinical Dementia Rating (CDR): current version and scoring rules. *Neurology*, 43:2412–2414.

Namenda™ Tablets, 2005. In: Physician's Desk Reference 2005. 59th edn. Montvale: Thomson Healthcare.

Panisset M, Roudier M, Saxton J, Boller F (1994) Severe Impairment Battery: a neuropsychological test for severely demented patients. *Archives of Neurology*, 51:41–45.

Peiper A (1963) Cerebral function in infancy and childhood. In: Wortis, J., ed., The International Behavioral Sciences Series. New York: Consultants Bureau, 147–210.

Reisberg B (1986) Dementia: a systematic approach to identifying reversible causes. *Geriatrics*, 41(4):30–46.

Reisberg B (1988) Functional assessment staging (FAST). *Psychopharmacology Bulletin*, 24:653–659.

Reisberg B, Ferris SH (1988) The Brief Cognitive Rating Scale (BCRS). *Psychopharmacology Bulletin*, 24:629–636.

Reisberg B, Saeed MU (2004) Alzheimer's disease. In: Sadovoy J, Jarvik LF, Grossberg GT, Meyers BS, eds. Comprehensive Textbook of Geriatric Psychiatry, 3rd edn. New York: W.W. Norton, 449–509.

Reisberg B, Ferris SH, de Leon MJ, Crook T (1982) The global deterioration scale for assessment of primary degenerative dementia. *American Journal of Psychiatry*, 139:1136–1139.

Reisberg B, Schneck MK, Ferris SH, Schwartz GE, de Leon MJ (1983) The brief cognitive rating scale (BCRS): findings in primary degenerative dementia (PDD). *Psychopharmacology Bulletin*, 19:47–50.

Reisberg B, Ferris SH, Anand R, de Leon MJ, Schneck MK, Buttinger C, Borenstein J (1984) Functional staging of dementia of the Alzheimer's type. *Annals of the New York Academy of Sciences*, 435:481–483.

Reisberg B, Ferris SH, Anand R, de Leon MJ, Schneck MK, Crook T (1985a) Clinical assessment of cognitive decline in normal aging and primary degenerative dementia: concordant ordinal measures. In: Pinchot, P., Berner, P., Wolf, R., and Thau, K., eds. Psychiatry (Vol. 5). New York: Plenum Press, 333–338.

Reisberg B, Ferris SH, de Leon MJ (1985b) Senile dementia of the Alzheimer type: diagnostic and differential diagnostic features with special reference to functional assessment staging. In: Traber J, Gispen WH, eds. Senile Dementia of the Alzheimer Type (Vol. 2). Berlin: Springer-Verlag, 18–37.

Reisberg B, Ferris SH, de Leon MJ, Kluger A, Franssen EH, Borenstein J, Alba R (1989a) The stage specific temporal course of Alzheimer's disease: functional and behavioral concomitants based upon cross-sectional and longitudinal observation. In: Iqbal, K., Wisniewski, H.M., and Winblad, B., eds. Alzheimer's Disease and Related Disorders: Progress in Clinical and Biological Research (Vol. 317). New York: Alan R. Liss, 23–41.

Reisberg B, Franssen EH, Sclan SG, Kluger A, Ferris SH (1989b) Stage specific incidence of potentially remediable behavioral symptoms in aging and Alzheimer's disease: a study of 120 patients using the BEHAVE-AD. *Bulletin of Clinical Neurosciences*, 54:95–112.

Reisberg B, Ferris SH, Torossian CL, Kluger A, Monteiro I (1992) Pharmacologic treatment of Alzheimer's disease: a methodologic critique based upon current knowledge of symptomatology and relevance for drug trials. *International Psychogeriatrics*, 4:9–42.

Reisberg B, Sclan SG, Franssen EH, de Leon MJ, Kluger A, Torossian CL, Shulman E, Steinberg G, Monteiro I, McRae T, Boksay I, Mackell JA, Ferris SH (1993) Clinical stages of normal aging and Alzheimer's disease: the GDS staging system. *Neuroscience Research Communications*, 13:551–554.

Reisberg B, Sclan SG, Franssen EH, Kluger A, Ferris SH (1994) Dementia staging in chronic care populations. *Alzheimer's Disease and Associated Disorders*, 8:S188–S205.

Reisberg B, Ferris SH, Franssen EH, Shulman E, Monteiro I, Sclan SG, Steinberg G, Kluger A, Torossian CL, de Leon MJ, Laska E (1996) Mortality and temporal course of probable Alzheimer's disease: a five-year prospective study. *International Psychogeriatrics*, 8:291–311.

Reisberg B, Auer SR, Monteiro I, Franssen E, Kenowsky S (1998) A rational psychological approach to the treatment of behavioral disturbances and symptomatology in Alzheimer's disease (AD) based upon recognition of the developmental age (DA). *International Academy for Biomedical and Drug Research*, 13:102–109.

Reisberg B, Franssen EH, Hasan SM, Monteiro I, Boksay I, Souren LEM, Kenowsky S, Auer LM, Elahi S, Kluger A (1999) Retrogenesis: clinical, physiologic and pathologic mechanisms in brain aging, Alzheimer's and other dementing processes. *European Archives of Psychiatry and Clinical Neuroscience*, 249:28–36.

Reisberg B, Franssen EH, Souren LEM, Auer SR, Akram I, Kenowsky S (2002) Evidence and mechanisms of retrogenesis in Alzheimer's and other dementias: management and treatment import. *American Journal of Alzheimer's Disease*, 17:202–212.

Reisberg B, Doody R, Stöffler A, Schmitt F, Ferris S, Mobius HJ (2003) Memantine in moderate to severe Alzheimer's disease. *New England Journal of Medicine*, 348:1333–1341.

Rockwood K, Howard K, Thomas VS, Mallery L, MacKnight C, Sangalang V, Darvish S (1998) Retrospective diagnosis of dementia using an informant interview based on the Brief Cognitive Rating Scale. *International Psychogeriatrics*, 10:53–60.

Sabbagh MN, Silverberg N, Bircea S, Majeed B, Samant S, Caviness JN, Reisberg B, Adler CH (2005) Is the functional decline in Parkinson's disease similar to the functional decline of Alzheimer's disease? *Parkinsonism and Related Disorders*, 11:311–315.

Sclan SG, Reisberg B (1992) Functional assessment staging (FAST) in Alzheimer's disease: reliability, validity and ordinality. *International Psychogeriatrics*, 4:55–69.

Shimada M, Hayat J, Meguro K, Oo T, Jafri S, Yamadori A, Franssen EH, Reisberg B (2003) Correlation between functional assessment staging and the 'Basic Age' by the Binet scale supports the retrogenesis model of Alzheimer's disease: a preliminary study. *Psychogeriatrics*, 3:82–87.

Souren LEM, Franssen EM, Reisberg B (1995) Contractures and loss of function in patients with Alzheimer's disease. *Journal of the American Geriatrics Society*, 43:650–655.

Souren LEM, Franssen EH, Reisberg B (1997) Neuromotor changes in Alzheimer's disease: implications for patient care. *Journal of Geriatric Psychiatry and Neurology*, 10:93–98.

Tanaka Institute for Education, 1987. Tanaka–Binet Intelligence Scale. Tokyo: Taken Publisher.

Tariot PN, Farlow M, Grossberg GT, Graham SM, McDonald S, Gergel I (2004) Memantine treatment in patients with moderate to severe Alzheimer Disease already receiving donepezil. *Journal of the American Medical Association*, 3:317–324.

Winblad B, Poritis N (1999) Memantine in severe dementia: results of the M-BEST Study (Benefit and efficacy in severely demented patients during treatment with memantine). *International Journal of Geriatric Psychiatry*, 14:135–146.

Clinical Features of Severe Dementia: Function

Serge Gauthier

Introduction

Decline in functional autonomy is a major component of symptoms in severe dementia. Very few instrumental activities of daily living (IADL) remain, and there is a gradual loss of self-care or basic ADL. Although by definition the functional impairment in dementia must be related to the cognitive decline, there are a number of other factors such as Parkinsonism (Franssen *et al.*, 1993) and comorbid disorders (Jones, 2004) that of themselves contribute significantly to the functional disability. Furthermore some patients are at home, others in institutions, with various levels of formal and informal care. Finally, there is a floor effect in many of the available ADL scales that have been developed for mild to moderate stages of dementia, where most of the randomised clinical trials (RCT) have taken place (Gauthier *et al.*, 1997).

This chapter will review the assessment of ADL in severe dementia, and the available RCT in that stage of Alzheimer's disease (AD), with comments on therapeutic benefits of donepezil and memantine on ADL.

Natural history of functional decline in severe dementia

The impact of severe dementia on individuals and on society at large have been highlighted, as well as the fact that there has been little attention paid to the development of staging and functional scales for severe dementia (Winblad *et al.*, 1999). Fortunately, pioneer work by Barry Reisberg and his team has led to the Functional Assessment Staging (FAST; Reisberg, 1988), which is the main staging measure across the different stages of AD. The stages on the FAST that are relevant to severe dementia are 5 to 7 (Table 1).

It is readily apparent, particularly though stage 7, that there is a hierarchic loss of basic skills learned as a child, which has lead Reisberg to propose the concept of 'retrogenesis'.

Another approach to the natural history of severe dementia has been the concept of milestones (Galasko *et al.*, 1995). For instance loss of two out of three residual basic ADL from the Blessed Dementia Scale, namely feeding, dressing and toileting, have been used to assess progression of AD in an RCT comparing tocopherol, selegiline and placebo (Sano *et al.*, 1997).

Measurement of ADL in severe dementia

In earlier stages of AD both caregiver and patient input is relevant (Ostbye *et al.*, 1997), but in severe dementia, only formal or informal caregivers can report on the patient's residual abilities. Interviews are usually preferred to performance-based tests (Kempen *et al.*, 1996). ADL scales

Severe Dementia. Edited by A. Burns and B. Winblad.
Copyright © 2006 John Wiley & Sons, Ltd. ISBN 0-470-01054-1

Table 1.   Functional assessment staging, in severe dementia (modified from Reisberg, 1988)

Stage 5. Deficient performance in basic ADL such as choosing proper clothing; need for
    reminders for bathing.

Stage 6. Decreased ability to dress, bathe and toilet independently.
    Substage 6(a) Decreased ability to put on clothing properly
    Substage 6(b) Decreased ability to bathe independently
    Substage 6(c) Decreased ability to perform mechanics of toileting independently
    Substage 6(d) Urinary incontinence
    Substage 6(e) Faecal incontinence

Stage 7. Loss of speech, locomotion and consciousness
    Substage 7(a) Fewer than a half-dozen words
    Substage 7(b) Single word
    Substage 7(c) Loss of ambulatory ability
    Substage 7(d) Loss of ability to sit
    Substage 7(e) Loss of ability to smile
    Substage 7(f) Loss of ability to hold head

identified as relevant to moderate and severe dementia have been identified (Gauthier *et al.*, 1999),
and are summarised in Table 2.

It is of note that most of these scales were established in the geriatric literature and listed as
instruments used to assess physical function (Applegate *et al.*, 1990), whereas the ADCS-ADL
and DAD were developed more recently and have questions relevant to initiation, planning and
execution of individual tasks. For example, the items of the Katz basic ADL are listed in Table 3,
and are answered as 'yes' or 'no' independence to perform, whereas the items of the DAD listed
in Table 4 are answered to 'during the past two weeks did the patient without help or reminder
undertake to…'. The scoring method of the DAD is designed to compensate for gender differences
by subtracting the number of non-applicable items (such as men who never cooked before) from the
denominator, and scores are expressed as a percentage of applicable items. All of the Katz items
and the first four items of the DAD are Basic ADL-related.

Some of these scales have been used in RCT (*vide infra*), some in studies of the natural history
of untreated dementia. For instance scores on the PSMS showed an average decline of 2.44 points
annually, with a curvilinear relationship of PSMS annual change with PSMS baseline in the severe
stage (Green *et al.*, 1993). This apparent movement into and out of disability may reflect a difficulty
in measuring ADL in severe dementia, when variable levels of care and patterns of reporting by

Table 2.   ADL scales for moderate to severe dementia (modified from Gauthier *et al.*, 1999)

Alzheimer Disease Cooperative Study ADL Scale (ADCS-ADL; Galasko *et al.*, 1997)
Barthel Index (Mahoney and Barthel, 1965)
D-scale in severe dementia (Fern, 1974)
Disability Assessment for Dementia (DAD; Gélinas *et al.*, 1999)
Katz ADL scale (Katz *et al.*, 1963)
Physical Self-Maintenance Scale (PSMS; Lawton and Brody, 1969)

Table 3.   Items of the Katz basic ADL scale

- Bathing
- Dressing
- Toileting
- Transferring
- Continence
- Feeding

different caregivers take place. Untreated patients at different stages of AD in Korea were assessed over one year using the DAD (Table 5; Suh *et al.*, 2004). Mild dementia was defined as MMSE more than 18, moderate as 10 to 18, and severe as below 10. Results are expressed as a percentage of ADL lost over one year, using only ADL items that were applicable to patients at a given time. It is readily apparent that IADL are lost early in AD, whereas Basic ADL are lost in severe stage. The apparent slower rate of decline on the total DAD score in severe stage reflects the fact that there are fewer ADL left to measure, leading to a nonlinear measure of functional decline in severe stage. Fortunately, ADL measures are linear over 12 months in the mild to moderate stages of AD (Feldman *et al.*, 2001), allowing for use of this outcome in one-year RCT looking at stabilisation of AD under experimental treatment. It is also likely that decline in Basic ADL would be linear, at least over 12 to 24 weeks.

Functional assessments in RCT for moderate to severe dementia

Most of the RCT in the moderate to severe stages of dementia have been performed in community-living patients with AD, although there have been a few RCT in nursing home settings. One such study compared donepezil to placebo over 24 weeks (Tariot *et al.*, 2001). The PSMS was used to measure changes in ADL, and both treatment groups showed a decline of one point over 24 weeks, in keeping with the 2.4-point annual decline found in untreated community-living patients (Green *et al.*, 1993). Another nursing home study compared memantine to placebo over 12 weeks using the D-scale as a functional outcome (Winblad and Poritis, 1999): significant differences were measured for eight of the 16 items of the scale on the treated per protocol analysis, including abilities to stand up, move, dress, eat, take in fluid, use the toilet.

Community-living patients with moderate to severe AD defined as MMSE below 14 were given memantine over 24 weeks, with (Tariot *et al.*, 2004) or without (Reisberg *et al.*, 2003) donepezil.

Table 4.   Items of the disability assessment for dementia scale

- Hygiene
- Dressing
- Continence
- Eating
- Meal preparation
- Telephoning
- Going on an outing
- Finance and correspondence
- Medications
- Leisure and housework

Table 5. Annual changes on the DAD at different levels of AD severity (modified from Suh *et al.*, 2004)

	Mild	Moderate	Severe
Mean decline of total DAD score	−16.6	−17.9	−13.8
Mean decline of IADL	−24.0	−17.1	−2.7
Mean decline of Basic ADL	−6.6	−18.0	−29.1

Both studies used a 19-item modified ADCS-ADL scale to measure functional changes. Placebo decline was 3.4 and 5.2 on the last observation carried forward (LOCF) populations, respectively, significantly worse than patients treated with memantine. A post hoc analysis of the monotherapy RCT showed statistical significance for 3 of the 19 items, making conversation, clearing a table, disposing of litter (Doody *et al.*, 2004).

Finally, an RCT compared donepezil to placebo over 24 weeks in community-living moderate to severe patients with AD, with MMSE of 5 to 17 (Feldman *et al.*, 2001). Using the DAD as functional outcome, the placebo group declined by 8.98% at week 24 LOCF, well in keeping with the DAD decline measured in untreated Koreans (Suh *et al.*, 2004). A statistically significant difference was found for patients treated with donepezil, with marked differences for three of the 10 DAD items, hygiene, dressing, leisure/housework (Feldman *et al.*, 2003). A sub-analysis of the more severe patients, defined as MMSE 12 or less, showed a steeper decline of DAD in the placebo group (>10.5%), with a statistically significant mean treatment difference of 7.18% in favour of donepezil (Feldman *et al.*, 2005).

Conclusions

There has been progress in measuring functional autonomy in severe dementia. Although many of the IADL have been lost, it is clear that both IADL and Basic ADL should be measured, particularly in RCT. IADL and Basic should be analysed separately, with more emphasis given to Basic ADL which are more likely to decline in a linear fashion over 12 to 24 weeks.

The natural history of functional decline, both in the community and in institutions, needs to be studied further, in order to measure rate of decline and impact on caregivers, both formal and informal.

References

Applegate WB, Blass JP, Williams TK (1990) Instruments for the functional assessment of older patients. *N Eng J Med*, 322:1207–1214.

Blessed G, Tomlinson RE, Roth M (1968) The association between quantitative measures of dementia and of senile change in the cerebral grey matter of elderly subjects. *Brit J Psychiatry*, 114:797–811.

Doody R, Wirth Y, Schmitt F, Möbius HJ (2004) Specific functional effects of memantine treatment in patients with moderate to severe Alzheimer's disease. *Dement Geriatr Cogn Disord*, 18:227–232.

Feldman H, Sauter A, Donald A *et al.* (2001) The Disability Assessment for Dementia scale. A 12 month study of functional ability in mild to moderate severity Alzheimer disease. *Alzheimer Dis Assoc Disord*, 15:89–95.

Feldman H, Gauthier S, Hecker J *et al.* (2001) A 24-week, randomised, double-blind study of donepezil in moderate to severe Alzheimer's disease. *Neurology*, 57:613–620.

Feldman H, Gauthier S, Hecker J *et al.* (2003) Efficacy of donepezil on maintenance of activities of daily living in patients with moderate to severe Alzheimer's disease and the effect on caregiver burden. *JAGS*, 51:737–744.

Feldman H, Gauthier S, Hecker J *et al.* (2005) Efficacy and safety of donepezil in patients with more severe Alzheimer's disease: a subgroup analysis from a randomised, placebo-controlled trial. *Int J Geriatr Psychiatry*, 20:559–569.

Fern L (1974) Behavioral activities in demented geriatric patients. *Gerontol Clin*, 16:185–194.

Franssen EH, Kluger A, Torossian CL, Reisberg B. (1993) The neurologic syndrome of severe Alzheimer's disease. *Arch Neurol*, 50:1029–1039.

Galasko D, Bennett D, Sano M *et al.* (1997) An inventory to assess activities of daily living for clinical trials in Alzheimer's disease. *Alzheimer Dis Assoc Disord*, 11(Suppl 2):S33–S39.

Galasko D, Edland SD, Morris JC *et al.* (1995) The Consortium to Establish a Registry for Alzheimer's Disease (CERAD). Part XI. Clinical milestones in patients with Alzheimer's disease followed over 3 years. *Neurology*, 45:1451–1455.

Gauthier S, Bodick N, Erzigkeit E *et al.* (1997) Activities of daily living as an outcome measure in clinical trials of dementia drugs. *Alzheimer Dis Assoc Disord*, 11(Suppl 3):6–7.

Gauthier S, Rockwood K, Gélinas I *et al.* (1999) Outcome measures for the study of activities of daily living in vascular dementia. *Alzheimer Dis Assoc Disord*, 13(Suppl 3):S143–S147.

Gélinas I, Gauthier L, McIntyre M, Gauthier S (1999) Development of a functional measure for persons with Alzheimer's disease: the Disability Assessment for Dementia. *Am J Occup Therapy*, 53:471–481.

Green CR, Mohs RC, Schmeidler J *et al.* (1993) Functional decline in Alzheimer's disease: a longitudinal study. *JAGS*, 41:654–661.

Jones R (2004) Management of comorbidity in Alzheimer's disease. In Alzheimer's Disease and Related Disorders Annual S. Gauthier, P. Scheltens, JL Cummings (Eds), 145–160.

Katz S, Ford AB, Moskowitz RW *et al.* (1963) Studies of illness in the aged: the index of ADL, a standardised measure of biological and psychological function. *JAMA*, 185:914–919.

Kempen G, Steverink N, Ormel J, Deeg D (1996) The assessment of ADL among frail elderly in an interview survey: self-report versus performance-based tests and determinants of discrepancies. *J Gerontology*, 51B:P254–P260.

Lawton MP, Bordy EM (1969) Assessment of older people: self maintaining and instrumental activities of daily living. *Gerontologist*, 9:179–186.

Mahoney F, Barthel DW (1965) Functional evaluation: the Barthel Index. *Md Med J*, 14:61–65.

Ostbye T, Tyas S, McDowell I, Koval J (1997) Reported activities of daily living: agreement between eldferly subjects with and without dementia and their caregivers. *Age and Aging*, 26:99–106.

Reisberg B (1988) Functional Assessment Staging (FAST). Psychopharmacol Bulletin, 24:653–659.

Reisberg B, Doody R, Stöffler A *et al.* (2003) Memantine in moderate-to-severe Alzheimer's disease. *N Engl J Med*, 348:1333–1341.

Sano M, Ernesto C, Thomas RG *et al.* (1997) A controlled study of selegiline, alpha-tocopherol, or both as treatment for Alzheimer's disease. *N Engl J Med*, 336:1216–1222.

Suh GH, Ju YS, Yeon BK, Shah A. (2004) longitudinal study of Alzheimer's disease: rates of cognitive and functional decline. *Int J Geriatr Psychiatry*, 19:817–824.

Tariot PN, Cummings JL, Katz IR *et al.* (2001) A randomised, double-blind, placebo-controlled study of the efficacy and safety of donepezil in patients with Alzheimer's disease in the nursing home. *JAGS*, 49:1590–1599.

Tariot PN, Farlow MR, Grossberg GT *et al.* (2004) Memantine treatment in patients with moderate to severe Alzheimer disease already receiving donepezil. *JAMA*, 291:317–324.

Winblad B, Wimo A, Möbius HJ, Fox JM, Fratiglioni L. (1999) Severe dementia: a common condition entailing high costs at individual and societal levels. *Int J Geriat Psychiatry*, 14:911–914.

Winblad B, Poritis N (1999) Memantine in severe dementia: results of the 9M-BEST Study (Benefit and Efficacy in Severely demented patients during Treatment with memantine). *Int J Geriat Psychiatry*, 14:135–146.

Management

10

Drug Treatment: Memantine

Anton P. Porsteinsson and Pierre N. Tariot

Introduction

As Alzheimer's disease advances, patients become progressively impaired in both cognitive and functional capacities, and the burden on caregivers increases. Behavioural symptoms such as apathy, agitation, aggression, disturbed mood, anxiety, and sleep–wake cycle disturbances are troubling to both patient and caregiver. This burden eventually results in the need for alternative care or nursing home placement (Cummings and Cole, 2002; Hebert *et al.*, 2003; Brookmeyer *et al.*, 1998; Alzheimer's Disease and Related Disorders Associations, 2003; Ernst and Hay, 1997). At present, no health care system or reimbursement plan exists in the United States that adequately addresses the extensive, long-term care required by most patients with AD.

The precise aetiology of AD is unknown. Studies indicate that it is a complex, heterogenous disorder involving numerous pathophysiological processes. Onset of the disease is gradual and marked by progressive decline in cognition and function. While a cascade of events typically produces the classic neuropathological features of neuritic plaques, neurofibrillary tangles and synaptic degeneration; genetic predisposition, and epidemiological factors such as age, gender and education contribute to the risk of developing AD as well as to the nature of its progression (Cummings and Cole, 2002; Butler *et al.*, 1996; Riley *et al.*, 2002). Data indicate that, in addition to the cholinergic neurotransmission pathway, various other neurotransmitter pathways such as glutamatergic, serotonergic, and dopaminergic systems as well as mechanisms of neuronal degeneration may also be involved in AD (Procter, 2000).

The Food and Drug Administration (FDA) and European Medicines Agency (EMEA) have approved memantine as the first treatment for patients with moderate-to-severe Alzheimer's disease.

Possible role of glutamate in AD

Glutamate is the principal excitatory neurotransmitter in the brain. It plays a central role in synaptic transmission in corticocortical association fibres and the majority of hippocampal pathways. Glutamate stimulates a number of postsynaptic receptors. There are two main classes of glutamate receptors: 'ionotropic', which control rapid synaptic activity by regulating the influx of cations (Na^+, K^+, and Ca^{++}) through ligand-gated ion channels into the cell; and 'metabotropic', which mediate slower and longer-lasting cellular effects via G-protein second messenger systems. There are three types of ionotropic receptors: N-methyl-D-aspartate (NMDA), α-amino-3-hydroxy-5-methyl-4-isoxalone propionic acid (AMPA), and kainate receptors, each with complex substructures. Each receptor type affords a possible means of modifying glutamatergic neurotransmission. NMDA receptors are present at high concentrations throughout the brain, especially in the neocortex and hippocampus. NMDA receptor activation plays an important part in memory encoding and storage via a mechanism of synaptic plasticity referred to as long-term potentiation (LTP) and has been

Severe Dementia. Edited by A. Burns and B. Winblad.
Copyright © 2006 John Wiley & Sons, Ltd. ISBN 0-470-01054-1

hypothesised to play a role in memory processes, dementia and the pathogenesis of Alzheimer's disease (AD) (Procter, 2000; Greenamyre *et al.*, 1988; Shimizu *et al.*, 2000).

Glutamatergic overstimulation may result in neuronal damage, a phenomenon that has been termed excitotoxicity (Rothman *et al.*, 1987). Under pathologic conditions, excessive activation of receptors by glutamate leads to neuronal calcium overload, impaired neuronal homeostasis and eventually cell death. Such excitotoxicity has been implicated in neurodegenerative disorders. Furthermore, beta-amyloid (Aβ) enhances the toxicity of glutamate, while activation of NMDA receptors appears to enhance production of pathologic forms of tau and Aβ, thus forming a vicious cycle (Procter, 2000; Greenamyre *et al.*, 1988).

Glutamate may both enhance cognitive function and be neurotoxic. While physiologic stimulation of NMDA receptors may improve memory, excessive stimulation is associated with neuronal injury. The glutamatergic system is therefore a logical target for both cognitive enhancement and for interrupting the pathophysiology of AD (Winblad *et al.*, 2002). Preclinical data indicate that the NMDA receptor is a particularly promising target for neuroprotective agents as the high Ca^{2+} permeability of this receptor probably underlies its neurotoxic potential. NMDA receptors are only activated following depolarisation of the postsynaptic membrane, which relieves their voltage-dependent blockade by Mg^{2+}. It is possible to counteract glutamate excitotoxicity by blocking the NMDA receptor and thus preventing neural cell death. However, if NMDA receptor activity is completely blocked, the physiological activity of the NMDA receptor (such as memory, learning activity and long-term potentiation) is blocked along with the pathological activity. High-affinity compounds such MK801 or phencyclidine (PCP), impair learning in animal models and can produce psychotomimetic effect. Approaches with moderate-affinity NMDA receptor antagonists have been more fruitful (Procter, 2000; Greenamyre *et al.*, 1988; Winblad *et al.*, 2002).

Memantine
Mode of action
Memantine (1–amino-3, 5-dimethyladamantane hydrochloride) is a moderate-affinity, non-competitive, NMDA receptor antagonist that exerts voltage-dependent effects with rapid blocking/unblocking kinetics. Memantine, acting at the NMDA receptor site, allows normal glutamatergic neurotransmission under physiological circumstances while inhibiting excitotoxicity under conditions of chronic glutamatergic stimulation (Parsons *et al.*, 1999; Danysz *et al.*, 1997, 2000).

Under physiological conditions, Mg^{2+} occupies the NMDA receptor channel and blocks Ca^{2+} entry into the neuron. During physiologic learning and memory processes, high concentrations of synaptic glutamate are transiently released and, owing to its strong voltage dependency, Mg^{2+} leaves the NMDA receptor and allows normal Ca^{2+} influx. On the other hand, the sustained, pathological release of glutamate from neurons and glia seen in neurodegenerative conditions such as AD generates a moderate prolonged depolarisation which displaces Mg^{2+} from the NMDA receptor channel, allowing continuous influx of Ca^{2+} into the neuron, thereby increasing the intraneuronal Ca^{2+} pool which can impede the promulgation of a physiological signal. The permanently increased intraneuronal Ca^{2+} concentration can also lead to neuronal degeneration. Memantine occupies the same NMDA receptor channel but is less voltage-dependent and does not leave the channel with minor depolarisation, thus preventing the sustained influx of Ca^{2+} during pathological release of glutamate. During physiological glutamate release, memantine leaves the channel and allows normal influx of Ca^{2+}. A signal is produced which can be recognised and processed owing to reduced intraneuronal noise. Memantine also blocks 5-HT$_3$ receptors at therapeutic concentrations. Antagonism at 5-HT$_3$ has been postulated to facilitate LTP, have antipsychotic and anti-nausea effects, as well as decreasing gastric hypermotility (Parsons *et al.*, 1999; Danysz *et al.*, 1997, 2000).

Memantine reduces acute excitotoxic damage *in vitro* and *in vivo* following administration of glutamate agonists and in models of global and focal ischaemia, confers protection against

Aβ-induced neurotoxicity and improves cognitive performance in rats (Parsons *et al.*, 1999; Danysz *et al.*, 1997, 2000).

Pharmacokinetics

Following oral administration, memantine is completely absorbed with a T_{max} of four to six hours and an oral bioavailability of 100%. Food does not affect its bioavailability. Memantine shows linear pharmacokinetics over the therapeutic dose range. It is extensively distributed in tissue and readily crosses the blood–brain barrier. Daily doses of 5 to 30 mg to patients resulted in a mean CSF/serum ratio of 0.52. Memantine is about 45% protein-bound. Terminal half-life of memantine is 60 to 80 hours. It undergoes little metabolism and is excreted largely unchanged in the urine. There are no therapeutically active metabolites. Memantine clearance is reduced with increasing degrees of renal impairment. The CYP450 system is minimally involved in the metabolism of memantine. These data indicate that no pharmacokinetic interactions with drugs metabolised by these enzymes are to be expected. Medications or conditions that raise urine pH may decrease the urinary elimination of memantine resulting in increased plasma levels (Memantine insert).

Data from preclinical trials, pharmacokinetic studies, pivotal trials and postmarketing studies suggest that the combined use of memantine and ChEI is safe and well tolerated (Periclou *et al.*, 2003; Wenk *et al.*, 2000; Hartmann and Möbius, 2003).

Pivotal clinical trials
MRZ9605

Study MRZ9605 was a randomised, double-blind, placebo-controlled, parallel arm trial of 28 weeks duration conducted at 32 centres in the United States. The objective was to demonstrate that memantine was superior to placebo as assessed by global and functional measures in treating community-residing patients with moderate-to-severe Alzheimer's disease (Reisberg *et al.*, 2003). It was followed by an optional 24-week open label study, during which all patients received the active drug (Ferris *et al.*, 2003). Two hundred and fifty-two patients (67% women; mean age 76 years) were enrolled. Of these, 181 (72%) completed the study and were evaluated at week 28. Seventy-one patients discontinued treatment prematurely, 42 (33% of total) taking placebo and 29 (23% of total) taking memantine. MMSE scores ranged from 3 to 14. The mean MMSE at baseline was 7.9. Memantine was dosed at 20 mg/day (10 mg b.i.d., starting dose 5 mg and increased by 5 mg weekly to the target dose). At endpoint, the decline in cognitive function, as measured by the change in Severe Impairment Battery (SIB) score was less in memantine patients compared with the deterioration seen in placebo patients ($p < 0.001$; LOCF). They also showed significantly greater levels of day-to-day functioning as measured by the ADCS-ADLsev as compared to the patients on placebo ($p = 0.02$; LOCF) and a marginally significant superiority of memantine over placebo in terms of global functioning observed for the CIBIC-plus on the LOCF analysis at endpoint ($p = 0.06$) with a statistically significant advantage for the OC analysis ($p = 0.03$). Analysis of resource utilisation and costs regarding the pharmacoeconomic impact of memantine treatment showed significant reduction in caregiver time burden and transition to an institution among those treated with memantine, indicating fewer costs to caregivers and society. There were no clinically important differences in adverse events between patients in the memantine or placebo group. There were also no clinically relevant differences between patients in the memantine and placebo group in baseline assessment of clinical laboratory values, electrocardiographic results, or measurement of vital signs (Reisberg *et al.*, 2003).

One hundred and seventy-five patients who completed the double-blind phase were enrolled in a subsequent six-month open label memantine extension study. The primary aim of this extension study was to assess the long-term safety and efficacy of memantine in this population of patients with AD. As in the double-blind phase, memantine dosing was 10 mg b.i.d. Outcome measures were unchanged. Inferences regarding efficacy are limited in open-label studies, but there is at least a suggestion that patients who were switched to memantine from placebo improved relative to the projected rate of continued decline on each of the efficacy measures. Patients treated continuously with memantine as well as those switched from placebo to open-label memantine continued to decline, however. There were no clinically important differences in adverse events between patients switched to memantine or maintained on memantine during the extension phase, suggesting that memantine therapy was well tolerated over the course of 52 week (Ferris *et al.*, 2003).

MEM-MD-02
Study MEM-MD-02 was a randomised, double-blind, placebo-controlled evaluation of the safety and efficacy of memantine in community-residing patients with moderate-to-severe dementia of the Alzheimer's type (Farlow *et al.*, 2003). MMSE scores ranged from 5 to 14 inclusive, the mean MMSE score at entry was 10. In contrast to the earlier monotherapy trial, in this case all subjects had to be on daily donepezil therapy for the past six months, and at a stable dose for the past three months. Average time on donepezil in enrolled subjects was approximately two years. Primary outcome measures were the SIB and ADCS-ADLsev. The CIBIC-plus was used as global assessment of response to treatment and was conducted by independent rater. Behaviour was assessed with the Neuropsychiatric Inventory (NPI). Of the 403 patients who were randomised (65% female; mean age 75.5 years) and treated with memantine 10 mg b.i.d. ($n = 202$) or placebo ($n = 201$), 85% of memantine/ChEI-treated patients and 75% of placebo/ChEI patients completed the trial; the dropout rate was significantly lower in the memantine/ChEI group ($p = 0.01$). At week 24, patients treated with memantine/ChEI showed a statistically significant improvement ($p < 0.001$) in cognitive function (SIB) compared to patients treated with placebo/ChEI, and showed significantly less decline ($p = 0.028$) in daily function (ADCS-ADLsev). A significant difference in favour of memantine/ChEI was also seen on the CIBIC-plus global assessment ($p = 0.027$) and NPI total score ($p = 0.002$). Subsequent post hoc analysis showed both delayed emergence of behavioural symptoms as well as some instances of symptom reduction, with significant improvements noted in domains of agitation/aggression, irritability/lability, and appetite/eating change compared to placebo/ChEI. Memantine/ChEI treatment was safe and well tolerated. The incidence of treatment emergent adverse event was similar in patients treated with memantine/ChEI or placebo/ChEI combination and premature discontinuation due to adverse events was numerically lower in the memantine/ChEI group (7%) compared to the placebo/ChEI group (12%). No clinically important differences between treatment groups were seen in the incidence of EKG abnormalities or potentially clinically significant laboratory parameters or vital signs (Farlow *et al.*, 2003).

These results further support the safety and efficacy of memantine therapy for patients with moderate-to-severe AD and demonstrated that treatment with memantine combined with a commonly used ChEI was superior to the ChEI alone on key indices of cognition, function, clinical global status, and behaviour in this trial. Importantly, treatment with memantine/ChEI resulted in improved cognitive performance at 24 weeks relative to baseline, whereas treatment with the ChEI alone was associated with continued cognitive decline.

MEM-MD-01
Study MEM-MD-01 had the same design as MEM-MD-02, except it was a monotherapy study with no concomitant ChEI allowed. The study failed to show superiority of memantine over placebo. The sponsoring company intends to eventually publish it on its clinical trials website.

M-Best study

The M-Best study was a double-blind study of 12 weeks duration conducted in a nursing home population with mixed dementias (AD and vascular dementia; VaD) (Winblad and Poritis, 1999). The 166 subjects had MMSE scores less than 10 (mean = 6.3) and Global Deterioration Scale staging of 5 to 7 and were randomised to either memantine ($n = 82$) or placebo ($n = 84$). Memantine treatment was initiated at 5 mg once daily and increased to 10 mg once daily after one week. The primary efficacy measures were the care-dependency subscale of the Behavioral Rating Scale for Geriatric Patients (BGP), a measure of day-to-day function; and the Clinical Global Impression of Change (CGI-C), a measure of overall clinical effect. Secondary efficacy variables were the D-scale, a descriptive measure of behavioural activities and functioning in patients with dementia; the GCI-S and BGP total score. Memantine showed significant improvement over placebo as measured by both primary efficacy measures; results were better for memantine- over placebo-treated patients on the secondary outcome measures. Regarding the safety profile, no significant differences between treatment groups were observed (Winblad and Poritis, 1999).

Conclusion

Alzheimer's disease is a serious public health concern. In terms of monetary cost and emotional and psychological toll, the burden of this disease on patients, caregivers and society at large is staggering. Cholinesterase inhibitors have been approved for treatment of patients with mild-to-moderate AD on the basis of cognitive, functional and behavioural outcome measures. Although, at least one cholinesterase inhibitor, donepezil, has demonstrated cognitive, functional and behavioural improvement in one study in patients with more advanced dementia, ChEIs are not FDA approved for this indication. Regrettably, cholinergic compounds are often limited by gastrointestinal side effects and there is no evidence of disease modification. Accordingly, there has been a surge in research to identify additional therapeutic strategies for all stages of illness.

Memantine has shown demonstrable benefit in patients with moderate-to-severe AD. Its mechanism of action may include enhanced neurotransmission in multiple systems as well as antiexcitotoxic effects. The safety, tolerability and efficacy of memantine alone or in combination with a ChEI have been supported by clinical trials, as well as by pharmacokinetic and German post-marketing data. These results provide evidence suggesting that modulation of NMDA receptors to reduce glutamate-induced excitotoxicity can alleviate the symptoms of Alzheimer's disease. The novel neurochemical approach is distinct from the cholinomimetic mechanism of all previously approved treatments for Alzheimer's disease. The side-effect profile of memantine is relatively benign. Memantine is the first treatment specifically FDA and EMEA approved for patients with moderate-to-severe Alzheimer's disease. Memantine will probably be used in both monotherapy and in combination with a ChEI. Future studies will need to further examine whether memantine treatment and cholinergic treatment may ultimately prove to be not only complementary but even synergistic.

References

Alzheimer's Disease and Related Disorders Associations: Statistics about Alzheimer's disease. February 1, 2003. Available at: www.alz.org. Accessed Nov 1, 2003.

Brookmeyer R, Gray S, Kawas C (1998) Projections of Alzheimer's disease in the United States and the public health impact of delaying disease onset. *Am J Public Health*, 88:1337–1342.

Butler SM, Ashford JW, Snowdon DA (1996) Age, education, and changes in the Mini Mental State Exam scores of older women: findings from the Nun Study. *J Am Geriatr Soc*, 44:675–681.

Cummings JL, Cole G (2002) Alzheimer disease. *JAMA*, 287(18):2335–2338.

Danysz W, Parsons CG, Kornhuber J, Schmidt WJ, Quack G (1997) Aminoadamantanes as NMDA receptor antagonists and antiparkinsonian agents – preclinical studies. *Neurosci Biobehav Rev*, 21(4):455–468.

Danysz W, Parsons CG, Möbius HJ, Stöfler A, Quack G (2000) Neuroprotective and symptomalogical action of memantine relevant for Alzheimer's disease – a unified glutamatergic hypothesis on the mechanism of action. *Neurotoxicity Res*, 2:85–98.

Ernst RL, Hay JW (1997) Economic Research on Alzheimer's disease: a review of the literature. *Alzheimer Dis Assoc Disord*, 11(suppl6):135–145.

Ferris SH, Schmitt FA, Doody RS, Möbius HJ, Stöffler A, Reisberg B (2003) Long-term treatment with the NMDA antagonist memantine: results of a 24-week, open-label extension study in moderate-to-severe Alzheimer's disease (abstract). *Neurology*, 60(suppl 1):A414.

Greenamyre JT, Maragos WF, Albin RL, Penney JB, Young AB (1988) Glutamate transmission and toxicity in Alzheimer's disease. *Prog Neuropsychopharmacol Biol Psychiatry*, 12(4):421–430.

Hartmann S, Möbius HJ (2003) Tolerability of memantine in combination with cholinesterase inhibitors in dementia therapy. *Int Clin Psychopharmacol*, 18(2):81–85.

Hebert LE, Scherr PA, Bienias JL, Bennett BD, Evans DA (2003) Alzheimer's disease in the US population. *Arch Neurol*, 60:1119–1122.

Memantine insert.

Parsons CG, Danysz W, Quack G (1999) Memantine is a clinically well tolerated N-methyl-D-aspartate (NMDA) receptor antagonist – a review of preclinical data. *Neuropharmacology* 38(6):735–767.

Periclou A, Ventura D, Sherman T, Rao N, Abramowitz W (2003) A pharmacokinetic study of the NMDA receptor antagonist memantine and donepezil in healthy young subjects (abstract). *J Am Geriatr Soc*, 51(s4): S225.

Procter A (2000) Abnormalities in non-cholinergic neurotransmitter systems in Alzheimer's disease. In: O'Brien J, Ames D, Burns A (eds). Dementia, 2nd edn, 433–442. United States: Oxford University Press.

Reisberg B, Doody R, Stöffler A, Schmitt F, Ferris S, Möbius HJ (2003) Memantine in moderate-to-severe Alzheimer's disease. *N Engl J Med*, 348(14):1333–1341.

Riley KP, Snowdon DA, Markesbery WR (2002) Alzheimer's neurofibrillatory pathology and the spectrum of cognitive function: findings from the Nun Study. *Ann Neurol*, 51:567–577.

Rothman SM, Thurston JH, Hauhart RE (1987) Delayed neurotoxicity of excitatory amino acids in vitro. *Neuroscience*, 22:471–480.

Schneider LS, Tariot PN (2003) Cognitive enhancers and treatments for Alzheimer's disease. In: Tasman A, Kay J, Lieberman JA, eds. Psychiatry, 2nd edn. Chichester, UK John Wiley.

Shimizu E, Tang YP, Rampon C, Tsien JZ (2000) NMDA receptor-dependent synaptic reinforcement is a crucial process for memory consolidation. *Science*, 290:1170–1174.

Tariot PN, Farlow MR, Grossberg GT, Graham SM, McDonald S, Gergel I for the Memantine Study Group (2004) Memantine Treatment in Patients with moderate to severe Alzheimer's disease already receiving donepezil. A randomized controlled trial. *JAMA*, 291:317–324.

Wenk GL, Quack G, Moebius H-J, Danysz W (2000) No interaction of memantine with acetylcholinesterase inhibitors approved for clinical use. *Life Sciences*, 66(12):1079–1083.

Winblad B, Poritis N (1999) Memantine in severe dementia: results of the M-BEST Study (Benefit and efficacy in severely demented patients during treatment with memantine). *Int J Geriatr Psychiatry*, 14(2):135–146.

Winblad B, Möbius HJ, Stöffler A (2002) Glutamate receptors as a target for Alzheimer's disease – are clinical results supporting the hope? *J Neural Transm*, (Suppl 62):217–225.

11

Drug Treatment: Cholinesterase Inhibitors

Michael Woodward and Howard H Feldman

Introduction

Alzheimer's disease (AD) is characterised by cholinergic deficits that correlate with cognitive deficits and are more marked as the disease progresses (Perry *et al.*, 1977). This is the justification for trialling cholinesterase inhibitors in more severe AD. There is also evidence for cholinergic deficits in vascular dementia (Erkinjuntti *et al.*, 2004; Bullock, 2004) and Dementia with Lewy bodies (DLB) (McKeith *et al.*, 2000). It is also likely that these cholinergic deficits increase with disease progression. In this chapter the discussion will concentrate on the treatment of severe AD with cholinesterase inhibitors, although it is possible that similar effects would be seen in the treatment of severe DLB, vascular dementia or mixtures of these dementias.

Severe Alzheimer's disease affects multiple domains – cognition, function, behaviour and caregiver burden. The cholinergic deficiency has been linked to neuropsychiatric symptoms in AD (Minger *et al.*, 2000; Cummings and Back, 1998; Mega *et al.*, 1999), where medial frontal and limbic cholinergic deficits have been identified (Craig *et al.*, 1996; Sultzer *et al.*, 1995).Compared to milder dementias, cognition may be a less important final therapeutic target in more severe dementia. In milder dementia the cholinesterase inhibitors have demonstrated efficiency across all these domains (Ritchie *et al.*, 2004; Lanctôt *et al.*, 2003; Hecker and Snellgrove, 2003) so these agents have the potential to provide benefit to those with more severe dementia, even if cognitive improvement is not sought as the primary outcome.

Therapy for severe dementia may occur in a range of settings – for example, in the community or in residential care such as nursing homes, as newly initiated or as ongoing therapy, to target a particular symptom requiring more urgent attention or in a more elective fashion, and in those with multiple comorbidities versus those who are otherwise relatively well. The very limited number of published trials of cholinesterase inhibitors for severe dementia have not provided sufficient evidence of efficacy across all these settings, and frequently the clinician is required to use clinical judgement in deciding whether and how to use these agents.

Acetylcholinesterase inhibitors in use

There are four acetylcholinesterase (AChE) inhibitors in use, with one, tacrine, only now available in a few countries due to inconvenient dosing (q.i.d.) and safety concerns (frequent liver enzyme elevations and isolated reports of more serious liver toxicity). All agents increase acetylcholine levels in the brain, but they differ substantially as shown in Table 1. These differences may be expected to influence efficacy and tolerability, and certainly some individuals who fail to tolerate one agent may tolerate another. However, in mild to moderate AD, clinical trials have not shown any substantial differences between agents (Ritchie *et al.*, 2004; Lanctôt *et al.*, 2003; Hecker and Snellgrove, 2003). Donepezil is a second-generation reversible cholinesterase inhibitor given once

Severe Dementia. Edited by A. Burns and B. Winblad.
Copyright © 2006 John Wiley & Sons, Ltd. ISBN 0-470-01054-1

Table 1. Pharmacology of cholinesterase inhibitors (adapted from Jones, 2003)

Properties	Cholinesterase inhibitor		
	Donepezil	Rivastigmine	Galantamine
AChE inhibitor type	Reversible, mixed	Pseudo-irreversible	Reversible, competitive
Selectivity	AChE ≫ BuChE	AChE = BuChE	AChE < BuChE
Plasma half-life	70 h	1–2 h	6 h
Dosage	Once daily	Twice daily	Twice daily
Dosage strengths	5 mg, 10 mg	1.5 mg, 3 mg, 4.5 mg, 6 mg (once daily patches soon)	4 mg, 8 mg, 12 mg – standard 8 mg, 16 mg, 24 mg – prolonged release
Plasma protein binding	High (95%)	Low (40%)	Minimal
Metabolism by cytochrome P450 (CYP) system	Yes (CYP2D6 and CYP3A4)	Minimal	Yes (CYP2D6 and CYP3A4)
Potential for drug interactions	Yes	Low	Moderate
Excretion	Urine/faeces	Urine	Urine

AChE = acetylcholinesterase; *BuChE* = butyrylcholinesterase.

daily at either 5 or 10 mg. It exhibits high selectivity for neuronal AChE as opposed to butyryl-cholinesterase (Ogura *et al.*, 2000). Each dose has been shown to be effective in trials in mild to moderate AD but greater efficacy has been associated with the 10-mg dose so this is the target dose. The dose should be increased no more frequently than four-weekly, to reduce the adverse effects found with all these agents. These adverse effects (predominantly gastrointestinal and including nausea, weight loss, vomiting and diarrhoea) affect about 10–20% of all people treated with an AChE inhibitor, but are usually mild and self-limiting.

Rivastigmine is a slowly reversible (pseudoirreversible) cholinesterase inhibitor that targets both acetyl- and butyrylcholinesterase. There is some evidence that in more severe dementia butyryl-cholinesterase becomes a more predominant pathway for acetylcholine breakdown, so inhibiting this enzyme may boost acetylcholine levels proportionally more in more severe dementia (Arendt, 1992). Rivastigmine also exhibits regional specificity for the hippocampus, amygdala and cerebral cortex, which are areas most affected by AD pathology (Polinsky, 1998). It is generally given twice daily, although pivotal trials in mild to moderate AD used a t.i.d. regime. Daily doses range from 3 to 12 mg, with slow titration upwards (four weeks between dose increases) recommended to reduce adverse effects. Only doses of 6 mg daily or more have shown efficacy in trials in mild to moderate AD and it is likely that lower doses will also be ineffective in more severe dementia. A once-daily rivastigmine patch is likely to soon become available in some countries and will increase convenience of administration.

Galantamine is a specific, competitive and reversible cholinesterase inhibitor that is also an allosteric modulator at nicotinic receptors. This additional mechanism may provide additional cholinergic effects beyond that of the drug's weak inhibition of AChE. It is administered at a starting dose of 8 mg a day. An increasing number of countries have a daily prolonged release preparation available, otherwise it is given as two divided daily doses. The starting dose has not shown efficacy in trials in mild to moderate AD and this too is likely to apply to more severe AD. The target dose is 24 mg daily – trials of 32 mg daily were initially reported but this higher dose is associated with a substantial increase in adverse effects and is now not recommended. The dosages should be increased no more frequently than four-weekly, to reduce adverse effects.

Measuring benefits of therapy

Assessing response to an anticholinesterase may be more difficult in more severely demented people. As stated above, these agents may affect a range of domains, and cognition may not be the primary target of therapy. The caregiver can be quite stressed by tending to a severely demented person. A main goal of therapy may therefore be to reduce caregiver burden and stress. This may be achieved by any of a number of changes in the patient such as them becoming less agitated, more interactive or more able to reach the toilet in time. Another goal of therapy may be to prevent or delay nursing home or other residential care admission. The target may be a specific behaviour or functional ability – e.g. reduced verbal aggression or the ability to dress themselves.

Trials of acetylcholinesterase inhibitors in severe dementia have endpoints that reflect those differing goals. The endpoints for mild to moderate dementia trials are less applicable to severe dementia. Whilst cognitive endpoints such as the MMSE are often included, they suffer from 'bottoming out' effects in severe dementia – they are so low on trial entry that it may be difficult to show a treatment effect (Reisberg *et al.*, 1996). Other endpoints are more appropriate to more severely demented people and more sensitive to change at this end of the dementia spectrum. Scales used in trials of cholinesterase inhibitors in more severe dementia are shown in Table 2. Other endpoints and measures include delay to nursing home admission and economic scales measuring resource utilisation.

One approach to the differing therapeutic goals across the dementia spectrum is to develop individualised treatment goals. Rockwood *et al.* (2002) have described a process of Goal Attainment Scaling that utilises this approach. A consensus is reached between physician, carer and patient – but patient input is often less appropriate in more severe dementia. This approach has not, however, yet been utilised as an endpoint in published trials of cholinesterase inhibitors, despite its attractiveness as a clinically relevant endpoint for this group.

Efficacy of anticholinesterases in severe Alzheimer's disease

In the absence of an agreed biomarker for severe dementia, including AD, and avoiding the issue of the nosology of severe dementia, this review will present evidence of efficacy in situations where severe AD may be found. This includes those with more severe dementia in the community, those wishing to delay the need for residential care, those in residential care and those who have had dementia for a longer period of time, even if the dementia was initially of more moderate severity.

Community

There are no published trials of a cholinesterase inhibitor commenced in severely demented people in a community setting. There is, however, one double-blind, randomised, placebo-controlled trial of donepezil on those with moderate to severe AD (MMSE 5 to 17) that included a largely community population with initially more severe AD (Feldman *et al.*, 2001a). There is also one published trial of galantamine in 'advanced moderate' AD (MMSE 11–14 or Alzheimer's Disease Assessment Scale-Cognitive subscale (ADAS-Cog) over 30) which is based on a subgroup analysis of pivotal trials in mild to moderate AD (Blesa *et al.*, 2003). Additionally, a similar subgroup analysis from

Table 2. Endpoints/scales used in severe dementia trials of cholinesterase inhibitors

Scale/endpoint	Domain measured	Range	Utility in severe AD (0 to 3+)
MMSE	Cognition	0 to 30	+
ADAS-Cog	Cognition	0 to 70	+
SIB	Cognition	0 to 100	+++
NP1	Neuropsychiatric disturbances	0 to 144	+++
NP1-NH	Neuropsychiatric disturbances	0 to 144	+++
CDR	Dementia severity	0 to 3	+
CDR-SB	Dementia severity	0 to 18	+
FRS	Global	0 to 40	+
CIBIC+	Global	1 to 7	++
DAD	Function	0 to 100%	+++
1ADL+	Function	0 to 100	++
PSMS/PSMS+	Function	6 to 30	+++
FAST	Function	0 to 7	++
BDRS	Function	1 to 17	+
Br ADL	Function	0 to 60	++
SCB	Caregiver burden	Number of items	++
CSS	Caregiver burden	Number of items	++

MMSE, Mini Mental State Examination;
ADAS-Cog, Alzheimer's Disease Assessment Scale, Cognitive subscale;
SIB, Severe Impairment Battery;
NPI, Neuropsychiatric Inventory;
NPI-NH, Neuropsychiatric Inventory, Nursing Home modification;
CDR, Clinical Dementia Rating;
CDR-SB, Clinic Dementia Rating – Sum of Boxes;
FRS, Functional Rating Scale;
CIBIC+, Clinician's Interview-Based Impression of Change;
DAD, Disability Assessment for Dementia;
IADL+, Modified Instrumental Activities of Daily Living Scale;
PSMS, Physical Self-Maintenance Scale;
FAST, Functional Assessment Staging Test;
BDRS, Blessed Dementia Rating Scale;
Br ADL, Bristol Activities of Daily Living;
SCB, Survey for Caregiver Burden;
CSS, Caregiver Stress Scale.

trials of rivastigmine in mild to moderate AD was performed for those with moderately severe AD – defined as those with a Global Deterioration Scale (GDS) (Reisberg *et al.*, 1982) of 5 or above at baseline (Doraiswamy *et al.*, 2002).

In the trial of donepezil in moderate to severe AD, 290 patients were treated for 24 weeks with either a target dose of 10 mg donepezil daily (144) or placebo (146). Patients with stable concomitant illnesses were included, and most concomitant medications were allowed except those with notable cholinergic or anticholinergic effects. The primary efficacy measure was the CIBIC, a global assessment of change. Other efficacy measures were the standardised MMSE (SMMSE), the severe impairment battery (SIB), a measure of cognition in more severely demented people, and other scales described in Table 2 including the DAD, IADL+, PSMS+, NPI, FRS and the CSS. An assessment of health care resource utilisation and work productivity, the Canadian Utilizations of Services Tracking (CAUST) was also utilised.

The majority of patients were community-dwelling (donepezil 87%, placebo 88%) with the remainder in assisted living situations. Completion rates were 84% in the donepezil group and 86% in the placebo group. The most common reasons for discontinuation were adverse events (8% donepezil, 6% placebo) and withdrawal of consent (3% donepezil, 5% placebo). The mean ages (and range) were 73.3 (52–92) in the donepezil group and 74.0 (48–92) in the placebo group.

There were significant drug–placebo differences in the CIBIC+ on all visits (mean treatment difference 0.54 at week 24, last observations carried forward (LOCF)) as shown in Figure 1. At week 24 LOCF, 63% of donepezil- and 42% of placebo-treated patients were rated as improved or unchanged ($p < 0.0001$). There were also mean improvements in cognition on both the SMMSE and the SIB, in the donepezil-treated group with mean differences from placebo that were significant at all visits throughout the trial (week 24 LOCF mean treatment difference = 1.79 on the SMMSE and 5.62 on the SIB; Figure 2).

The functional measures also improved significantly and were analysed in more detail in a subanalysis (Feldman *et al.*, 2003). In all of the DAD, IADL+ and PSMS+, there were significant differences in favour of donepezil treatment compared with placebo at week 24 LOCF. On the DAD, the donepezil-treated group remained stable throughout the study with a mean decline of only 0.74 points compared with the 8.98-point decline in the placebo group at week 24 LOCF ($p < 0.0001$, mean treatment difference = 8.23; Figure 3). Subanalysis of the DAD (into basic ADL

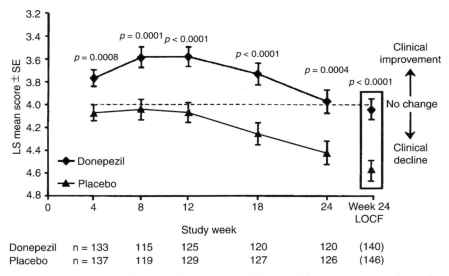

Figure 1. Clinician's interview-based impression of change with caregiver input. Least Squares (LS) mean±SE scores for donepezil- and placebo-treated patients through 24 weeks of treatment. LOCF = Last Observation Carried Forward. From Feldman *et al.* (2001). A 24-week, randomised, double blind study of donepezil in moderate to severe Alzheimer's disease. *Neurology*, 57, 613–20. Reproduced by permission of Lippincott, Williams & Wilkins.

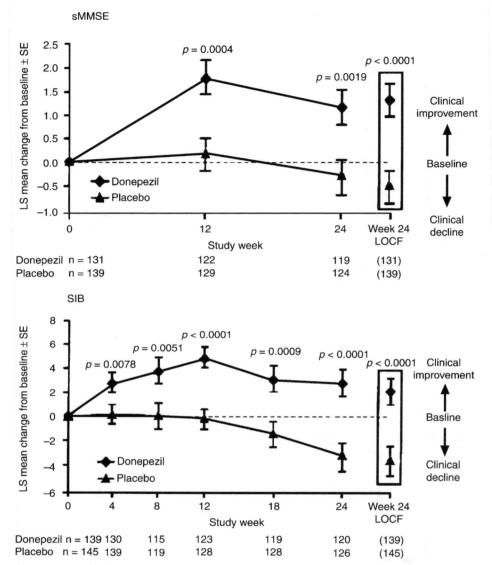

Figure 2. Cognition. Least Squares (LS) means±SE change from baseline scores for donepezil- and placebo-treated patients through 24 weeks of treatment, as measured using the standardised Mini Mental State Examination (sMMSE) and Severe Impairment Battery (SIB). LOCF = Last Observation Carried Forward. From Feldman *et al.* (2001). A 24-week, randomised, double blind study of donepezil in moderate to severe Alzheimer's disease. *Neurology*, 57, 613–20. Reproduced by permission of Lippincott, Williams & Wilkins.

only or instrumental ADL only) as well as the components of initiation, planning and organisa- tion, and effective performance for all ADLs showed differences between the groups in favour of donepezil-treated patients at week 24 LOCF ($p < 0.002$). Similarly, the results of the IADL+ and PSMS+ showed less mean decline in the donepezil-treated group than placebo (week 24 LOCF,

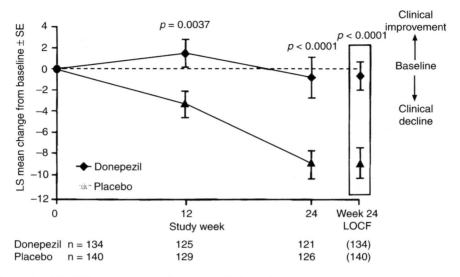

Figure 3. Disability Assessment for Dementia (DAD). Least Squares (LS) mean±SE change for baseline scores for donepezil- and placebo-treated patients through 24 weeks of treatment. LOCF = Last Observation Carried Forward. From Feldman *et al.* (2001). A 24-week, randomised, double blind study of donepezil in moderate to severe Alzheimer's disease. *Neurology*, 57, 613–20. Reproduced by permission of Lippincott, Williams & Wilkins.

mean treatment difference = 6.83 on the IADL+ $p < 0.0001$, and 1.32 on the PSMS+ ($p = 0.0015$)). The FRS, a global multidomain scale evaluating cognition and function, showed a stabilisation of global function in the donepezil-treated group, with a mean decline of 0.38 sum of the boxes compared with the 1.66 sum of the boxes decline in the placebo group at week 24 LOCF (mean treatment difference = 1.28, $p = 0.0002$).

The benefit on function is clinically important. The loss of ADLs typically occurs in a hierarchical fashion, beginning with more complex functions (instrumental ADLs such as housekeeping and finances) and progressing to basic functions such as bathing, dressing and toileting. In one study in milder AD, individuals with greater cognitive impairment showed a more rapid decline in overall functional ability than did those with less cognitive impairment (Feldman *et al.*, 2001b). Other data shows that the rate of decline in basic ADLs is greater in patients with more advanced AD (Schmeidler *et al.*, 1998). To be able to maintain function in more advanced AD is likely to improve quality of life and reduce caregiver burden.

Behavioural and neuropsychiatric symptoms improved from baseline with donepezil by 4.6 points on the NPI total score at week 24 LOCF, and were analysed in a further subanalysis (Gauthier *et al.*, 2002). There were fluctuations in the mean NPI total scores in the placebo group with a decline of one point at week 24 LOCF (Figure 4). The mean differences in NPI total scores were significant at weeks 4, 24 and week 24 LOCF (treatment difference 5.64). At baseline, the most common symptoms were apathy/indifference (67%), aberrant motor behaviour (53%), depression/dysthymia (52%), anxiety (49%) and agitation/aggression (45%). NPI individual items change from baseline scores to week 24 LOCF showed benefits with donepezil treatment compared with placebo for all items, with significant treatment differences for depression/dysthymia, anxiety, and apathy/indifference ($p < 0.05$ for each). Symptoms present at baseline that improved significantly for donepezil- compared with placebo-treated patients at week 24 LOCF were anxiety, apathy/indifference and irritability/lability ($p < 0.05$ for each). In patients who were

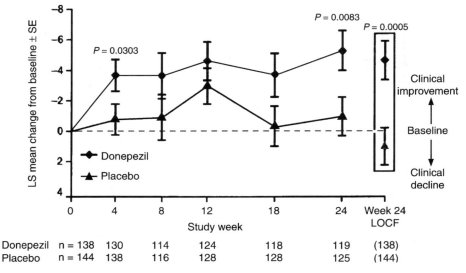

Figure 4. Neuropsychiatric Inventory (NPI). Least Squares (LS) mean±SE change for baseline scores for donepezil- and placebo-treated patients through 24 weeks of treatment. LOCF = Last Observation Carried Forward. From Feldman *et al.* (2001). A 24-week, randomised, double blind study of donepezil in moderate to severe Azheimer's disease. *Neurology*, 57, 613–20. Reproduced by permission of Lippincott, Williams & Wilkins.

receiving psychoactive medications at baseline (45% in donepezil- and 36% in placebo-treated patients), differences between the groups favoured donepezil on NPI total scores at weeks 4, 18, 24 and 24 LOCF but were not significant. For non-users of psychoactive medications at baseline, there were significant differences between the two treatment groups in favour of donepezil on NPI total scores at all visits and at week 24 LOCF.

Behavioural disturbances in AD increases with disease progression (Haupt *et al.*, 2000; Mega *et al.*, 1996), and 95% of this cohort had at least one symptom at baseline. This efficacy of donepezil on behavioural disturbances in more severe dementia is thus very encouraging. The results should be extrapolated to the general population with some caution, as patients were not selected on the basis of the presence of particular behavioural disturbances. It is, however, encouraging that the study also showed a reduction in caregiver burden, as this burden is significantly affected by behavioural disturbances (Coen *et al.*, 1997; Kaufer *et al.*, 1998; Teri, 1997). Behavioural disturbances are also important factors involved in the decision to institutionalise a patient (Haupt and Kurz, 1993).

At baseline, caregivers of patients treated with donepezil did not differ significantly from caregivers of patients treated with placebo with respect to demographics or mean total scores on the CSS, a scale which assesses caregiver hardships, stress, level of fatigue and the source of these feelings. At week 24 LOCF, the overall distribution of caregiver ratings on each of the three-caregiver diary items favoured donepezil-treated patients over placebo-treated patients ($p < 0.005$). At week 24 LOCF, mean change from baseline scores for CSS total and individual domain scores (all domains except caregiver competence, personal gains, and management of distress) were better for caregivers of donepezil-treated patients (CSS total, mean treatment difference = 1.82). Caregivers of donepezil-treated patients also reported spending less time assisting with ADLs than caregivers of placebo-treated patients (mean difference 52.4 minutes per day at week 24 LOCF, $p = 0.004$).

Adverse events were experienced by 83.3% of the donepezil group and 80.1% of the placebo group.The donepezil group had substantially more diarrhoea (12.5% compared to 4.8%), headache (11.8% compared to 4.1%), arthralgia (6.9% compared to 1.4%), nausea (6.9% compared to 4.1%), vomiting (6.9% compared to 2.7%), and weight loss (6.9% compared to 4.1%).Weight loss as a decrease of at least 7% of baseline body weight at any time in the trial occurred in 7% of donepezil- and 8% of placebo-treated patients. There was a single death – it occurred in the donepezil-treated group and was due to myocardial infarction considered unrelated to treatment. Clinically meaningful bradycardia (below 60 beats per minute and a reduction from baseline of at least 20% at any assessment during the trial) was experienced by 1% of the donepezil-treated patients and 7% of those who received placebo. Parkinsonism, as measured by the Unified Parkinsons Disease Rating Scale, occurred insignificantly more frequently in the placebo group ($p = 0.062$).

The economic evaluation (Feldman *et al.*, 2004) used the Canadian Utilization of Services, the CAUST, and evaluated costs for patients and caregivers in each group based on resource utilisation multiplied by the unit prices for each resource. A cost was assigned to unpaid time that caregivers spent assisting the patient with activities of daily living. After adjusting for baseline total costs per patient, the mean total societal cost per patient for the 24-week trial period was donepezil Can$9,904 and placebo Can$10,236.This net cost saving of Can $332 (US$224) included the average 24-week cost of donepezil treatment. Most of the cost-saving with donepezil treatment was due to less use of residential care, and caregivers spending less time assisting patients with daily activities. At the very least, this analysis suggests that donepezil costs were covered by other savings, in the economically developed countries where this study was carried out (Canada, France and Australia).

The analysis of galantamine efficacy in advanced moderate AD (Blesa *et al.*, 2003) was a post hoc analysis. In this study the subject numbers were small and results at 12 months compare the treatment group with an historic rather than concurrent placebo group. The 12 months data are based on those completing a six-month open-label extension to the initial randomised, placebo-controlled, double-blind trial, with consequent survivor effects. For the group with baseline ADAS-Cog above 30 (a higher score indicating more cognitive impairment), there were 69 galantamine-treated and 96 placebo-treated patients. For those with a baseline MMSE of 14 or below, there were 26 galantamine- and 46 placebo-treated patients. These two groups overlapped – they were not mutually exclusive.

At 12 months the ADAS-Cog score had been maintained (i.e. returned to baseline after an initial improvement, of nearly 6 points) in the group with initial ADAS-Cog above 30, and the same cognitive maintenance was also seen in the group with initial MMSE of 14 or below. This compares with a historical placebo group deterioration in the ADAS-Cog of 9 and 10 points respectively, in the two groups. This difference would reflect a clinically significant improvement in cognition.

The DAD deteriorated in those with ADAS-Cog initially above 30 by 6.3 points at 12 months in the galantamine-treated patients compared to 20.3 points in the historic placebo group ($p < 0.001$). It is interesting to compare the six month data, which used a concurrent placebo group, with the six month donepezil data. In the galantamine group the DAD declined by approximately 1 point compared to 7 points in the placebo group; in the donepezil study the declines were 0.74 points and 8.98 in the two respective groups. The results are thus very similar and lend support to the methodology of the galantamine analysis. Again, this maintenance of function, as opposed to decline in the placebo-treated groups, is clinically important and should contribute to a reduction in caregiver burden, although this was not reported on in the galantamine study.

Galantamine was well tolerated in this 'advanced moderate' AD group. Indeed gastrointestinal adverse events had similar or lower rates in those with initial ADAS-Cog above 30 and those with initial MMSE at or below 14 when compared to the total trial population (nausea 27.5% 15.4% and 38.1% respectively, vomiting 10.1%, 11.5% and 18.3% respectively, diarrhoea 17.4%, 23.1% and 18.6% respectively and weight loss 11.6%, 15.4% and 10.5% respectively). This suggests that this more severely demented group are no more prone to common adverse events from therapy than those with milder dementia.

The post hoc analysis of rivastigmine (Doraiswamy *et al.*, 2002) includes 158 patients. This analysis too follows these patients out to 12 months, but compares them with a projected placebo rather than the historical placebo used in the galantamine 12-month analysis. The 158 patients are derived from the 206 with GDS of 5 or above at baseline, who successfully completed the double-blind phase then entered the six-month extension. There was only one patient with a GDS above 5 – the remainder in this analysis were GDS 5.The main reason for dropping out of the double-blind phase was adverse events. The study assesses three treatment groups – those treated in the initial 26 weeks with lower rivastigmine doses(1–4 mg per day),those treated over the first 26 weeks with higher doses (6–12 mg/day),and those initially treated with placebo then crossed over to rivastigmine after 26 weeks. All three groups received 2–12 mg rivastigmine per day after week 26.

In each group the ADAS-Cog declined at week 52, but more so in those initially placebo-treated (5.5 ± 1.42 points).In the initial higher-dose rivastigmine group the ADAS-Cog decline was 1.2 ± 1.29 points and in the initial lower-dose rivastigmine group the ADAS-Cog decline was intermediate (3.4 ± 0.98 points).For all three groups, the ADAS-Cog decline was less than that of the projected 12-month placebo group (12.5 ± 1.6 points) and this difference was significant for each group ($p < 0.001$ for each comparison). The highest initial dose group performed similarly over the 12 months to the two galantamine groups, and the ADAS-Cog difference between the high-dose rivastigmine group and the projected placebo group (11.3 points) was also similar to the difference between the two galantamine groups and the historical placebo (9 and 10 points for each of the two galantamine groups).These similar results may suggest similar treatment efficacy of the two medications, and tends to support the validity of these post hoc analyses.

There is no analysis of other, non-cognitive, endpoints in the rivastigmine study. With respect to safety, the incidence of adverse events in the open-label phase was noted to be similar to that reported in the double-blind phase. During weeks 27 to 52, the main adverse events were gastrointestinal, with nausea experienced by 40%, vomiting 27% and anorexia 25%. These rates were similar to those seen in patients with initially milder AD (GDS below 5), suggesting that those with initially more severe AD are no more prone to (longer-term) adverse events from rivastigmine therapy – a finding similar to that of the galantamine analysis. Laboratory parameters, ECG findings and vital signs were within the normal range and were stable during the week 27–52 stage.

Delay to nursing home admission

Because of the long duration required of studies where admission to nursing home is a primary endpoint, there are as yet no prospective, randomised placebo-controlled trials, but less methodologically rigorous observational trials are very consistent in demonstrating a delay in such admission. These trials, however, suffer a number of potential biases including survivor effects and an associated selective and increasingly large dropout rate as the trial progresses. The first such study (Knopman, 1996) was of patients treated with tacrine and showed higher (therapeutic) doses were associated with a reduced probability of nursing home placement. A further study compared those treated with varying doses of donepezil in clinical trials and open-label extensions and followed them for up to five years (Geldmacher *et al.*, 2003). The four dose groups were 'minimal dose' (less than 5 mg a day at any time), 'early moderate-use' (initially 5 mg a day or above but did not enter an open-label extension, or dropped out early), 'delayed start' (received less than 5 mg daily during a double-blind clinical trial but then received 5 mg or more in the extension) and 'maximal use' (received 5 mg a day or more throughout). There was a clear dose-effect on time to nursing home placement, which was resilient when a number of concerns were factored out of the final analysis using case models (e.g. excluding those who entered nursing home early in the first 48 weeks). In the 'minimal use' group, the median time to first nursing home placement was 44.7 months, compared to 66.1 months in the 'maximal use' group (a difference of 21.4 months). This difference was not statistically significant but the relative risk for nursing home placement was significantly lower in the 'maximal use' group than in the 'minimal use' group.

Whilst delay to nursing home placement does not equate to therapeutic efficacy in severe dementia, it does again suggest a delay in progression to the more severe stages of dementia, and perhaps on-going therapeutic efficacy in those more severe stages. Similar data has been presented for galantamine and rivastigmine in posters, but not published.

Use in nursing home patients

The only cholinesterase inhibitor to be evaluated in a randomised, double-blind, placebo-controlled trial in the nursing home setting is donepezil (Tariot *et al.*, 2001). Other cholinesterase inhibitors have been evaluated in open-label studies but these trials have not been published. The donepezil nursing home study included 208 nursing home patients in the USA. They had a diagnosis of probable or possible AD, or AD with cerebrovascular disease. To be eligible they were required to have a reported frequency of at least one symptom from the NPI-NH occurring at least several times a week. The primary measure of efficacy was the NPI-NH, a modified version of the NPI that has been developed as a tool to assess the neuropsychiatric disturbances exhibited by nursing home residents with dementia. Secondary efficacy measured included the MMSE, CDR-SB and the PSMS. Patients were randomised to donepezil, 5 mg daily for 4 weeks then 10 mg daily if tolerated, or placebo. The study duration was 24 weeks.

At baseline the mean MMSE was 14.4 (range 5–26), reflecting the relatively moderate severity of USA nursing home residents with dementia. By comparison, in a study of Australian and New Zealand nursing home residents with dementia treated with risperidone for behavioural disturbance, the mean MMSE was 5.5 (Brodaty *et al.*, 2003). In the Tariot study one-quarter of patients had an MMSE below 10. Patients completing the 24 weeks of therapy received an average daily dose of 9.5 mg/day during the last four weeks of the study. Some 46 patients discontinued the study, 30 because of adverse events (19 in the placebo group and 11 in the donepezil group). The mean age of all patients was 85.7. Patients had considerable comorbidity at baseline, with over 50% having at least one of musculoskeletal/skin disorders, disorders of the eyes/ears/nose/throat, heart or vascular disease. Eighty two per cent of placebo- and 81% of donepezil-treated patients had at least one comorbid medical condition scored at a severity of at least 2 (moderate disability or morbidity requiring first-line therapy).

The primary efficacy endpoint, the NPI-NH, showed no difference after 24 weeks between the two groups and both improved from baseline. The mean±SE improvements at week 24 endpoint were -4.9 ± 1.9 and -2.3 ± 1.9 for placebo- and donepezil-treated patients, respectively. A planned secondary analysis of changes in behaviour on each category in the NPI-NH revealed a significant difference in response patterns for one item only, agitation/aggression, which favoured donepezil ($p = 0.044$). When considering only patients who had agitation/aggression at baseline, the percentage of patients improving was 46% (29/63) for placebo- and 67% (46/69) for donepezil-treated ($p = 0.017$).

The authors note that both treatment groups improved on the NPI-NH, as opposed to an average decline of almost 4 points in NPI 10-item score in a study of outpatients receiving placebo for 26 weeks (Morris *et al.*, 1998). This difference between placebo-groups in the two studies may have been explained by behavioural management in the nursing home, and extensive use of concomitant pyschotrophics (61% in this trial). The improvement in one category, agitation/aggression, may be explained by testing multiple variables, but if it is a true donepezil effect it is encouraging as it may lead to improvement in patient management and quality of life. However, other approaches (non-pharmacological and pharmacological) may be more appropriate before considering donepezil therapy.

Differences in the mean change from baseline MMSE favoured donepezil at all time-points but were not statistically significantly different at the 24-week endpoint, and did not differ significantly between the two groups at that endpoint. In the subgroup of older patients (≥ 85), those treated with donepezil showed a similar pattern of response on the MMSE to the full population. The MMSE, as noted earlier in this chapter, is less able to show changes in more severely demented people and may not have been an appropriate endpoint in this population.

The CDR-SB total score was significantly improved ($p < 0.05$) compared to placebo at 24 weeks and also improved significantly at week 24 in the subgroup over age 85. This improvement in overall dementia severity, as measured by CDR-SB, in the donepezil-treated group – an effect not lost in the older subgroups – is potentially clinically important. On the PSMS there were no statistically significant differences between the donepezil- and placebo-treated groups at any time-point. This failure of function to improve may have reflected the baseline severity of functional impairment of the total group – for instance 46% were unable to ambulate without assistance. The PSMS differs from the CDR as the latter assigns functional scores based on impairment due to cognitive loss, so is a more reliable measure of function in this setting.

Gastrointestinal adverse events, such as diarrhoea, nausea and anorexia, predictably occurred more frequently in donepezil-treated patients, but the incidence and severity of diarrhoea, vomiting and nausea were similar in subgroups above and below 85 years of age. Weight loss occurred in 19% of the donepezil- and 10% of the placebo-treated patients ($p < 0.05$), and more frequently in the older donepezil-treated patients (23% vs. 10% placebo) than in younger donepezil-treated patients (13% vs. 8% placebo). In those who experienced weight loss as an adverse event, the means loss was 3 kg. These gastrointestinal effects are as expected from a cholinesterase inhibitor and are similar to those seen in outpatient trials in patients with mild to moderate AD. However, the weight loss is concerning in a frail nursing home population, especially as it was more frequent in the older subgroup.

Vital signs were similar for both the donepezil- and placebo-treated groups and showed no significant changes with treatment. Bradycardia, defined as a heart rate of 60 beats per minute and a decrease by at least 20% from baseline at any time-point, occurred in 5% of placebo- and 6% of donepezil-treated patients. Three donepezil- and seven placebo-treated patients died during the study. This suggests the medication was not associated with significant cardiovascular adverse effects, or excess mortality, in this population.

The lack of a significant improvement in the primary endpoint makes this a negative study, but the subanalyses may offer significant insights into the effects of cholinesterase inhibitors in severe AD. This trial has suggested some positive benefits from donepezil therapy in this setting, and shows donepezil has an acceptable safety profile. It is particularly encouraging that those over age 85 seemed to respond similarly to younger patients. Donepezil clearance is unaffected by age (Ohnishi *et al.*, 1993) and the same 10 mg daily target dose seems appropriate in both older and younger people.

Two open-label trials of rivastigmine in nursing home populations have been published in abstract form. One 24-week trial of 173 patients with probable AD was conducted in 13 USA centres (Cummings *et al.*, 2000). The mean baseline MMSE was 9.2, considerably less than in the donepezil trial and more reflective of nursing home populations in other countries. Some 81% of patients had at least one baseline behavioural symptom on the NPI-NH, and the baseline mean score on the NPI-NH was 15.8. After 26 weeks there was an average 3.25-point reduction in the total NPI-NH score, similar to the 2.3-point improvement in the donepezil study. For patients who had behavioural symptoms at baseline and who completed 26 weeks of treatment, 58% demonstrated improvement, with 50% showing an improvement of at least 30%. There was also a slight improvement, of 0.5 points, in the mean MMSE score.

The other nursing home study with rivastigmine (Bullock *et al.*, 2001) was performed in Europe. After 26 weeks of (open-label) treatment 40% of all patients showed at least 30% improvement in total NPI-NH score from baseline, similar to the US study. For patients with behavioural symptoms present at baseline, 53% showed improvement in each of the 12 items of the NPI-NH except depression. Only a minority (not specified) had no symptoms at baseline, and a little over 70% of these did not develop behavioural symptoms during treatment with rivastigmine. There was also a slight improvement (not specified) in cognition over the 24 weeks.

In both these rivastigmine nursing home studies the target dose was 6 mg b.i.d. although it is not specified what percentage achieved this. Safety and tolerability were stated to be reflective of that previously reported with rivastigmine, despite the multiple comorbidities present in these nursing home patients.

Long-term studies

There have been two published double-blind, randomised, placebo-controlled trials on donepezil over 12 months. Whilst these studies were conducted in those with initially mild to moderate AD, it can be expected that over 12 months some patients would have reached a more severe stage of dementia. This is supported by a recent population study, which showed overall survival from time of initial diagnosis of AD was 4.2 years for men and 5.7 years for women (Larson *et al.*, 2004). In a 12-month study conducted in Nordic countries (Winblad *et al.*, 2001), a primary composite end-point called the Gottfries–Brane–Steen scale showed significant improvement in donepezil-treated as opposed to placebo-treated patients. In a separate 12-month study (Mohs *et al.*, 2001) which followed participants to a predetermined level of functional decline, significantly more donepezil- than placebo-treated patients reached 48 weeks without experiencing that decline (51% vs. 35%, $p = 0.002$). Again, the appropriateness of extrapolating these studies to severe dementia is somewhat limited, but they suggest a positive benefit of cholinesterase inhibitors even as dementia becomes more severe.

It is possible that long-term therapy with cholinesterase inhibitors may influence the longer-term symptoms and milestones of AD. A non-randomised, non-blinded study included 135 patients treated with cholinesterase inhibitors,and compared them with 135 patients from the same AD research Centre who were never treated with a cholinesterase inhibitor (Lopez *et al.*, 2002). Over years change in cognitive and functional performance were estimated. The likelihood of arriving at four endpoints was estimated over an average 36.7 months of observation:

(1) MMSE of nine or lower
(2) Blessed dementia rating scale (BDRS) for ADLs of 12 or higher
(3) Nursing home admission
(4) Death

The one-year follow-up data showed a significant effect of time but not of drug use on the MMSE. However, over the 12 months the MMSE rate of change was significantly greater in the non-drug than in the drug users, deteriorating from 18.8 to 14.8 in the non-drug using group, and from 18.7 to 16.3 in the drug-using group. This four-point deterioration in the non-treated group is similar to that of 3.3 seen in a natural untreated population of AD patients (Han *et al.*, 2000) and twice that seen in the treatment group. The treated group showed a significantly lower score on the BDRS at 12 months compared to the untreated group (4.7 versus 7.3) and a significantly lower rate of change ($p < 0.001$) in the treated versus untreated patients. A survivor analysis revealed a greater proportion of patients who never used cholinesterase inhibitors reached any of the four endpoints, including nursing home admission, than the proportion of those who had used such treatment (Table 3).

Whilst this study was not randomised, it does suggest that in a 'real world' population cholinesterase inhibitors may delay progression to more severe AD or to death.

Table 3. Number of patients reaching endpoint

Outcome measure	Patients on ChEI (%)	Patients who never used a ChEI (%)	χ^2(p-value)
Death	17 (13)	52 (39)	23.8 (< 0.0001)
BDRS > 12	35 (26)	62 (46)	13.1 (< 0.0001)
MMSE < 9	38 (28)	67 (49)	11.7 (< 0.001)
Institutionalisation	8 (6)	56 (47)	47.1 (< 0.0001)

BDRS = Blessed Dementia Rating Scale; MMSE = Mini Mental State Examination.

Add-on therapy

No studies have yet evaluated the potential benefits of adding a cholinesterase inhibitor to other therapy. A study on memantine (Tariot *et al.*, 2004) showed a benefit from adding this to established cholinesterase inhibitor therapy in those with more severe dementia, and is described elsewhere in this book. It is possible that, as memantine is increasingly used as initial monotherapy for severe dementia (Winblad and Poritis, 1999; Reisberg *et al.*, 2003), the benefit of secondarily adding a cholinesterase inhibitor will be evaluated. Cholinesterase inhibitors may also be of benefit as add-on therapy to those with severe dementia treated with other agents such as atypical antipsychotics for agitation or psychosis, and to complementary and alternative therapies such as *Ginkgo biloba* – but this remains untested.

Head-to-head studies

There is a need for head-to-head studies of cholinesterase inhibitors in those with severe dementia. Whilst several head-to-head studies have been conducted, the majority of patients had mild to moderate AD, in accordance with local prescribing guidelines and regulations. The only published longer term (12 months) randomised parallel-groups study compared galantamine with donepezil (Wilcock *et al.*, 2003). Raters were blinded to treatment groups, but patients and prescribers were not. This study did not exclude people with more severe dementia and the baseline mean MMSE was 15.1 in the galantamine group ($N = 94$, mean age 74.1) and 14.8 in the donepezil group ($N = 88$, mean age 72.8). This compares with baseline mean MMSE scores of around 19–20 in most trials in mild to moderate AD. There were 13 galantamine-treated and 12 donepezil-treated patients with an initial MMSE below 12, but no analysis of this subgroup was provided. There are analyses of those with baseline MMSE from 12 to 18. Only one patient in each group had a baseline MMSE above 18. It is thus possible to deduce how those with initial MMSE below 12 fared. 71.1% of patients achieved the target of 24 mg daily of galantamine, and 69.2% achieved the target of 10 mg daily donepezil.

The study showed therapeutic equivalence between the two treatment groups on the primary endpoint, the Br ADL, at 52 weeks and as the subgroup with MMSE from 12 to 18 performed similarly to the whole group, it is likely that for those with MMSE initially below 12 there was also no difference between the treatment groups. The MMSE scores remained at baseline, after 52 weeks of galantamine treatment, and declined by 1.6 points in the donepezil group. The differences between groups at 52 weeks whilst clinically insignificant, were statistically significantly different (LOCF analysis) for those with initial MMSE 12–18 ($p < 0.005$), but not for the whole group ($p < 0.1$). It is thus unlikely that galantamine was more effective, as measured by the MMSE, than donepezil in those with initial MMSE below 12. This demonstration of probable therapeutic equivalence was also seen for the NPI. The SCB (caregiver burden scale) showed more than two-thirds of caregivers of galantamine patients reported maintenance or improvement in objective (67.1%, $n = 57$) and subjective (68.3%, $n = 85$) caregiver burden compared with rates of 51.3% ($n = 41$) and 49.4% ($n = 79$), respectively, for caregivers of donepezil patients but no subgroup analysis is provided.

Safety analysis shows similar rates of adverse events in the two groups: 13.4% of galantamine-treated and 13.2% of donepezil-treated patients withdrew because of adverse events. Nausea affected 19.6% of galantamine- and 17.6% of donepezil-treated patients, vomiting 17.5% and 14.3% respectively, agitation 18.6% versus 12.1%, headache 16.5% versus 12.1% and a fall occurred in 16.5% of galantamine- versus 8.8% of donepezil-treated patients.

It would thus seem that there might be little to choose between galantamine and donepezil in the treatment of more severe dementia, although the best trial data to date is from studies with donepezil. The recent availability in some countries of a once-daily preparation of galantamine will increase the convenience of the medication towards that of donepezil, particularly as more severely demented patients may be less compliant with more complicated medication regimes. A long-term, randomised, blinded study comparing rivastigmine with donepezil in more severe dementia has been recently completed and is the only completed head-to-head study in more severe dementia; results are expected soon.

Predictors of response

Given the likely efficacy of cholinesterase inhibitors in the treatment of severe dementia, is it possible to predict response and are there modulators of response? Again, there is almost no data in this more severe group, and even for those with mild to moderate AD it has proved very difficult to predict response. One study has shown that serum cholesterol may modulate the long-term efficacy of cholinesterase inhibitors in AD – probably through to more severe dementia (Borroni *et al.*, 2003). High cholesterol levels correlated with faster decline at one year. This may be related to an effect of high cholesterol on amyloid production (Fassbender *et al.*, 2001, 2002). Studies on the effect of apolipoprotein E states on response to cholinesterase inhibitors have produced variable results and none have specifically looked at severe dementia. Possibly the best marker of response is the severity of the dementia – for instance, the six-month treatment difference of 10 points in the ADAS-Cog in the 'advanced moderate' galantamine trial (Blesa *et al.*, 2003) is almost three times the six-month effect seen in the overall trial in mild to moderate AD.

When and how should a cholinesterase inhibitor be trialled in severe dementia?

In community-residing patients, the above studies suggest it is appropriate to consider a trial of a cholinesterase inhibitor whatever the severity of AD. The main goals may be to improve behaviour or function, to reduce caregiver burden or to delay nursing home admission. The main contraindications are as for mild to moderate AD – severe bradycardia, severe asthma and active peptic ulceration. Also, the medication may need to be ceased in the presence of severe adverse effects that do not settle with time and supportive therapy (e.g. slower dose titration or anti-emetic drugs for nausea and vomiting). It is reassuring, however, that adverse affects do not seem to be more common in more severely demented people. Intolerance of one cholinesterase inhibitor does not necessarily mean that another will not be tolerated. There is no need to routinely use a slower titration up to target dose in more severely demented people. Also, the above studies do not suggest that a cholinesterase inhibitor should be ceased as dementia progresses to more severe stages.

In a residential care population, including those in nursing homes, one may choose to be more circumspect in initiating a cholinesterase inhibitor. Cessation of such therapy upon entering such care may lead to a decline which may not be fully reversible upon reintroducing the medication and so cannot be justified as a routine practice. Cognitive improvement may not be a primary goal of therapy. Behavioural disturbances should initially be managed non-pharmacologically but, if persistent, a cholinesterase inhibitor should be considered, either as initial therapy or after antipsychotic and related agents have been trialled. In the donepezil nursing home study only agitation/aggression responded better to donepezil than placebo, and this may be first treated pharmacologically with an atypical antipsychotic such as risperidone. However, recent concerns about the safety of atypical antipsychotic agents (CSM, 2004; FDA, 2005) may sway the prescriber to a trial of a cholinesterase inhibitor first. It is also possible that a cholinesterase inhibitor may prevent the emergence of unwanted behaviours but in placebo-controlled published trials this has to date only been shown with mild to moderate AD (Trinh et al., 2003; Cummings, 2004). The donepezil nursing home study showed no benefits of such therapy on function so function may not be an appropriate target in this functionally impaired population. If a cholinesterase inhibitor is used, careful attention should be paid to the patient's weight as the weight loss reported in the donepezil nursing home study is of some concern.

Most clinicians would agree that it is not appropriate to initiate cholinesterase inhibitors in those with end-stage dementia. Patients who are immobile and incontinent and have very limited or no language as a result of severe Alzheimer's disease are unlikely to benefit from such therapy. However, progressively more patients are reaching this stage of their illness after long periods of cholinesterase inhibitor therapy, and withdrawal of therapy may be seen as a sign of abandonment by the physician – in this case, on-going therapy may be appropriate even though providing no benefit to the more usual endpoints. A frank end-of-life discussion with relatives and other carers should, however, routinely include the option of ceasing the cholinesterase inhibitor.

Future developments

There is an identified need for more studies of cholinesterase inhibitors in severely demented people across a range of settings, as monotherapy, as add-on therapy and in those who have inadequately responded to other therapies such as memantine. One randomised controlled study of donepezil as monotherapy for community-dwelling people with severe dementia is in progress in the USA. We also need better markers and predictors of therapeutic efficacy. It is possible that neuroimaging (e.g. FDG-PET) and other markers such as CSF-Aβ and tau levels (Stefanova et al., 2003) may be useful predictors and markers of clinical response, as well as useful endpoints in research trials. Other assessment scales may also become more routinely used to evaluate a severely demented individual's response – these may include the SIB or other more specific scales not yet used in trials in severe dementia such as the EXIT-25, an assessment of executive function (Royall et al., 1992). Pending this extra information the use of cholinesterase inhibitors in severely demented people appears to be justified and may well be beneficial to an individual.

References

Arendt T, Buckner MK, Lange M, Bigl V (1992) Changes in acetylcholinesterase and butyrylcholinesterase in Alzheimer's disease resemble embryonic development- a study of molecular forms. *Neurochem Int*, 21:381–96.

Blesa R, Davidson M, Kurz A, et al. (2003) Galantamine provides sustained benefits in patients with 'advanced moderate' Alzheimer's disease for at least 12 months. *Dementia and Geriatric Cognitive Disorders*, 15:79–87.

Borroni B, Pettenati C, Bordonali T, et al. (2003) Serum cholesterol levels modulate long-term efficacy of cholinesterase inhibitors in Alzheimer's disease. *Neuroscience Letters*, 343:213–215.

Brodaty H, Ames D, Snowdon J, et al. (2003) A randomized placebo-controlled trial of risperidone for the treatment of aggression, agitation and psychosis of dementia. *Journal of Clinical Psychiatry*, 64:134–143.

Bullock R, (2004) Cholinesterase inhibitors and vascular dementia:another string to their bow?. *CNS Drugs*, 18:79–92.

Bullock R, Moulias R, Steinwachs KC, *et al.* (2001) Effects of rivastigmine on behavioural symptoms in nursing home patients with Alzheimer's disease: a European,open-label,multi-centre study [abstract]. *International Psychogeriatrics*, 13(Suppl 2): P. 248.

Coen RF, Swanwick GRJ, O'Boyle CA, Coakley D (1997) Behavioural disturbance and other predictors of carer burden in Alzheimer's disease. *International Journal of Geriatric Psychiatry*, 12:331–336.

Craig AH, Cummings JL, Fairbanks L, Itti L, Miller BI, *et al.* (1996) Cerebral blood flow correlates of apathy in Alzheimer disease. *Archives of Neurology*, 53:1116–1120.

CSM (2004) Atypical antipsychotic drugs and stroke: message from Professor Gordon Duff, Chairman, Committee on Safety of Medicines (CEM/CMO/2004/1).

Cummings J, Anand R, Koumaras B, *et al.* (2000) Rivastigmine provides behavioural benefits in AD patients residing in a nursing home:findings from a 26-week trial [abstract]. *Neurology*, 54:A468.

Cummings JL, Back C, (1998) The cholinergic hypothesis of neuropsychiatric symptoms in Alzheimer's disease. *American Journal of Geriatric Psychiatry*, 6(Suppl. 1):S64–S78.

Cummings JL (2004) Drug therapy: Alzheimer's disease. *New England Journal of Medicine*, 351:56–57.

Davis KL, Mohs RC, Marin D, *et al.* (1999) Cholinergic markers in elderly patients with early signs of Alzheimer's disease. *Journal of American Medical Association*, 281:1401–1406.

De Kosky ST, Ikonomovic MD, Styren SD, *et al.* (2002) Up regulation of choline acetyltransferase activity in hippocampus and frontal cortex of elderly subjects with mild cognitive impairment. *Annals of Neurology*, 51:145–155.

Doraiswamy PM, Krishan KRR, Anand R, *et al.* (2002) Long-termeffects of rivastigmine in moderately severe alzheimer's disease. Does early initiation of therapy offer sustained benefits? *Progress in Neuro-Psychopharmacology and Biological Psychiatry*, 26:705–712.

Erkinjuntti T, Roman G, Gauthier S, Feldman H, Rockwood K (2004) Emerging therapies for vascular dementia and vascular cognitive impairment. *Stroke*, 35:1010–1017.

Fassbender K, Simons M, Bergmann C, *et al.* (2001) Simvastatin strongly reduces level of Alzheimer's disease beta-amyloid peptides A beta 42 and A beta 40 in vitro and in vivo. *Proceedings of the National Academy of Sciences USA*, 98:5856–5861.

Fassbender K, Stroick M, Bertsch T, *et al.* (2002) Effects of statins on human cerebral cholesterol metabolism and secretions of Alzheimer's amyloid peptide. *Neurology*, 59:1257–1258.

FDA (2005) At http://www.fda.gov/cder/drug/advisory/antipsychotics.htm

Feldman H, Gauthier MD, Hecker J, *et al.* (2001a) A 24-week, randomized, double-blind study of donepezil in moderate to severe Alzheimer's disease. *Neurology*, 57:613–620.

Feldman H, Sauter A, Donald A, *et al.* (2001b) A 12-month study of functional ability in mild to moderate severity Alzheimer's disease. *Alzheimer's Disease and Associated Disorders*, 15:89–95.

Feldman H, Gauthier S, Hecker J, *et al.*, (2003) Efficacy of donepezil on maintenance of activities of daily living in patients with moderate to severe Alzheimer's disease and the effect on caregiver burden. *Journal of the American Geriatrics Society*, 51:737–744.

Feldman H, Gauthier S, Hecker, J, *et al.* (2004) Economic evaluation of donepezil in moderate to severe Alzheimer disease. *Neurology*, 63:644–50.

Gauthier S, Feldman H, Hecker J, *et al.* (2002) Efficacy of donepezil on behavioural symptoms in patients with moderate to severe Alzheimer's disease. *International Psychogeriatrics*, 14:389–404.

Geldmacher DS, Provenzano G, McRae T, Mastey V, Ieni JR (2003) Donepezil is associated with delayed nursing home placement in patients with Alzheimer's disease. *Journal of the American Geriatrics Society*, 51:937–944.

Han L, Cole M, Bellavance F, McCusker J, Primeau F (2000) Tracking cognitive decline in Alzheimer's disease using the Mini-Mental State Examination:a meta-analysis. *International Psychogeriatrics*, 12:231–247.

Haupt M, Kurz A (1993) Predictors of nursing home placement in patients with Alzheimer's disease. *International Journal of Geriatric Psychiatry*, 8:741–746.

Haupt M, Kurz A, Jänner M (2000) A 2-year follow-up of behavioural and psychological symptoms in Alzheimer's diseasse. *Dementia and Geriatric Cognitive Disorders*, 11:147–152.

Hecker JR, Snellgrove CA (2003) Pharmacological Management of Alzheimer's disease. *Journal of Pharmacy Practice and Research*, 33:24–29.

Hope T, Keene J, Gedling K, Fairburn CG, Jacoby R (1998) Predictors of institutionalization for people with dementia living at home with a carer. *International Journal of Geriatric Psychiatry*, 13:682–690.

Jones RW (2003) Have cholinergic therapies reached their clinical boundary in Alzheimer's disease?. *International Journal of Geriatric Psychiatry*, 18:S7–S13.

Kaufer RI, Catt K, Pollock DG, Lopez OM, DeKosky ST (1998) Donepezil in Alzheimer's disease: relative cognitive and neuropsychiatric responses and impact on caregiver distress. *Neurology*, 50:A89.

Knopman D, Schneider L, Davis K, *et al.* (1996) Long term tacrine (Cognex) treatment. Effects on nursing home placement and mortality. *Neurology*, 47:166–177.

Lanctôt KL, Herrmann N, Yau K, *et al.* (2003) Efficacy and safety of cholinesterase inhibitors in Alzheimer's disease: a meta-analysis. *Canadian Medical Association Journal*, 169:557–64.

Larson B, Shadlen M-F, Wang L, *et al.* (2004) Survival after initial diagnosis of Alzheimer's disease. *Annals of Internal Medicine*, 140:501–509.

Lopez OL, Becker JT, Wisniewski S, *et al.* (2002) Cholinesterase inhibitor treatment alters the natural history of Alzheimer's disease. *Journal of Neurology, Neurosurgery and Psychiatry*, 72:310–314.

McKeith I, Del Ser T, Spano P, *et al.* (2000) Efficacy of rivastigmine in dementia with Lewy bodies:a randomised,double-blind,placebo-controlled international study. *Lancet*, 356:2031–2036.

Mega MS, Cummings JL, Fiorello T, Gorbein J (1996) The spectrum of behavioural changes in Alzheimer's disease. *Neurology*, 46:130–135.

Mega MS, Masterman DM, O'Connor SM, Barclay TR, Cummings JL (1999) The spectrum of behavioural responses to cholinesterase inhibitor therapy in Alzheimer's disease. *Archives of Neurology*, 56:1388–1393.

Minger SL, Esiri MM, McDonald B, *et al.* (2000) Cholinergic deficits contribute to behavioural disturbances in patients with dementia. *Neurology*, 55:1460–1467.

Mohs R, Doody RS, Morris JC, *et al.* (2001) A one-year placebo-controlled preservation of function survival study of donepezil in AD patients. *Neurology*, 57:481–488.

Morris JC, Cyrus PA, Orazem J, *et al.* (1998) Metrifonate benefits cognitive, behavioural and global function in patients with Alzheimer's disease. *Neurology*, 50:1222–1230.

Ogura H, Kosasa T, Kuriga Y, *et al.* (2000) Comparison of inhibitory activities of donepezil and other cholinesterase inhibitors on acetylcholinesterase and butyrylcholinesterase in vitro. *Methods and Findings in Experimental and Clinical Pharmacology*, 22:609–613.

Ohnishi A, Mihara M, Kamaskura H, *et al.* (1993) Comparison of the pharmacokinetics of E2020, a new compound for Alzheimer's disease, in healthy young and elderly subjects. *Journal of Clinical Pharmacology*, 33:1086–1091.

Perry EK, Perry RH, Blessed G, *et al.* (1977) Necropsy evidence of central cholinergic deficits in senile dementia *Lancet*, 1:189.

Polinsky RJ (1998) Clinical pharmacology of rivastigmine:a new generation acetylcholinesterase inhibitor for the treatment of Alzheimer's disease. *Clinical Therapeutics*, 20:634–647.

Reisberg B, Ferris SH, de Leon MJ, Crook T (1982) The Global Deterioration Scale for assessment of primary degenerative dementia. *American Journal of Geriatric Psychiatry*, 139:1136–1139.

Reisberg B, Franssen EH, Bobinsk M, *et al.* (1996) Overview of methodologic issues for pharmacological trials in mild, moderate and severe Alzheimer's disease. *International Psychogeriatrics*, 8:159–193.

Reisberg B, Doody R, Stöffler A, *et al.* (2003) Memantine in moderate-to-severe Alzheimer's disease. *New England Journal of Medicine*, 348:1333–1341.

Ritchie CW, Ames D, Clayton T, Lai R (2004) Meta-analysis of randomized trials of the efficacy and safety of donepezil, galantamine, and rivastigmine for the treatment of Alzheimer's disease. *American Journal of Geriatric Psychiatry*, 12:358–69.

Rockwood K, Graham JE, Fay S, Acadie Investigators (2002) Goal setting and attainment in Alzheimer's disease patients treated with donepezil. *Journal of Neurology, Neurosurgery and Psychiatry*, 73:500–507.

Royall DR, Mahurin RK, Gray K (1992) Bedside assessment of executive dyscontrol:The Executive Interview(EXIT 25). *Journal of the American Geriatrics Society*, 40:1221–1226.

Schmeidler J, Mohs RC, Aryan M (1998) Relationships of disease severity to decline on specific cognitive and functional measures in Alzheimer's disease. *Alzheimer's Disease and Associated Disorders*, 12:146–151.

Stefanova E, Blennow K, Almkvist O, Hellström-Lindahl E, Nordberg A (2003) Cerebral glucose metabolism, cerebrospinal fluid $-\beta$-amyloid 1-42 (CSF-Aβ42), tau and apolipoprotein E genotype in long-term rivastigmine and tacrine treated Alzheimer's disease (AD) patients. *Neuroscience Letters*, 338:159-163.

Sultzer DL, Mahler ME, Mandelkern MI (1995) The relationship between psychiatric symptoms and regional cortical metabolism in Alzheimer's disease. *Journal of Neuropsychiatry and Clinical Neuroscience*, 7:476–484.

Tariot PN, Cummings JL, Katz IR, *et al.* (2001) A randomized, double-blind, placebo-controlled study of the efficacy and safety of donepezil in patients with Alzheimer's disease in the nursing home setting. *Journal of the American Geriatrics Society*, 49:1590–1599.

Tariot PN, Farlow MR, Grossberg GT, *et al.* (2004) Memantine treatment in patients with moderate to severe Alzheimer's disease already receiving donepezil: a randomized controlled trial. *Journal of the American Medical Association*, 291:317–324.

Teri L (1997) Behaviour and caregiver burden: behavioural problems in patients with Alzheimer's disease and its association with caregiver distress. *Alzheimer's Disease and Associated Disorders*, 11(Suppl. 4): S35–S38.

Trinh N-H, Hoblyn J, Mohanty S, Yaffe K (2003) Efficacy of cholinesterase inhibitors in the treatment of neuropsychiatric symptoms and functional impairment in Alzheimer's disease. A metaanalysis. *Journal of the American Medical Association*, 289:210–216.

Wilcock G, Howe I, Coles H, *et al.* (2003) A long-term comparison of galantamine and donepezil in the treatment of Alzheimer's disease. *Drugs and Ageing*, 20:777–789.

Winblad B, Poritis N (1999) Memantine in severe dementia: results of the 9M-Best Study (Benefit and efficacy in severely demented patients during treatment with memantine). *International Journal of Geriatric Psychiatry*, 14:135–146.

Winblad B, Engedal K, Soininen H, *et al.* (2001) A one year randomized, placebo-controlled, study of donepezil in patients with mild to moderate AD. *Neurology*, 57:489–495.

12

Drug Treatment: Treatment of Behavioural and Psychological Symptoms of Dementia with Neuroleptics

Peter Paul De Deyn

Introduction

Dementia, regardless of its cause, is a clinical syndrome that expresses itself in three domains: (1) neuropsychological, or cognitive deficits such as memory loss, aphasia, apraxia, and agnosia; (2) psychiatric and behavioural disturbances, also known as behavioural and psychological symptoms of dementia (BPSD); and (3) difficulties in carrying out activities of daily living. The incidence of dementia generally increases, leading to growing humanitarian and economic concerns for countries with ageing populations. Treatment of behavioural and psychological symptoms of dementia should follow the following process: first, to identify and whenever possible treat the cause; second, to use non-pharmacological treatment techniques; and third, to try medication that modulates behavioural disturbances and neurospychiatric symptomatology.

Until recently, the main focus of pharmacological research related to dementia was on the improvement of cognitive functioning. However, BPSD are among the most predominant and pervasive features of dementia, and increasingly form a target for therapeutic intervention in this cognitively impaired population (Reisberg *et al.*, 1986, 1987; Jost and Grossberg, 1996). Aggression and other behavioural symptoms of dementia (e.g. agitation, purposeless activity, wandering, pacing and psychotic symptoms) are important features of the illness and have a severe impact on the quality of life of patients and caregivers, thus complicating effective medical management (Reisberg *et al.*, 1987; Tariot *et al.*, 1994, 1995). Behavioural symptoms have been described as the primary predictor of caregiver burden (Coen *et al.*, 1997; Donaldson *et al.*, 1997; McKhann, 1984). In fact, the behavioural symptoms of dementia (in particular, aggression and agitation) may be the most common reason for patients being admitted to hospital or residential care (Ferris *et al.*, 1987).

A variety of pharmacological agents have been evaluated for the treatment of BPSD, including cholinergic agents, anticonvulsants, antidepressants, anxiolytics, hormonal preparations and neuroleptic drugs. Unfortunately, the reports often rely on anecdotal observations and/or open-label clinical trials (Porsteinsson *et al.*, 1997; Mintzer *et al.*, 1998).

Neuroleptics have been studied more intensively than other agents. Until the mid-1990s, conventional neuroleptic drugs such as haloperidol were the primary pharmacological treatment for BPSD. Although available evidence supports the efficacy of the conventional neuroleptics, side effects, including the risk of irreversible movement disorders, extrapyramidal symptoms (EPS), anticholinergic effects and adverse drug interactions, are particularly problematic in this elderly patient population (Schneider *et al.*, 1990).

Severe Dementia. Edited by A. Burns and B. Winblad.
Copyright © 2006 John Wiley & Sons, Ltd.   ISBN 0-470-01054-1

Recent research has assessed the effects of the newer generation of atypical antipsychotic drugs on BPSD. When compared with conventional neuroleptics, these drugs are associated with significantly fewer extrapyramidal side effects (Jeste *et al.*, 1999a) and a lower incidence of tardive dyskinesia in elderly patients (Jeste *et al.*, 1999b). Nevertheless, recent analysis indicated increased incidence of cerebrovascular adverse events with atypical antipsychotics in this patient population. In this chapter, we will focus on the treatment of neuropsychiatric symptoms of dementia. Major advances have been achieved during the previous decade in the field of Alzheimer's disease which will therefore be the main topic of this chapter. Nevertheless, whenever applicable, we will also refer to other dementias such as vascular dementia, mixed dementia and Parkinson's disease dementia. We will not give a review of all published clinical trials or substances investigated in this field, nor present formal guidelines.

First, we will give a general description of efficacy and safety of typical and atypical antipsychotic agents in the treatment of neuropsychiatric symptoms of dementia. In this section, we will further elaborate on the safety profile of the atypical antipsychotics in view of the recent safety warnings related to those substances in this indication.

Secondly, we will give a rather detailed overview of the available data on atypical antipsychotics in BPSD; BPSD with aggression; dementia with psychosis, agitation and aggression; and finally in psychosis of AD (PAD). This section illustrates the evolution in the clinical pharmacological research in this field and also contains a brief overview of frequently used outcome measures.

In a third section we briefly refer to indicative data related to atypical antipsychotics and their potential benefit on sleep disturbances associated to dementia.

General description of efficacy and safety of typical and atypical antipsychotics

Antipsychotics are active on psychotic signs, agitation and aggressive behaviour when they are subtended by a delusional process. The meta-analysis by Schneider *et al.* in 1990 (Schneider *et al.*, 1990) revealed the poor efficacy of conventional neuroleptics versus placebo (18%) and their poor tolerability in dementia: disabling extrapyramidal effects related to the action of dopaminergic D2 receptor inhibition, confusion, risk of urinary retention and constipation (especially with phenothiazines) (Schneider, 1996). The impact of these products on acceleration of cognitive decline has subsequently been demonstrated on several occasions (McShane *et al.*, 1997; Bennet *et al.*, 1992; De Deyn *et al.*, 1999). Hypersensitivity to neuroleptics related to dopaminergic D2 receptor dysregulation has also been demonstrated in Lewy body dementia, the second most frequent cause of degenerative dementia in the elderly (Piggott *et al.*, 1998).

Benzamides such as tiapride appear to have fewer harmful effects; at low doses (less than 300 mg/day), this molecule is useful in states of agitation with or without aggressive behaviour related to AD (Robert and Allain, 2001). Based on limited data (duration of treatment of 21 days), this product appears to be well tolerated in terms of motor and cognitive functions (Allain *et al.*, 2000). In an earlier RCT, tiapride administered at a dose of 400 mg/day was as effective and safe as melperone 100 mg/day in the treatment of restlessness in dementia (Gutzmann *et al.*, 1997).

The new-generation antipsychotics, whose serotoninergic-blocking action predominates over the dopaminergic action, may be very useful in the treatment of psychotic signs with associated behavioural disorders, as they present fewer side effects, especially extrapyramidal effects related to dopaminergic inhibition particularly of the nigrostriatal pathway (Jeste *et al.*, 1999a). Clozapine, one of the most extensively studied atypicals in Parkinsonian psychoses, is not recommended in AD because its adverse effects, especially the risk of neutropaenia, limit the prescription.

Published placebo-controlled, double-blind studies in neuropsychiatric symptoms of dementia are available for risperidone, olanzapine and aripiprazole (Katz *et al.*, 1999; De Deyn *et al.*, 1999, 2004; Jeste *et al.*, 2000; Street *et al.*, 2000; Clark *et al.*, 2001, De Deyn *et al.*, in press a).

Risperidone at dosages of 0.25 mg to 1 mg per day has a demonstrated efficacy in the treatment of the psychotic signs, agitation and aggressive behaviour of AD (Katz *et al.*, 1999; De Deyn *et al.*, 1999). Although it induces fewer extrapyramidal effects than haloperidol (De Deyn *et al.*, 1999), at higher doses it causes extrapyramidal effects without being more effective. Like clozapine, it can induce clinically significant extrapyramidal effects in patients with Lewy body dementia (Jeste *et al.*, 2000). On the other hand, short-term use of risperidone (mean dosage, 1.1 mg per day) was found to improve the psychotic symptoms of patients with PD who have dopamine-induced psychosis without adversely affecting the symptoms of PD (Mohr *et al.*, 2000).

The second atypical antipsychotic agent that has been demonstrated to have beneficial effects in the treatment of BPSD, is olanzapine (Street *et al.*, 2000; Clark *et al.*, 2001; Edell and Tunis, 2001; De Deyn *et al.*, 2004). Street *et al.* (2000) conducted a multi-centre, double-blind, placebo-controlled, six-week study in 206 elderly US nursing home residents with AD who exhibited psychotic and/or behavioural symptoms. Patients were randomly assigned to placebo or a fixed dose of 5, 10 or 15 mg/d of olanzapine. The primary efficacy measure was the sum of the Agitation/ Aggression, Hallucinations, and Delusions items (Core Total) of the Neuropsychiatric Inventory – Nursing Home version. Low-dosages of olanzapine (5 and 10 mg/d) produced significant improvement compared with placebo while 15 mg/d failed to do so. The Occupational Disruptiveness score, reflecting the impact of patients' psychosis and behavioural disturbances on the caregiver, was significantly reduced in the 5-mg/d olanzapine group compared with placebo. Somnolence was significantly more common among patients receiving olanzapine (25.0–35.8%), and gait disturbance occurred in those receiving 5 or 15 mg/d (19.6% and 17.0%, respectively). No significant cognitive impairment, increase in extrapyramidal symptoms, or central anticholinergic effects were found at any olanzapine dose relative to placebo.

While 5 and 10 mg a day were initially shown to be efficacious (Street *et al.*, 2000), a later trial indicated that 7.5 mg a day had a beneficial effect (De Deyn *et al.*, 2004). Olanzapine was again shown to have a lower risk of extrapyramidal side effects, but was found to possibly have a more harmful impact on cognitive functions owing to its sedative effect, which was shown in some but not all trials.

Recently, the novel antipsychotic agent aripiprazole, a partial agonist at dopamine D_2 receptors, has been shown to be beneficial in the control of psychotic symptoms in outpatients and inpatients with AD psychosis (De Deyn *et al.*, in press a; Streim *et al.*, 2004; Breder *et al.*, 2004).

Although atypical antipsychotics are generally accepted to have a more favourable safety profile – substantially lower risk of extrapyramical symptoms, substantially lower risk of tardive dyskinesia, less or no anticholinergic side effects, better tolerated in patients with BPSD, Lewy body dementia and Parkinson's disease, less cognitive impairment – than typical antipsychotics (Bullock and Saharan, 2002), analyses of large data sets of a series of randomised clinical trials comparing atypicals to placebo have raised some concerns with regard to increased mortality and incidence of cerebrovascular adverse events.

Initial analyses on pooled datasets have indeed shown increased risks for cerebrovascular adverse events (CAEs) under treatment with olanzapine, risperidone and aripiprazole. Based on six double-blind, placebo-controlled clinical trials in elderly patients with dementia (including the three represented in this publication, one currently being evaluated, one small pilot trial, and one terminated early), an increased risk for CAEs was observed with risperidone treatment. Results from these studies showed a threefold increased risk of CAEs, including stroke as well as transient ischaemic attacks, with risperidone (3.3%) compared to placebo (1.2%) (Wooltorton, 2004a; Greenspan *et al.*, 2003). A comparable three-fold increased risk of CAEs in elderly patients with dementia was observed with olanzapine as well (Wooltorton, 2004b; Zyprexa (olanzapine) US prescribing information, 2004).

Recently the FDA shared the results of a meta-analysis on overall mortality of 17 placebo-controlled clinical trials ($n = 5106$) (http://www.fda.gov/bbs/topics/ANSWERS/2005/ANS01350. html, as accessed on April 11, 2005) including four atypical antipsychotics (aripiprazole, olanzapine, quetiapine, and risperidone) in elderly patients with dementia-related psychosis. FDA requested that the manufacturers of all of these kinds of drugs add a boxed warning to their drug labelling describing this risk and noting that these drugs are not approved for the treatment of behavioural symptoms in elderly patients with dementia. Patients receiving these drugs for treatment of behavioural disorders associated with dementia should have their treatment reviewed by their health care providers. In these analyses of 17 placebo-controlled studies of four drugs in the class of atypical antipsychotics, the rate of death for those elderly patients with dementia was about 1.6 to 1.7 times that of placebo. Although the causes of death were varied, most seemed to be either heart-related (such as heart failure or sudden death) or from infections (pneumonia). The atypical antipsychotics fall into three drug classes based on their chemical structure. Because the increase in mortality was seen with atypical antipsychotic medications in all three chemical classes, the agency has concluded that the effect is probably related to the common pharmacologic effects of all atypical antipsychotic medications, including those that have not been studied in the dementia population. In addition, the agency is considering adding a warning to the labelling of older antipsychotic medications because limited data also suggest a similar increase in mortality for these drugs. The review of the data on these older drugs, however, is still on-going according to the April 11 2005 FDA note. An overall 4.5% incidence of mortality for atypical antipsychotics versus 2.6% for placebo was observed in the combined dataset of the 17 included placebo-controlled clinical trials.

In the six included clinical dementia trials of risperidone ($n = 1,721$), one of the best-studied antipsychotics in this indication, the incidence of mortality during or within 30 days after the trial end was 4.0% with risperidone and 3.1% with placebo (Katz *et al.*, 2005). The mortality incidences for evaluated trials were 3.5% vs. 1.5% for olanzapine vs. placebo and 3.9% vs. 1.7% for aripiprazole vs. placebo.

In order to assess the risk of strokes associated to the usage of atypical antipsychotics and other drugs often used in this indication, two retrospective cohort studies in dementia patients have been conducted. Herrmann *et al.*, (2004) conducted a retrospective, population-based cohort study of patients over the age of 66 by linking administrative health care databases. Three cohorts – users of typical antipsychotics, risperidone, and olanzapine – were compared. Subjects treated with typical antipsychotics ($N = 1,015$) were compared with those given risperidone ($N = 6,964$) and olanzapine ($N = 3,421$). On the basis of epidemiological studies, the authors stated it was likely that the majority of the antipsychotic users were treated for dementia and not schizophrenia-related behaviours. Model-based estimates adjusted for covariates hypothesised to be associated with stroke risk revealed relative risk estimates of 1.1 (95% CI = 0.5–2.3) for olanzapine and 1.4 (95% CI = 0.7–2.8) for risperidone. The authors concluded that olanzapine and risperidone use were not associated with a statistically significant increased risk of stroke compared with typical antipsychotic use. However, assuming for example the relative risk of stroke in risperidone-treated patients was 1.4, this would translate into approximately two extra strokes per thousand patient-years.

In their retrospective, population-based cohort study, Gill *et al.* (2005) compared the incidence of admissions to hospital for stroke among older adults with dementia receiving atypical or typical antipsychotics (17,845 dispensed an atypical antipsychotic and 14,865 dispensed a typical antipsychotic). Main outcome measure was admission to hospital with the most responsible diagnosis (single most important condition responsible for the patient's admission) of ischaemic stroke. After adjustment for potential confounders, participants receiving atypical antipsychotics showed no significant increase in risk of ischaemic stroke compared with those receiving typical antipsychotics (adjusted hazard ratio 1.01, 95% confidence interval 0.81 to 1.26). This finding was consistent in a series of subgroup analyses, including ones of individual atypical antipsychotic drugs (risperidone, olanzapine and quetiapine) and selected subpopulations of the main cohorts.

Atypical antipsychotics in BPSD; BPSD with aggression; dementia with psychosis, agitation and aggression; and PAD

Table 1 lists the published large Phase III RCTs evaluating efficacy and safety of atypical antipsychotics. A series of reliable and sensitive scales have been applied in order to demonstrate clinical efficacy and safety of pharmacological agents in the treatment of BPSD (De Deyn and Wirshing, 2001). The Behaviour Pathology in Alzheimer's Disease Rating Scale BEHAVE-AD is a 25-item scale that measures behavioural symptoms in a total of seven clusters: paranoid and delusional ideation; hallucinations; activity symptoms; aggressiveness; diurnal rhythm symptoms; affective symptoms; anxieties and phobias (Reisberg *et al.*, 1987). All items are scored on a four-point scale of increasing severity. The BEHAVE-AD global score is a measure of behaviour deemed to be disturbing or dangerous to the patient or to those in their environment. The Cohen–Mansfield Agitation Inventory (CMAI) is a rating scale used in nursing homes to assess a total of 29 agitated behaviours on a seven-point scale of increasing frequency (Cohen–Mansfield *et al.*, 1989). The cluster scores include physical, verbal and total aggression, and physical, verbal and total non-aggressive scores. CGI ratings by the investigator measured behavioural symptoms on a seven-point scale of increasing severity. The Neuropsychiatric Inventory (NPI) scores a somewhat wide range of psychopathology and may help distinguish between different causes of dementia. It also records severity and frequency separately. The behavioural disturbances assessed by the NPI (Cummings *et al.*, 1994) are delusions, hallucinations, agitation, dysphoria, anxiety, apathy, irritability, euphoria, disinhibition, aberrant motor behaviour, nighttime behaviour disturbances and appetite and eating abnormalities. The Brief Psychiatric Rating Scale (BPRS; Overall and Gorham, 1962) consists of 18 items, each rated on a scale from 1 (symptom not present) to 7 (symptom extremely severe). It allows a rapid assessment of global psychiatric symptomatology. The Clinical Global Impression of Change scale (CGI-C; National Institute of Mental Health 1976), a global patient-status rating scale ranging from 1 to 7 (1 referring to marked improvement and 7 corresponding to marked worsening).

The first phase III clinical trials evaluating efficacy and safety of atypical antipsychotics in dementia focused on BPSD in general, resulting in rather heterogeneous groups with a variety of behavioural and psychological symptoms (De Deyn *et al.*, 1999; Katz *et al.*, 1999). Later trials included patients with BPSD and aggression (Brodaty *et al.*, 2003) and patients with psychosis, agitation and aggression in AD (Street *et al.*, 2000).

Post hoc analyses of data on subpopulations from some of the abovementioned studies, have been performed. A post hoc analysis of a subgroup of Alzheimer's disease patients with PAD, from a clinical trial that originally included dementia patients with more general BPSD (Katz *et al.*, 1999) demonstrated significant reductions in the severity of psychosis with fixed doses of risperidone (1 or 2 mg), compared to placebo (Schneider *et al.*, 2003; Grossman *et al.*, 2004). Brodaty *et al.* (in press) performed a post hoc analysis of efficacy and safety of low-dose risperidone in treating psychosis of Alzheimer's disease (AD) and mixed dementia (MD) in a subset of nursing-home dementia patients suffering from more general behavioural and psychological symptoms associated with dementia that participated in a controlled clinical trial of risperidone for aggression (Brodaty *et al.*, 2003). This post hoc analysis included only patients diagnosed with AD or MD with psychosis, defined by a score of ≥ 2 on any item of the Behavioural Pathology of Alzheimer's Disease (BEHAVE-AD) psychosis subscale at both screening and baseline. Co-primary efficacy endpoints were changes in scores on BEHAVE-AD psychosis subscale and Clinical Global Impression of Change (CGI-C). Mean change at endpoint in BEHAVE-AD psychosis subscale with risperidone was superior to placebo (-5.2 vs. -3.3; $P = 0.039$). Distribution of CGI-C at endpoint also favoured risperidone ($P < 0.001$). At endpoint, 59% of risperidone-treated patients were responders (i.e. were 'very much' or 'much' improved) compared with 26% of patients receiving placebo. The mean risperidone dose was 1.03 ± 0.61 mg/day.

Table 1. Trial design, selection criteria and primary efficacy assessments for the individual placebo-controlled, double-blind clinical trials on atypical antipsychotics (published or in press) on neuropsychiatric symptoms in (severe) dementia

Trial	Trial design	Patients (n)	Inclusion criteria (behaviour)	Dosing schedule	Primary efficacy assessment	Patient characteristics
Katz et al., 1999	12-week, Phase IIIA, double-blind, placebo-controlled, parallel-group	RIS: 462 PLA: 163	A score of at least 1 on the global rating of the BEHAVE-AD and a total of at least 8 on the BEHAVE-AD total score	Fixed dose of 0.25, 0.5 and 1.0 mg tablets b.i.d.	30% improvement from baseline at endpoint in BEHAVE-AD total score	73% AD 15% VaD 12% Mixed Nursing Home MMSE: 6.6 [6.3] BPSD
De Deyn et al., 1999	12-week, Phase IIIA, double-blind, placebo-controlled, parallel-group with haloperidol as internal reference	RIS: 115 PLA: 114	A score of at least 1 on the global rating of the BEHAVE-AD and a total of at least 8 on the BEHAVE-AD total score	Flexible dose of 0.25–2.0 mg oral solution (1 mg/ml) b.i.d.	30% improvement from baseline at endpoint in BEHAVE-AD total score	67% AD 26% VaD 7% Mixed Nursing Home MMSE: 8.4 [7.7] BPSD
Brodaty et al., 2003	12-week, Phase IIIB, double-blind, placebo-controlled, parallel-group	RIS: 167 PLA: 170	A total score of at least 4 on at least one aggression item, or a score of 3 on at least two aggression items, or a score of 2 on at least three aggression items, or two aggression items occurring at a frequency of 2 and one at a frequency of 3 on the CMAI total aggression subscale	Flexible dose of 0.25–1.0 mg oral solution (1 mg/ml) b.i.d.	Change from baseline at end point in CMAI total Aggression score	58% AD 29% VaD 13% Mixed Nursing Home MMSE: 5.5 [5.7] BPSD + aggression

Study	Design	Treatment groups	Inclusion criteria	Dose	Outcome measure	Population
Street et al., 2000	6 weeks, Phase IIIa, double-blind, placebo-controlled, parallel group	OLZ:159 PLA:47	A score at least 3 on any of the agitation/aggression, hallucinations, or delusions items of the NPI/NH	Fixed dose of 5, 10 or 15 mg (o.i.d.)	Sum of 3 NPI/NH core symptoms (agitation/aggression, hallucinations, delusions)	100% AD Nursing Home MMSE: 6.7 [6.4] psychosis, agitation and aggression
De Deyn et al., 2004	10 weeks, Phase IIIb, double-blind, placebo-controlled, parallel group	OLZ:520 PLA:129	NINCDS-ADRDA and DSM-IV-TR criteria for possible or probable Alzheimer's disease (AD). Clinically significant psychotic symptoms (delusions or hallucinations) due to AD	Fixed dose of 1, 2, 5 or 7.5 mg(o.i.d.)	NPI/NH Psychosis Total scores (sum of delusions, hallucinations items) + CGIC	100% AD Nursing Home MMSE: 13.7 [5.1] [31% of the study population was severely cognitively impaired (score: <10). pAD
De Deyn et al., in press	10 weeks, Phase IIIb, double-blind, placebo-controlled, parallel group	ARI:106 PLA:102	DSM-IV criteria for possible or probable Alzheimer's disease (AD). Clinically significant psychotic symptoms (delusions or hallucinations) due to AD	Flexible dose: 2–15 mg/day(mean dose at endpoint: 10mg/day) o.i.d.	NPI Psychosis subscale score (delusions, hallucinations)	100% AD Outpatients MMSE: 14.2 [6.2] pAD

Legend: RIS: risperidone. OLZ: olanzapine. ARI: aripiprazole. PLA: placebo. BEHAVE-AD: Behavioral Pathology in Alzheimer's Disease rating scale. CMAI: Cohen–Mansfield Agitation Inventory. AD = Alzheimer disease. VaD = Vascular dementia. Mixed = dementia with features of both Alzheimer and vascular dementia. MMSE = Mini Mental State Examination. BPSD = behavioural and psychological symptoms of dementia. pAD = psychosis of dementia. MMSE scores are given as the mean±SD.

In addition, an analysis of a pooled data set of patients of suffering from BPSD and BPSD with aggression, yielded additional insights in the therapeutic efficacy of the atypical antipsychotic agent risperidone (De Deyn et al., in press b). The efficacy data (risperidone $n = 722$, placebo $n = 428$) were obtained from the Cohen–Mansfield Agitation Inventory (CMAI) and Behavioural Pathology in Alzheimer's Disease (BEHAVE-AD) total and subscales (De Deyn and Wirshing, 2001). Additionally, Clinical Global Impression (CGI) assessments were performed. Subgroup analyses were performed by type of dementia, severity of dementia, presence or absence of somnolence as an adverse event, and presence or absence of psychosis at baseline. The mean dose of risperidone at endpoint was 1.0 mg/day (0.02 SE). The observed mean change at endpoint was significantly higher for risperidone than for placebo on CMAI total score (-11.8 vs. -6.4, respectively; $p < 0.001$), total aggression score (-5.0 vs. -1.8, respectively; $p < 0.001$), BEHAVE-AD total score (-6.1 and -3.6, respectively; $p < 0.001$), and psychotic symptoms score (-2.1 and -1.3, respectively; $p = 0.003$). The main treatment effects of risperidone were similar in all subgroup analyses. Additionally, risperidone-treated patients scored significantly better than placebo-treated patients on the CGI scales at endpoint. The incidence of treatment-emergent adverse events was comparable between risperidone (84.3%) and placebo (83.9%). More patients discontinued due to adverse events in the risperidone-treated group (17.2%) than in the placebo group (11.2%). Differences in adverse event incidences between placebo and risperidone were observed for extrapyramidal symptoms (EPS), mild somnolence and the less common cerebrovascular adverse events (CAE). Cerebrovascular adverse events were reported more frequently in the risperidone group than in the placebo group. The incidence of CAEs did not appear to be dose-dependent. In all, 1.6% patients who received risperidone and 0.7% of patients who received placebo (all aged >85 years) experienced a serious cerebrovascular event. All patients who suffered CAEs had one or several preexisting risk factors, including atrial fibrillation, prior stroke, hypertension and diabetes. Risperidone induced neither orthostatic, nor anticholinergic side effects, nor falls, nor cognitive decline.

Psychosis of Alzheimer's Disease (PAD) has rather recently been recognised as a distinct entity as defined by Jeste and Finkel (2000). The characteristic features of PAD and other dementias include delusions, misidentifications and hallucinations, frequently associated with agitation, and aggression and depression. The criteria for PAD as put forward by Jeste and Finkel can be summarised as follows: (1) characteristic delusions or hallucinations in the presence of possible or probable AD; (2) onset of psychotic symptoms after onset of other dementia symptoms, which are present at least intermittently for at least one month; and (3) symptoms severe enough to disrupt patients' functioning, not better accounted for by another psychotic disorder, medical condition or effects of a drug, and not occurring during the course of a delirium. The US Food and Drug Administration has adopted this definition of PAD as a distinct and definable entity, which can be viewed as an unique target for treatment (Laughren, 2001). New claims for this entity would require two independent, adequate and well-controlled trials, each of which would need to show an effect on two primary outcomes, one focused on the defining criteria for the entity, and a second focused more on functional and global improvement (Laughren, 2001).

In line with this conceptual evolution, the most recent studies concentrated on patients suffering from PAD (De Deyn et al., 2004, in press a; Streim et al., 2004; Breder et al., 2004; Mintzer et al., 1998).

De Deyn et al. (2004) conducted a study to compare the efficacy of olanzapine versus placebo in patients with psychotic symptoms associated with AD in long-term or continuing-care settings. Patients ($N = 652$) with AD and delusions or hallucinations were randomly assigned to 10 weeks of double-blind treatment with placebo or fixed-dose olanzapine (1.0, 2.5, 5.0, 7.5 mg/day). Repeated-measures analysis showed significant improvement from baseline in NPI/NH Psychosis Total scores (sum of Delusions, Hallucinations items – primary efficacy measure) in all five treatment groups ($p < 0.001$), but no pairwise treatment differences were seen at the 10-week endpoint. However, under LOCF analysis, improvement in the 7.5-mg olanzapine group (-6.2 ± 4.9) was significantly greater than with placebo (-5.0 ± 6.1, $p = 0.008$), while endpoint CGI-C scores showed the greatest improvement in the Olz2.5 olanzapine group (2.8 ± 1.4, $p = 0.030$) relative to placebo (3.2 ± 1.4). There were significant overall treatment-group differences in increased weight, anorexia and urinary incontinence, with olanzapine showing numerically higher incidences. However, neither the incidence of any other individual events, including extrapyramidal symptoms, nor that of total adverse events occurred with significantly higher frequency in any olanzapine group relative to placebo. No clinically relevant significant changes were seen across groups in cognition or any other vital sign or laboratory measure, including glucose, triglyceride and cholesterol.

Another Phase IIIb randomised clinical trial compared the efficacy, safety and tolerability of aripiprazole with placebo in patients with PAD (De Deyn *et al.*, in press a). This 10-week, double-blind, multi-centre study randomised 208 outpatients. This was a flexible dose trial with mean aripiprazole dose at endpoint of 10.0 mg/day. Evaluations included Neuropsychiatric Inventory (NPI) Psychosis subscale and Brief Psychiatric Rating Scale (BPRS), adverse event (AE) reports, extrapyramidal symptoms (EPS) rating scales, and body weight. The NPI Psychosis subscale score showed improvements in both groups (aripiprazole, -6.55; placebo, -5.52; $p = 0.17$ at endpoint). Aripiprazole-treated patients showed significantly greater improvements from baseline in BPRS Psychosis and BPRS Core subscale scores at endpoint compared with placebo. Adverse events were generally mild to moderate in severity and included urinary tract infection and mild somnolence not associated with falls or accidental injury.

The final results of the RIS-USA-232 trial, which is another double-blind, Phase IIIb, randomised, placebo-controlled, parallel-group, eight-weeks-lasting trial in nursing-home-residing PAD patients, have not been published yet. In this trial, risperidone was administered in a flexible dose regimen (1.0–1.5 mg/day). Co-primary efficacy endpoints were: changes in scores on BEHAVE-AD Psychosis subscale and Clinical Global Impression of Change (CGI-C). Both treatment groups improved significantly on BEHAVE-AD Psychosis subscale and CGI-C scales, with no significant difference between groups. In patients with more severe dementia (MMSE <10), the distribution of the CGI-C ratings showed significant differences at endpoint favouring risperidone treatment.

Possible effects of atypical antipsychotics on sleep-wake disturbances in dementia

Atypical antipsychotic drugs, affecting both the dopaminergic and serotonergic systems, may influence sleep–wake cycle disturbances in patients with dementia. Early indications of a positive influence of risperidone on sleep–wake cycle disturbances in elderly patients with dementia came from a clinical trial reporting improvement in nighttime sleep as well as a decrease in daytime somnolence (Goldberg and Goldberg, 1997). Since then, several other trials in community-based settings have shown improvements in sleep–wake cycle disturbances in elderly patients with dementia (Arriola and Diago, 2002; Schwalen and Kurz, 2002). However, the positive effect of risperidone on sleep–wake cycle disturbances in the demented patient may be an indirect effect secondary to the reduction of agitation, wandering and psychosis (De Deyn *et al.*, 1999; Katz *et al.*, 1999; Brodaty *et al.*, 2003), all potential underlying causes of sleep–wake cycle disturbances. Further research in this field is indicated.

Conclusions

It is concluded that the efficacy and safety of atypical antipsychotics (in contrast to the typical antipsychotics) have been very well studied in the treatment of neuropsychiatric symptoms of dementia. Although several of the large Phase III studies failed to reach their primary endpoints, several others were positive. Analysis of pooled datasets further confirmed the favourable efficacy and safety profile. Beneficial effects were demonstrated on agitation, aggression and psychotic features. In addition, there are some indications that atypical antipsychotics may have a beneficial impact on sleep–wake disturbances in dementia. Overall, the improved safety profile was characterised by limited or no extrapyramidal symptomatology, lower risk of tardive dyskinesia, less or no anticholinergic side effects, and less or no cognitive impairment.

Analyses of 17 placebo-controlled studies of four drugs in the class of atypical antipsychotics (risperidone, olanzapine, aripiprazole and quetiapine) have shown that the rate of death for elderly patients with dementia was about 1.6 to 1.7 times that of placebo. Available data indicate that this increased mortality is also the case for typical antipsychotics. These findings should be an important consideration when choosing treatment with this class of drugs and should be incorporated into the benefit/risk assessment of treatment for each patient. Needless to say, when balancing risks versus benefit, one should take into account the severity of and burden related to BPSD presenting in individual patients.

The use of antipsychotics, including risperidone, should be targeted towards the treatment of those patients in whom psychological and behavioural symptoms of dementia such as psychosis, agitation and aggression are prominent and associated with significant distress, functional impairment or danger to the patient.

Acknowledgements

We acknowledge support by the Fund for Scientific Research-Flanders (FGWO grant G.0038.05), agreement between Institute Born-Bunge and University of Antwerp, and the Medical Research Foundation Antwerp.

References

Allain H, Dautzenberg PHJ, Maurer K, Schuck S, Bonhomme D, Gérard D (2000) Double blind study of tiapride versus haloperidol and placebo in agitation and agressiveness in elderly patients with cognitive impairment. *Psychopharmacology*, 148:361–366.

Arriola E, Diago JI (2002) Risperidone in demented patients and its impact on caregiver stress. *J Clin Psychiatry*, 63:1056.

Bennet D, Gilley DW, Wilson RS (1992) Rate of cognitive decline and neuroleptic use in Alzheimer's disease. *Neurology*, 42(Suppl 3):276.

Breder C, Swanink R, Marcus R, Kostic D, Iwamato T, Carson W, McQuade R (2004) Dose-ranging study of aripiprazole in patients with dementia of Alzheimer's Disease. *Neurobiology of Aging*, 25:S2, 190.

Brodaty H, Ames D, Snowdon J, Woodward M, Kirwan J, Clarnette R, Lee E, Greenspan A. Risperidone for psychosis of Alzheimer's disease and mixed dementia: results of a double-blind, placebo-controlled trial. *Int J Geriatr Psychiatry*, (in press).

Brodaty H, Ames D, Snowdon J, Woodward M, Kirwan J, Clarnette R, Lee E, Lyons B, Grossman F (2003) A randomised placebo controlled trial of risperidone for the treatment of aggression, agitation and psychosis of dementia. *J Clin Psychiatry*, 64:134–143.

Bullock R, Saharan A (2002) Atypical antipsychotics: experience and use in the elderly. *Int J Clin Pract*, 56:515–525.

Clark WS, Street JS, Feldman PD, Breier A (2001) The effects of olanzapine in reducing the emergence of psychosis among nursing home patients with Alzheimer's disease. *J Clin Psychiatry*, 62(1):34–40.

Coen RF, Swanwick GRJ., O'Boyle CA, Coakley D (1997) Behavior disturbance and other predictors of carer burden in Alzheimer's disease. *Int J Geriatr Psychiatry*, 12:331–336.

Cohen–Mansfield J, Marx MS, Rosenthal AS (1989) A description of agitation in a nursing home. *J Gerontol*, 44:M77–M84.

Cummings JL, Mega M, Gray K, Rosenberg-Thompson S, Carusi DA, Gornbein J (1994) The Neuropsychiatric Inventory: comprehensive assessment of psychopathology in dementia. *Neurology*, 44:2308–2314.

De Deyn PP, Carrasco MM, Deberdt W, Jeandel C, Hay DP, Feldman PD, Young CA, Lehman DL, Breier A (2004) Olanzapine versus placebo in the treatment of psychosis with or without associated behavioral disturbances in patients with Alzheimer's disease. *Int J Geriatr Psychiatry*, 19(2):115–126.

De Deyn PP, Jeste DV, Swanink R, Kostic D, Breder C (in press a) Aripiprazole for the treatment of psychosis in patients with Alzheimer's disease: a randomised, placebo-controlled study. *J Clin Psychopharmacol*.

De Deyn PP, Katz IR, Brodaty H, Lyons B, Greenspan A, Burns A (in press b) Management of agitation, aggression, and psychosis associated with dementia: a pooled analysis including three randomised, placebo-controlled double-blind trials in nursing home residents treated with risperidone. *Clinical Neurology and Neurosurgery*.

De Deyn PP, Rabheru K, Rasmussen A, Bocksberger JP, Dautzenberg PL, Eriksson S, *et al.* (1999) A randomised trial of risperidone, placebo, and haloperidol for behavioral symptoms of dementia. *Neurology*, 53(5):946–955.

De Deyn PP, Wirshing WC (2001) Scales to assess efficacy and safety of pharmacologic agents in the treatment of behavioral and psychological symptoms of dementia. *J Clin Psychiatry* 62 (Suppl 21):19–22.

Donaldson C, Tarrier N, Burns A (1997) The impact of the symptoms of dementia on caregivers. *Br. J. Psychiatry*, 170:62–68.

Edell WS, Tunis SL (2001) Antipsychotic treatment of behavioral and psychological symptoms of dementia in geropsychiatric inpatients. *Am J Geriatr Psychiatry*, 9(3):289–297.

Ferris SH, Steinberg G, Shulman E, Kahn R, Reisberg B (1987) Institutionalisation of Alzheimer's disease patients: reducing precipitating factors through family counseling. *Home Health Care Services Quarterly*, 8:23–51.

Gill S, Rochon PA, Nathan Herrmann, Lee PE, Sykora K, Gunraj N, Normand SLT, Gurwitz JH, Marras C, Wodchis WP, Mamdani M (2005) Atypical antipsychotic drugs and risk of ischaemic stroke: population based retrospective cohort study. *BMJ*, 330:445.

Goldberg RJ, Goldberg J (1997) Risperidone for dementia-related disturbed behavior in nursing home residents: a clinical experience. *Int Psychogeriatr*, 9:65–68.

Greenspan A, Eerdekens M, Mahmoud R (2003) Risk of cerebrovascular adverse events, including mortality, with risperidone in elderly patients. *Int Psychogeriatrics*, PB-041(Suppl 2):261–262.

Grossman F, Okamoto A, Turkoz I, Gharabawi G (2004) Risperidone in the treatment of elderly patients with psychosis of Alzheimer's disease and related dementias. *J Am Geriatr Soc*, 52:852–853.

Gutzmann H, Kühl K-P, Kanowski S, Khan-Boluki J (1997) Measuring the efficacy of psychopharmacological treatment of psychomotoric restlessness in dementia: clinical evaluation of tiapride. *Pharmacopsychiatry*, 30:6–11.

Herrmann N, Mamdani M, Pharm.D., Lanctôt KL (2004) Atypical antipsychotics and risk of cerebrovascular accidents. *Am J Psychiatry*, 161:1113–1115.

Jeste DV, Finkel SI (2000) Psychosis of Alzheimer's disease and related dementias. Diagnostic criteria for a distinct syndrome. *Am J Geriatr Psychiatry*, 8(1):29–34.

Jeste DV, Rockwell E, Harris MJ, Lohr JB, Lacro JP (1999a) Conventional vs newer antipsychotics in elderly patients. *Am J Geriatr Psychiatry*, 7:70–76.

Jeste DV, Lacro JP, Bailey A, Rockwell E, Harris MJ, Caligiuri MP (1999b) Lower incidence of tardive dyskinesia with risperidone compared with haloperidol in older patients. *J Am Geriatr Soc*, 47:716–719.

Jeste DV, Okamoto A, Napolitano J, Kane JM, Martinez RA (2000) Low incidence of persistent tardive dyskinesia in elderly patients with dementia treated with risperidone. *Am J Psychiatry*, 157(7):1150–1155.

Jost BC, Grossberg GT (1996) The evolution of psychiatric symptoms in Alzheimer's disease: a natural history study. *J Am Geriatr Soc*, 144:1078–1081.

Katz IR, Jeste DV, Mintzer JE, Clyde C, Napolitano J, Brecher M (1999) Comparison of risperidone and placebo for psychosis and behavioral disturbances associated with dementia: a randomised, double-blind trial. Risperidone Study Group. *J Clin Psychiatry*, 60(2):107–115.

Katz IR, Brodaty H, De Deyn PP, Mintzer J, Greenspan A (2005) Risperidone in the treatment of psychosis of Alzheimer's Disease (PAD). A pooled analysis of 4 controlled trials. Poster presented at the Annual Scientific Meeting of the American Geriatrics Society (AGS), May 11–15, Orlando, Florida, USA, C109.

Laughren T (2001) A regulatory perspective on psychiatric syndromes in Alzheimer disease. *Am J Geriatr Psychiatry*, 9(4):340–345.

McKhann G, Drachman D, Folstein M, Katzman R, Price D, Stadlan EM (1984) Clinical diagnosis of Alzheimer's disease: report of the NINCDS-ADRDA Work Group under the auspices of the Department of Health and Human Services Task Force on Alzheimer's Disease. *Neurology*, 34:939–944.

McShane R, Keene J, Gedling K, Fairburn C, Jacoby R, Hope T (1997) Do neuroleptic drugs hasten cognitive decline in dementia? Prospective study with necropsy follow up. *BMJ*, 314(7076):266–270.

Mintzer JE, Hoernig KS, Mirski DF (1998) Treatment of agitation in patients with dementia. *Clinics in Geriatric Medicine*, 14:147–175.

Mohr E, Mendis T, Hildebrand K, De Deyn PP (2000) Risperidone in the treatment of dopamine-induced psychosis in Parkinson's disease: an open pilot trial. *Mov Disord*, 15(6):1230–1237.

National Institute of Mental Health (1976) Clinical global impressions. In ECDEU Assessment Manual for Psychopharmacology, Revised, GuyW(ed.). US Department of Health, Education, and Welfare: Bethesda, MD 217–222.

Overall JE, Gorham DR (1962) The Brief Psychiatric Rating Scale. *Psychol Rep*, 10:799–812.

Piggott MA, Perry EK, Marshall EF, McKeith IG, Johnson M, Melrose HL, *et al.* (1998) Nigrostriatal dopaminergic activities in dementia with Lewy bodies in relation to neuroleptic sensitivity: comparisons with
Parkinson's disease. *Biol Psychiatry*, 44(8):765–774.

Porsteinsson AP, Tariot PN, Erb R, Gaile S (1997) An open trial of valproate for agitation in geriatric neuropsychiatric disorders. *Am J Geriatr Psychiatry*, 5:344–351.

Reisberg B, Borenstein J, Franssen E, Shulman E, Steinberg G, Ferris SH (1986) Remediable behavioral symptomatology in Alzheimer's disease. *Hosp. Community Psychiatry*, 37:1199–1201.

Reisberg B, Borenstein J, Salob SP, Ferris SH, Franssen E, Georgotas A (1987) Behavioral symptoms in
Alzheimer's disease: phenomenology and treatment. *J Clin Psychiatry*, 48(5-Suppl):S9–S15.

Reisberg B, Borenstein J, Salob SP, Ferris SH, Franssen E, Georgotas A (1987) Behavioral symptoms in
Alzheimer's disease: phenomenology and treatment. *J Clin Psychiatry*, 48(5-Suppl):S9–S15.

Robert PH, Allain H (2001) Clinical management of agitation in the elderly with tiapride. *Eur Psychiatry*,
16(Suppl 1):42s–47s.

Schneider LS, Katz IR, Park S, Napolitano J, Martinez RA, Azen SP (2003) Psychosis of Alzheimer disease:
validity of the construct and response to risperidone. *Am J Geriatr Psychiatry*, 11:414–425.

Schneider LS, Pollock VE, Lyness SA (1990) A meta analysis of controlled trials of neuroleptic treatment of
Dementia. *J Am Geriatr Soc*, 38:553–563.

Schneider LS (1996) Meta-analysis of controlled pharmacologic trials. *Int Psychogeriatr*, 8(Suppl 3):375–379;
discussion 381–382.

Schwalen S, Kurz A (2002) Risperidone for the treatment of behavioural disorders in dementia. *Nerven-
heilkunde*, 21:208–213.

Street JS, Clark WS, Gannon KS, Cummings JL, Bymaster FP, Tamura RN, *et al.* (2000) Olanzapine treatment of psychotic and behavioral symptoms in patients with Alzheimer disease in nursing care facilities:
a double-blind, randomised, placebo-controlled trial. The HGEU Study Group. *Arch Gen Psychiatry*,
57(10):968–976.

Streim J, Breder C, Swanink R, McQuade R, Iwamoto T, Carson W, Stock E (2004) Flexible-dose aripiprazole
in psychosis of Alzheimer's Disease. *Neurobiology of aging*, 25(S2):191.

Tariot PN, Mack JL, Patterson MB, Edland SD, Weiner MF, Fillenbaum G, Blazina L, Teri L, Rubin E, Mortimer JA, Stern Y, the Behavioral Pathology Committee of the Consortium to Establish a Registry for Alzheimer's Disease (1995) The behavior rating scale for dementia of the consortium to establish a registry for
Alzheimer's disease. *Am J Psychiatry*, 152:1349–1357.

Tariot PN, Erb R, Leibovici A, Podgorski CA, Cox C, Asnis J, Kolassa J, Irvine C (1994) Carbamazepine
treatment of agitation in nursing home patients with dementia: a preliminary study. *J Am Geriatr Soc*,
42:1160–1166.

Wooltorton E: Risperidone (Risperdal) (2004a) increased rate of cerebrovascular events in dementia trials.
Can Med Assoc J, 167(11):1269–1270.

Wooltorton E: Olanzapine (Zyprexa) (2004b) increased incidence of cerebrovascular events in dementia trials.
Can Med Assoc J, 170(9):1395.

Zyprexa (olanzapine) US prescribing information: http://pi.lilly.com/us/zyprexapi.pdf, as accessed on 23 April
2004. Eli Lilly and Company 2004.

13

Non-pharmacological Treatment of Severe Dementia: An Overview

Ross Overshott and Alistair Burns

Introduction

The choice of intervention to treat BPSD (Behavioural and Psychological Symptoms of Dementia) must be taken considering which specific symptoms are present as treatments' effectiveness varies between the groups of symptoms. Specific symptoms are common at different stages of dementia. Agitation has a higher prevalence in people with severe dementia while depression is most common in people with mild dementia and it has been reported that delusions arise most frequently in those with moderate dementia (Margallo-Lana *et al.*, 2001). The first line treatment for BPSD is often psychotropic medication, particularly antipsychotic drugs. There have been no trials specifically examining the efficacy of psychotropic medication in the treatment of BPSD in severe dementia. Trials for treatments of BPSD in people with mild dementia have shown a moderate improvement although there is a high placebo response of approximately 40% (Schneider *et al.*, 1990). Psychotropic medication can also cause side effects such as Parkinsonism and drowsiness which can lead to falls and other adverse events. They also possibly hasten cognitive decline (McShane *et al.*, 1997). The recent concerns of increased cerebrovascular events following the use of risperidone and olanzapine (Hermann *et al.*, 2004) for the treatment of agitation have increased the emphasis on finding safe, effective treatment for all types of BPSD. People with severe dementia are particularly sensitive to these effects and their quality of life can be significantly reduced by the commencement of these medications, rather than enhanced.

Non-pharmacological interventions

Non-pharmacological interventions offer a first-line alternative to pharmacological treatments for BPSD and have several advantages. They are associated with fewer, and less serious, side effects and the implementation of many of the interventions increases the interaction with the patient. Their safety is especially beneficial in treating BPSD in people with severe dementia, who often cannot tolerate pharmacological treatments.

There are a variety of forms of non-pharmacological interventions for BPSD, with an increasing evidence base for their efficacy. Many studies, however, do not concentrate on people with severe dementia and BPSD and include participants with mild and moderate dementia. When considering non-pharmacological interventions for BPSD in people with severe dementia it must be remembered that most of the evidence available is not specific to this group.

There are a number of methodological problems with the studies that have been conducted examining non-pharmacological interventions for BPSD. Many studies have tried to replicate the methods used in controlled drug trials, despite many of them being unsuitable for non-pharmacological

Severe Dementia. Edited by A. Burns and B. Winblad.
Copyright © 2006 John Wiley & Sons, Ltd.   ISBN 0-470-01054-1

interventions. The nature of many interventions (e.g. behavioural and education programmes, re-ality orientation) is such that it is impossible to compare the intervention against a placebo. This makes it too difficult to determine whatever it is in the intervention that is effective rather than any positive changes being secondary to increased attention and interaction (Woods, 2002). Several interventions aim to alter caregiver interactions with the patient and modify their environment, which makes it very difficult to have a control group as carer interactions with patients cannot be controlled and environmental changes affect all patients in the vicinity. To avoid this, some studies have randomised their interventions by nursing home populations rather than individual patients. This, however, gives rise to a potential bias as any difference in outcome may be due to the varia-tion in care between nursing homes rather than the study intervention and control.

Many non-pharmacological interventions do not address the aetiology of BPSD but instead try to modify observed behaviours. They are therefore frequently aimed at people with different types of dementia with a range of BPSD. There is currently a lack of information available to guide which interventions are effective for which dementias and symptoms. There is also a great variation be-tween studies on reporting how interventions should be delivered, who should deliver them, what training they need and the regime of the treatment. There is a dearth of information regarding the cost–benefit of non-pharmacological interventions, an issue which has led to concerns about phar-macological treatments and consequently interest in increasing the usage of non-pharmacological ones. Until the method of intervention is more clearly defined it will be difficult to expand the use of non-pharmacological interventions.

Types of non-pharmacological intervention

Non-pharmacological interventions include a wide range of therapies; some have similarities while others share few common properties. The interventions can be broadly described as either nonver-bal or verbal therapies. Nonverbal therapies generally offer sensory stimulation and include music therapy, aromatherapy and bright light therapy. Verbal therapies (e.g. validation therapy, reality ori-entation, reminiscence therapy) rely on the patient having adequate comprehension and language skills. Depending on their specific cognitive deficit, patients with severe dementia may be unable to engage in verbal therapies.

Nonverbal interventions

- Aromatherapy
- Bright light therapy
- Music therapy
- Snoezelen
- Exercise

Aromatherapy uses essential oils to provide sensory stimulation and reduce agitation and aggres-sive behaviour (Thorgrimsen *et al.*, 2003). They can be administered through several routes includ-ing inhalation, massage, bathing and topical application. The two main essential oils that have been used in dementia are melissa balm and lavender which are thought to be relaxants (Worwood, 1996). Lavender has been shown to be effective for the use of depression and anxiety in cancer patients (Kite *et al.*, 1998). The mechanism of action of aromatherapy is unclear. The essential oils may have cholinergic activity, the act of massage may be relaxing and increase socialisation or the aromas may evoke the memory of a more pleasant and relaxed time (Ballard *et al.*, 2001).

Bright light therapy (BLT) has been found to be effective for various psychiatric conditions including sleep disorders and seasonal affective disorder (Lam, 1998). It aims to reestablish cir-cadian rhythms and reduce sleep disturbance. In dementia, BLT is thought to be useful in not only improving sleep but also reducing 'sun downing syndrome', the phenomenon of a recurrent increase in restlessness in late afternoon and evening, which is thought to have a circadian origin (Martin *et al.*, 2000). Patients usually have a light box placed in their visual field, approximately 1 metre from them, or a light visor approximately 3 or 4 cm from their eyes. There are currently no guidelines for the use of BLT in dementia and studies have used a variety of light intensities, from 2,000 to 10,000 lux. The regimes for exposure have also differed, with patients receiving treatment from 30 minutes to two hours, once or twice a day, for up to eight weeks.

Music therapy can increase communications with patients with severe dementia who are unable to understand verbal language. It may be helpful in reorientation, rebuilding social links, eliciting memory and raising the morale of patients (Lou, 2001). Music therapy can be active, with patients participating in singing or dancing, or passive by using musicians, therapists or pre-recorded music.

Snoezelen is a multi-sensory stimulation therapy which aims to stimulate the primary sense of sight, touch, hearing and smell, through the use of lighting effects, tactile surfaces, meditative music and the odour of relaxing essential oils (Pinkney, 1997). It was originally used for people with learning disability but has been adapted for use in dementia to provide a sensory environment which places fewer demands on cognitive abilities but maximises residual sensorimotor abilities (Chung, 2002).

Exercise and activities-based interventions have been utilised as a method of reducing agitation and improving mood and sleep. The complication for people with severe dementia is that they are more likely to have impaired mobility and are at risk of falling so such interventions may not be appropriate.

Verbal interventions

- Behavioural and education programmes
- Reality Orientation
- Reminiscence Therapy
- Validation Therapy

Behavioural and education programmes aim to give carers of people with severe dementia the knowledge and skills to manage the patient's BPSD. Caregiver interventions have been shown to enhance feelings of competence, reduce negative affect in carers and improve communication with the patient (Green and Brodaty, 2002). Formal and informal caregivers are given information concerning dementia and its symptoms to help understanding of the patient and their behaviour. They are taught to identify specifics about the BPSD under consideration, define the factors that lead up to and sustain the occurrence and systematically alter those factors to reduce the BPSD. Behavioural techniques utilised can include extinction, differential reinforcement and stimulus control.

Reality Orientation (RO) helps people with dementia by reminding them of facts about themselves and their environment. The aim is to reorientate them in time, person and place, and thus reduce anxiety. RO can be conducted in any setting, and by formal or informal carers. RO is delivered either in a sessional, formal way or in a 24-hour, informal approach. Sessions of RO are usually conducted in groups where orientating information is given and current events are discussed. They are usually one hour long, up to five times a week. The 24-hour method uses clear orientating signposts, notices and other memory aids. Carers reinforce the information and consistently orientate the patient.

Reality Orientation mainly focuses on the here an now while Reminiscence Therapy (RT) encourages patients to relive their past and recall the positive events in their life. Like RO, it can be conducted individually or in groups, informally or formally. The recall of past events is stimulated by photographs, music, artefacts and other aids. RT hopes to provide socialisation and memory stimulation and allows carers to learn more about the lives of their patients.

Validation Therapy (VT) was developed by Naomi Feil in the 1960s. It was originally called 'Fantasy Therapy' as Feil believed that patients with dementia retreated into an inner, fantasy world to escape from their current, painful existence. VT aims to validate the feelings the person with dementia has and assumes that their behaviours and actions have meaning. VT incorporates specific techniques to aid communication and reduce anxiety and distress.

Agitation

Agitation is an inappropriate verbal, vocal or motor activity judged by an outsider as not resulting directly from the person's needs or as confusion of a person (Cohen-Mansfield and Billig, 1986). Agitation is more common in people with severe dementia and has a negative impact on quality of life of the patient and carers and affects the quality of social interactions (Chou *et al.*, 1990; Mungas *et al.*, 1989).

Nonverbal interventions

The nonverbal intervention which has the strongest evidence for treatment of agitation in severe dementia is aromatherapy. Ballard *et al.* (2002) conducted a randomised controlled trial of aromatherapy for dementia in the UK which included 72 participants, from eight nursing homes, who had severe dementia. A lotion with 10% melissa oil was applied to the arms and face for one to two minutes a day, for four weeks. The control group received the same intervention using sunflower oil. Sixty per cent of the melissa group and 14% of the placebo-treated group experienced a 30% reduction of the Cohen-Mansfield Agitation Inventory (CMAI) ($\chi^2 = 16.3$, $p < 0.0001$), the threshold generally defined as clinically significant in BPSD intervention trials. The number needed to treat was reported to be 4.2, which compares well to previous pharmacological studies of BPSD in less impaired patients (Ballard and O'Brien, 1999). There was an overall improvement in agitation (mean reduction in CMAI score) of 35% in patients receiving melissa balm essential oil and 11% in those treated with placebo.

This is one of the few double-blind, placebo-controlled trials of a non-pharmacological intervention specifically examining BPSD in people with severe dementia. It does, however, have a number of weaknesses: no account was taken of changes in medication. Nursing homes rather than individuals were randomised, allowing the possibility that group difference were produced by differences between institutions. Holmes *et al.* (2002) conducted a placebo-controlled trial, using a blinded observer rater, for lavender oil aromatherapy in the treatment of BPSD in severe dementia. The communal area of a long-stay dementia ward was diffused with 2% lavender oil for a two-hour period alternated with placebo (water) every other day for 10 treatment sessions. The study included 15 patients with severe dementia: four with Alzheimer's disease, seven with vascular dementia, three with dementia with Lewy bodies and one patient with fronto-temporal lobe dementia. For each participant 10 total Pittsburgh Agitation Scale (PAS) scores were obtained: five during treatment and five during placebo periods. Nine patients showed an improvement, five showed no change and one patient showed a worsening of agitated behaviour during aromatherapy compared with placebo. Interestingly, none of the patients with dementia with Lewy bodies were in the group that showed improvement.

There has also been one randomised controlled trial which has compared aromatherapy massage, plain oil massage and conversation and aroma disseminated by diffuser (Smallwood *et al.*, 2001). Only 21 patients with severe dementia were studied and the type of aroma used was not reported. There was reduction in agitation in all three groups with a trend towards a more consistent reduction following aromatherapy massage although this was not statistically significant. In all the studies aromatherapy was well tolerated with no adverse effects. It has been reported that lavender oil can increase agitation (Brooker *et al.*, 1997).

BLT has mainly been successful in treating sleep disturbance although there is some evidence that it can also reduce agitation. Trials in people with severe dementia that have shown a significant reduction in agitation have been small and have used a range of treatment regimes. Skjerve *et al.* (2004a) gave 10 patients with severe dementia BLT at 5,000–8,000 lux for 45 minutes each morning for four weeks whilst Satlin *et al.* (1992) administered a week's course in the evening. Haffmans *et al.* (2001) showed in a double-blind, placebo-controlled, crossover trial that BLT reduced agitation but adding in melatonin had no positive effects. Evidence from randomised controlled trials (RCT) has shown a reduction in agitation (Allen *et al.*, 2003) and no effect on either behaviour or sleep (Lyketsos *et al.*, 1999). Ancoli-Israel *et al.*'s (2003a) study had a majority of subjects with severe dementia and showed that BLT was associated with improved caregiver's ratings but had little effect on observational ratings of agitation. BLT is thought to be generally safe, although there have been reports of increased agitation and development of delusional symptoms (Schindler *et al.*, 2002) and irritation of the eye (Fetveit *et al.*, 2003). There are still concerns over the practicality of administering BLT as most studies reported that patients were unable to sit in front of lights for long periods; this may be particularly a problem for people with severe dementia.

The quality of evidence for music therapy for treating agitation is also reduced by small sample size and different treatment regimes between studies. Clark *et al.*'s (1998) RCT showed that playing the patients preferred music on an audio tape recorder during bathing reduced aggressive behaviour compared to the control of playing no music. Gerdner (2000) conducted a randomised crossover trial of 39 patients with agitation assigned to preferred music or standard classical music over six weeks. The results suggest significantly less agitation during and after the preferred music intervention. A meta-analysis of music therapy concluded that it is effective for decreasing agitation in people with dementia (Koger *et al.*, 1999). The analysis included observational studies, and methods used varied greatly, e.g. listening/playing music, live/taped music.

The Cochrane Review of Snoezelen for dementia (Chung *et al.*, 2002) included an RCT (Baker *et al.*, 1997) and a crossover trial (Kragt *et al.*, 1997). The RCT included patients with moderate and severe dementia and found a slight deterioration in behaviours with treatment. Kragt's study found Snoezelen significantly reduced incidents of disturbed behaviour. The review was unable to draw a firm conclusion as data from the two trials was limited and they had different methodology and control conditions (Chung *et al.*, 2004).

Exercise and physical activity is thought to reduce agitation in patients with severe dementia by distracting and stimulating them. There are many observational studies which have found a positive effect for a wide range of activities and types of exercises. Rovner *et al.*'s (1996) RCT found that group activities led by a group therapist reduced agitation significantly compared to control group. Another RCT (Alessi *et al.*, 1999) compared age-appropriate exercises and walking activity combined with sleep hygiene measuring to sleep hygiene measures only. Observations of agitation decreased by 22% in the 15 intervention subjects but increased by 150% in the control group.

Although there have been positive findings from different types of activities in studies it has been suggested that it is the timing of the activities, and not the type, that its important in reducing agitation. Kovach *et al.* (2004) found a significant improvement in agitation with Balancing Arousal Controls Excesses (BACE) interventions in a pre-test–post-test, double-blinded experimental study with random assignment. The BACE intervention controls the daily activity schedule so that there is a balance between the time a person is in a high-arousal and a low-arousal state. This reflects the model of 'Imbalance in Sensoristasis', which suggests that agitated behaviours may be initiated or exacerbated when there is an imbalance between sensory-stimulating and sensory-calming activity. The study was specific for patients with severe dementia as subjects with moderate dementia were included although it was found that response was not dependent on cognitive level or verbal ability.

Verbal interventions

Behavioural approaches utilise conditioning and social-learning theory to modify behaviours seen in dementia. In patients with severe dementia, because of level of cognitive impairment, it is often necessary to involve caregivers with the treatment. Many interventions combine behavioural techniques with psychoeducation for caregivers. This provides caregivers with information and knowledge about dementia and BPSD. Caregivers can be taught behavioural techniques such as ABC – where the Antecedents, Behaviours and Consequences are recorded using a chart or diary. This process provides understanding of behaviours and gives a focus for behavioural techniques which caregivers can also learn.

Behavioural management techniques' (BMT) effectiveness has been examined compared to common pharmacological interventions for BPSD, haloperidol and trazodone (Teri *et al.*, 2000). In this RCT, BMT consisted of eight weekly and three bi-weekly structured sessions that provided information on AD, strategies for decreasing agitated behaviours and structured assignments. One hundred and forty-nine patients with Alzheimer's disease with agitation, from 21 sites, were randomised to 16 weeks of treatment. The maximum dose of haloperidol was 3 mg/day while for trazodone it was 300 mg/day. There was a reduction in agitation in 34% of patients relative to baseline, although there was no significant difference between the three treatments and placebo. There was no difference in specific symptom reduction across the active treatments. In this study the magnitude of improvements was small but BMT did have significantly fewer adverse events than the pharmacological treatments. The same behavioural intervention was used in another RCT which looked at caregivers delivering the intervention in their homes to patients with moderate and severe dementia (Teri *et al.*, 2005). Not only was there a significant reduction in the frequency and severity of the patient's behaviour but also improvements in quality of life and caregiver depression and burden.

There have been other RCTs evaluating similar behavioural programmes in the treatment of aggression in moderate and severe dementia. A short behavioural programme of four sessions over eight weeks conducted with 62 caregivers revealed a trend towards a reduction in aggressive behaviours in the experimental group when compared in the group after adjusting for baseline scores (Gormley *et al.*, 2001). The programme provided education and training to identify precipitating and maintaining factors as well as behavioural interventions, based on communication and distraction, to modify them. The sample size was small and no impact on carer burden was observed. A three-month group intervention for caregivers, which included psychoeducative training, non-specific psychotherapeutic strategies and specific cognitive behavioural techniques to develop problem-solving and implement behaviour medication, has also been shown to significantly improve agitation (Haupt *et al.*, 2000).

The evidence-base for the effectiveness of reminiscence therapy largely consists of descriptive and observational studies. A Cochrane Review of reminiscence theory (Woods *et al.*, 2005) included five RCTs, although most of the studies were small and did not concentrate on change in behaviour. Some of the smaller studies did find some improvement in behaviour on standardised rating scales, but the largest study (Lai *et al.*, 2004) showed fewer benefits. One hundred and one nursing home residents were randomised to either individualised reminiscence therapy, social support or no treatment; no differences were found between the two active groups, although a small significant improvement was demonstrated compared to placebo. Baillon *et al.* (2004) assigned 16 patients, in a randomised, controlled, crossover trial, to a reminiscence therapy group or a Snoezelen group. Both interventions had beneficial effects but no significant difference was found between them. Large variations in response between patients were noted.

A Cochrane Review of Reality Orientation (Spector *et al.*, 2000) identified six RCTs but only three studies used behavioural outcomes measures, which were all different. The analysis was conducted on data from 48 subjects and showed a significant improvement in behaviour with Reality Orientation.

The evidence for validation therapy is unconvincing. Neal and Briggs (2003) reported on three small randomised studies in which only one found significant behavioural improvements. A number of methodological concerns were highlighted included a lack of clarity in some cases of whether participants had dementia. An RCT which investigated the effectiveness of emotion-oriented care, a combination mainly based on Validation Therapy but also including reminiscence as sensory stimulus approaches, found no significant improvement on behavioural outcome measures (Schrijnemaekers *et al.*, 2002).

There is less available evidence for non-pharmacological interventions for apathy, depression and sleep disturbance in severe dementia. Most studies are small and are not primarily evaluating these aspects of BPSD. They also usually include subjects with moderate dementia, as well as severe.

Apathy

Apathy is the most common BPSD reported to occur in up to 92% patients with dementia (Mega *et al.*, 1996), but is under-diagnosed. It is commonly described as a lack of interest, emotion and motivation. Compared to patients with depression, patients with apathy are emotionally indifferent rather than dysphoric, although they may both lack spontaneity and be socially withdrawn.

Nonverbal interventions

It is perhaps expected for sensory stimulating interventions to be the most effective non-pharmacological measures in reducing apathy. There is, however, little evidence to support this. In an RCT, which included 60 nursing home residents, listening to 'big band' music for 30 minutes a day was found to have beneficial effects on apathy, alertness and social interaction when compared to doing puzzle exercises and a control group (Lord and Garner, 1993). One of the two studies included in Chung *et al.*'s (2002) Cochrane Review of Snoezelen reported significantly fewer apathetic behaviours in patients who received three half sessions of Snoezelen over three days. The study group only included 16 patients. There is no published evidence that BLT is effective in treating apathy in severe dementia while a single case study suggests that aromatherapy can improve motivational behaviour (McMahon and Kermode, 1996).

Verbal interventions

There are currently no published studies addressing the potential benefits of caregiver-based behavioural interventions for reducing apathy in severe dementia. Apathy is, however, often unrecognised and patients are frequently labelled as lazy or awkward. Educated caregivers may be more able to understand the patient's symptoms and cope better with the difficulties that arise. Once recognised, apathetic patients can be encouraged to partake in pleasurable activities, helped with initiating goal-directed behaviours and provided with stimulating environments. These simple measures may improve the patient's social functioning and quality of life.

Current evidence would suggest that VT and RO do not provide significant benefits in the treatment of apathy. An RCT of reminiscence therapy and a time and attention control condition showed a reduction in apathy as measured by the Neuropsychiatric Inventory, for both interventions; this suggests that any contact with the patient may produce beneficial effects on apathy (Politis *et al.*, 2004).

Depression

Depression can be very difficult to diagnose in people with severe dementia as they may have difficulty recognising and expressing their feelings. Assessment is therefore likely to rely more on observed behaviours and collateral history. Diagnostic tools which have been validated in people with dementia, such as the Carnell Scale for Depression in Dementia (CSDD) (Alexopoulos *et al.*, 1988) can be extremely helpful. Studies examining the effectiveness of non-pharmacological treatments for depression in severe dementia have many flaws. Many studies do not establish a diagnosis of depression in their sample and instead refer to 'depressive symptoms'. Well-recognised, validated rating scales are not consistently used to measure change which questions the clinical relevance of any reported improvements. There is also again the problem that most studies do not concentrate on people with severe dementia but largely include patients with mild and moderate dementia. It cannot be presumed that a successful intervention for depressed people with mild dementia will be equally, if at all, effective for people with severe dementia and depression.

Nonverbal interventions

There is little evidence to support the efficacy of sensory stimulating interventions in the treatment of depressive symptoms in severe dementia. Aromatherapy has no reported effect on depression, while the findings for BLT are limited. A crossover, double-blind, controlled trial comparing BLT with a control condition of lower light found a significant improvement in Geriatric Depression Scale (Sumaya *et al.*, 2001) but Lyketsos *et al.*'s RCT of BLT showed no significant improvement on the CSDD (Lyketsos *et al.*, 1999). Music therapy has been reported to improve the observed mood of people with dementia (Lord and Garner, 1993) but there have been no studies assessing whether it is effective for treating depression.

Baillon *et al.*'s (2004) crossover, randomised, controlled study of Snoezelen compared reminiscence therapy showed improvement in patient's mood, for both interventions as measured on Interact Scale. The difference between the two therapies was small, although Snoezelen had a slightly more positive effect. Snowden *et al.*'s (2003) review reported on four RCTs of exercise or activity programmes which were shown to improve ratings on depression scales. The studies, however, mainly included people with mild dementia. One study (Fitzsimmons, 2001) instituted therapeutic recreation activity of staff members taking depressed nursing home residents around the grounds with the resident seated in a wheelchair attached in tandem to the front of a bicycle. The activity lasted one hour every day for five days a week and showed a significant reduction in Geriatric Depression Scale scores when compared to the control (45% reduction vs. 8% increase in controls). This is a simple intervention which could easily be applied to people with severe dementia.

Verbal interventions

Cognitive behavioural therapy has been shown to be effective for the treatment of depression in people with dementia. An RCT compared two behavioural treatments with a typical care control group and waiting-list control groups (Teri *et al.*, 1997). The two active interventions consisted of nine 60-minute sessions of either a treatment where caregivers were taught behavioural strategies for improving the patients' depression by increasing pleasant events or a problem-solving focus therapy which utilised a systematic approach to behaviours. Seventy-two patient–caregiver dyads were randomised, with all patients, and 76% of caregivers, meeting the criteria for major or minor depressive disorder. Both behavioural interventions showed significant improvement in depression symptoms and diagnosis as compared with patients in the two control groups. Sixty per cent of patients in the active treatment groups showed clinically significant improvement and none deteriorated, while only 20% of the control group showed improvement and 10% deteriorated, with 70% showing no change. Caregivers in each behavioural intervention group also showed significant improvement in their depressive symptoms while caregivers in the two control groups did not. All the gains demonstrated in the trial were maintained at six-month follow-up. Behavioural management techniques combined with physical exercise programmes implemented by caregivers in an RCT resulted in reduced scores on the CSDD when compared to a treatment as usual group (Teri *et al.*, 2003). There is also evidence that staff of nursing and residential homes can implement behavioural management interventions to reduce depression in their residents (Proctor *et al.*, 1999).

The Cochrane Review of RT (Woods *et al.*, 2005) reported that an RCT studying patients with mild to moderate dementia found that RT significantly improved depression while another RCT found that RT significantly increased depression. There have been a few small RCTs which indicate a trend for positive effects of VT on depression (Neal and Briggs, 2003).

Sleep

The prevalence of sleep problems increases with age and includes difficulties in initiating and maintaining sleep and decrease in total sleep time. The sleep changes seen in dementia appear to be an exacerbation of normal age-related changes, which increase in magnitude with the severity of dementia (Vitiello *et al.*, 1991).

Nonverbal interventions

BLT is regarded as a promising treatment for sleep disturbance in dementia as it is thought to affect the generation and regulation of sleep–wake circadian rhythm. Non-RCT studies, by and large, show the expected improvement in sleep with BLT but these have not been consistently replicated in RCTs (Skjerve *et al.*, 2004b). In an RCT trial Mishima *et al.* (1998) reported a group of patients with vascular dementia who received BLT showed a reduction in nighttime activity level and nighttime relative to daytime activity level, but this was not seen in a group of patients with Alzheimer's disease. In a RCT of 15 patients who received one hour per day, for at least two weeks, of BLT or dim light therapy, BLT was shown to significantly improve nocturnal sleep from a mean of 6.4 hours/night to 8.1 hours/night (Lyketsos *et al.*, 1999). The participants of this study had a mean MMSE score of 6.4 (standard deviation 6.8). The majority of subjects in Ancoli-Israel *et al.*'s RCT of 71 nursing home residents also had severe dementia (MMSE mean 5.7, range 0–27) (Ancoli-Israel *et al.*, 2003b). In this study patients received either morning BLT, morning red light (comparison group) or evening BLT. BLT did not improve total sleep time or percentage sleep but did increase the duration of maximum sleep bouts. This increase was by over 30 minutes for the morning BLT group and over 20 minutes for the evening BLT group. The evening BLT, but not the morning BLT, showed improvement in circadian rhythm activity. Two weeks of BT, for two hours a day, has also been shown to improve duration of sleep and latency in nursing home residents with dementia. Interestingly the effect was more positive during winter months (Allen *et al.*, 2003). There have, however, been other RCTs which have not had positive findings and the Cochrane Systematic review (Forbes *et al.*, 2004) concluded that there is insufficient evidence of the efficacy of BLT in managing sleep.

It has been proposed that music therapy and aromatherapy, using camomile oil, can promote sleep although there are no RCTs to substantiate this.

Exercise and sleep hygiene measures are the mainstay of non-pharmacological interventions for sleep disturbance in dementia. They are easy to implement and cheap, and have no discernible side effects. A combination of a light physical exercise programme and sleep hygiene strategies (e.g. keeping patients out of bed during the day and decreasing noise at night) can significantly improve sleep (Alessi *et al.*, 1999).

Verbal interventions

Receiving just information on sleep hygiene, however, may not be enough for caregivers to be effective in implementing a sleep hygiene programme. A RCT compared two groups of caregivers who both received written material describing age- and dementia-related changes in sleep and standard principles of good sleep hygiene, but the study group also received specific recommendations on how to set up and implement a programme (McCurry *et al.*, 2003). Caregivers who received active assistance were more successful in setting goals related to sleep scheduling, daytime napping and walking goals. The experimental group had significantly better consistent bedtimes (83% vs. 38%), rising times (96% vs. 59%), napped less (70% vs. 28%) and walked daily (86% vs. 7%). A similar RCT included 36 community-dwelling patients in AD, some of which had severe dementia (mean MMSE 11.8, standard deviation 8.4), and their family caregivers (McCurry *et al.*, 2005). All participants received written materials describing sleep changes and principles of good sleep hygiene and again the experimental group received specific recommendations on implementing a sleep hygiene programme. They were also instructed to walk daily and increase daytime light exposure using a light box. The control subjects received general dementia education and caregiver support. The experimental group showed significantly greater reduction in the number of nighttime awakenings, total time awake at night, depression and increases in weekly exercise days. The treatment gains were maintained at six-month follow-ups. The findings from this study suggest that several non-pharmacological interventions can be effective in treating sleep disturbance in dementia.

Summary

The current evidence base for non-pharmacological interventions is small. The RCTs that have been conducted have usually involved small numbers of patients with different types of dementia and a range of severity. In some areas of treatment there are only one or two studies, which usually have different methodologies, which makes comparison, or accumulation, of results nearly impossible. It is therefore difficult to draw strong conclusions from what is available when considering the treatment of BPSD in people with severe dementia. People with severe dementia could, however, potentially benefit the most from increased use of non-pharmacological interventions as this would reduce the reliance on pharmacological treatments, which frequently induce adverse effects in this frail, vulnerable patient group. There is encouraging evidence for the treatment of agitation and sleep disorders particularly and, as there are virtually no side effects, non-pharmacological interventions should be considered first-line treatment for these symptoms in people with severe dementia. There is, however, an urgent need to improve the support of their use. Future studies must address the issues of small, sample sizes, differing methodology, poor descriptions of the intervention and a lack of control groups.

References

Alessi CA, Yoon EJ, Schnelle JF, Al-Samarrai NR, Cruise PA (1999) A randomised trial of a combined physical activity and environmental intervention in nursing home residents: do sleep and agitation improve? *J Am Geriatr Soc*, 47(7):784–791.

Alexopoulos GS, Abrams RC, Young R C, Shamoian CA (1988) Cornell Scale for Depression in dementia. *Biol Psychiatry*, 23(3):271–284.

Allen J, Byrne EJ, Sutherland D, Tomenson B, Butler S, Burns A (2003) Bright light therapy, diurnal rhythm and sleep on dementia. *Int Psychogeriatr*, 15(Suppl 12):97–98.

Ancoli-Israel S, Martin JL, Gehrman P, Shochat T, Corey-Bloom J, Marker M, Nolan S, Levi L (2003a) Effect of light on agitation in institutionalised patients with severe Alzheimer's disease. *Am J Geriatr Psychiatry*, 11(2):194–203.

Ancoli-Israel S, Gehrman P, Martin JL, Shochat T, Marler M, Corey-Bloom J, Levi L (2003b) Increased light exposure consolidated and strengthens circadian rhythms in severe Alzheimer's disease patients. *Behave Sleep Med*, 1(1):22–36.

Baillon S, Van Deiepen E, Prettyman R, Redman J, Rooke N, Campbell R (2004) A comparison of the effects of Snoezelen and reminiscence therapy on the agitated behaviour of patients with dementia. *Int J Geriatr Psychiatry*, 19(11):1047–1052.

Baker R, Dowling Z, Wareing LA, Dawson J, Assey J (1997) Snoezelen: its long-term and short-term effects on older people with dementia. *Br J Occupational Therapy*, 60(5):213–218.

Ballard CG, O'Brien J (1999) Pharmacological treatment of behavioural and psychological signs in Alzheimer's disease: how good is the evidence for current pharmacological treatments? *Br Med J*, 319:138–139.

Ballard CG, O'Brien J, James I, Swann A (2001) Dementia: Management of Behavioural and Psychological Symptoms. Oxford University Press.

Ballard CG, O'Brien JT, Reichelt K, Perry EK (2002) Aromatherapy as a safe and effective treatment for the management of agitation in severe dementia: the results of a double-blind placebo in controlled trial with Melissa. *J Clin Psychiatry*, 63(7):553–558.

Brooker DJ, Snape M, Johnson E, Ward D, Payne M (1997) Single case evaluation of the effects of aromatherapy and massage on disturbed behaviour in severe dementia. *Br J Clin Psychol*, 36(2):287–296.

Chou KR, Kaas MJ, Ritchie MF (1990) Assaultive behaviour in geriatric patients. *Journal of Gerontol Nursing*, 22(11):31–38.

Chung JCC, Lai CKY, Chung PMD, French HP Snoezelen for Dementia *The Cochrane Database of Systematic Reviews*, 2002, Issue 4.

Clark ME, Lipe AW, Bilbrey M (1998) Use of music to decrease aggressive behaviours in people with dementia. *J Gerontol Nurs*, 24(7):10–17.

Coen RF, Swanwick GR, O'Boyle CA, Coakley D (1997) Behaviour disturbance and other predictors of carer burden in Alzheimer's disease. *Int J Geriatr Psychiatry*, 12(3):331–336.

Cohen-Mansfield J, Billig N (1986) Agitated behaviours in the elderly. *J Am Geriatr Soc*, 34(10):711–721.

Fetveit A, Skjerve A, Bjorvatn B (2003) Bright light treatment improves sleep in institutional elderly – an open trial. *Int J Geriatr Psychiatry*, 18(6):520–526.

Finkel SI, Costa e Silva J, Cohen G *et al.* (1996) Behavioural and psychological signs and symptoms of dementia: a consensus statement on current knowledge and implications for research and treatment. *Int Psychogeriatr*, 8(Suppl 3):497–500.

Fitzsimmons S (2001) Easy rider wheelchair biking. A nursing-recreation therapy clinical trial for the treatment of depression. *J Gerontol Nurs*, 27(5):14–23.

Forbes D, Morgan DG, Bangma J, Peacock S, Pelletier N, Adamson J (2004) Light Therapy for Managing, Sleep, Behaviour and Mood Disturbances in Dementia. *The Cochrane Database of Systematic, Reviews* 2004; Issue 2.

Gerdner LA (2000) Effects of individualised versus classical relaxation music on the frequency of agitation in elderly persons with Alzheimer's disease and related disorders. *Int Psychogeriatr*, 12(1):49–65.

Gilley DW, Whalen ME, Wilson RS, Bennett DA (1991) Hallucinations and associated factors in Alzheimer's disease. *J Neuropsychiatry Clin Neurosci*, 3:371–376.

Gormley N, Lyons D, Howard R (2001) Behavioural management of aggression in dementia: a randomised controlled trial. *Age Ageing*, 30(2):141–145.

Green A, Brodaty H (2002) Caregiver interventions. In: Evidence-based Dementia Practice, Eds Qizilbash N, Schneider L, Chui H, Tariot P, Brodarty H, Kaye J, Erkinjunthi T. Blackwell Science, Oxford, UK.

Haffmans PMJ, Sival RC, Lucius SAP, Cats Q, van Gelder LV (2001) Bright light therapy and melatonin in motor restlessness behaviour in dementia: a placebo-controlled study. *Int J Geriatr Psychiatry*, 16(1):106–110.

Haupt M, Karger A, Janner M (2000) Improvement of agitation and anxiety in demented patients after psychoeducatative group intervention with their caregivers. *Int J Geriatr Psychiatry*, 15(12):1125–1129.

Hermann KM, Mandoni KM, Lancrot KL (2004) Atypical antipsychotics and risk of cerebrovascular accidents. *Am J Psychiatry*, 16:1113–1115.

Holmes C, Hopkins V, Hensford C, MacLaughlin V, Wilkinson D, Rosenvinge H (2002) Lavender oil as a treatment for agitated behaviour in severe dementia: a placebo controlled study. *Int J Geriatr Psychiatry*, 17(4):305–308.

Kite SM, Maher EJ, Anderson K, Young T, Young J, Wood J, Howells N, Bradburn J (1998) Development of an aromatherapy service at a Cancer Centre. *Palliat Med*, 12(3):177–180.

Koger SM, Chopin K, Brotons M (1999) Is music therapy an effective intervention for dementia? A meta-analytic review of literature. *J Music Ther*, 36(1):2–15.

Kovach CR, Taneli Y, Dohearty P, Schliat AM, Cashin S, Silva-Smith AL (2004) Effect of the BACE intervention on agitation of people with dementia. *The Gerontologist*, 44(6):797–806.

Kragt K, Holtkamp CC, van Dongen MC, van Rossum E, Salentiyn C (1997) The effect of sensory stimulation in the sensory stimulation room on the well-being of demented elderly. A cross-over trial in residents of the RC, Care Center Bernardus in Amsterdam. *Verplecgkunde*, 12(4):227–236.

Lai CK, Chi T, Kayser-Jones J (2004) A randomised controlled trial of a specific reminiscence approach to promote the well-being of nursing home residents with dementia. *Int Psychogeriatr*, 1(1):33–49.

Lam RW (1998) Seasonal and Affective Disorder and Beyond: Light Treatment for SAD and non-SAD conditions. American Psychiatric Press, Washington, DC.

Lord TR, Garner JE (1993) Effects of music therapy on Alzheimer patients. *Percept Mot Skills*, 76(2):451–455.

Lou MF (2001) The use of music to decrease agitated behaviour of the demented elderly: the state of the science *Scand J Caring Sci*, 15(2):165–173.

Lyketsos CG, Lindell Veiel L, Baker A, Steele C (1999) A randomised, controlled trial of bright light therapy for agitated behaviours in dementia patients residing in long-term care. *Int J Geriatr Psychiatry*, 14(7):520–525.

Margallo-Lana M, Swann A, O'Brien J *et al.* (2001) Prevalence and pharmacological management of behavioural and psychological symptoms amongst dementia sufferers living in care environments. *Int J Geriatr Psychiatry*, 16(1):39–44.

Martin J, Marler M, Scochat T, Ancoli-Israel S (2000) Circadian rhythms of agitation in institutional patients with Alzheimer's disease. *Chronobiol Int*, 17(3):405–418.

McCurry SM, Gibbons L, Logsdon RG, Vitiello MV, Teri L. (2003) Training caregivers to change the sleep hygiene practices of patients with dementia: the NITE-AD project. *J Am Geriatr Soc*, 51(10):1455–1460.

McCurry SM, Gibbons LE, Logsdon RG, Vitiello MV, Teri L (2005) Night-time insomnia treatment and education for Alzheimer's disease: a randomised controlled trial. *J Am Geriatr Soc*, 53(5):73–802.

McMahon S, Kermode S (1996) A clinical trial of the effect of aromatherapy on motivational behaviour in a dementia care setting using a single subject design. *Aust J Hollist Nurs*, 5(2):47–49.

McShane R, Keene J, Gedling K, Fairburn C, Jacoby R, Hope T (1997) Do neuroleptic drugs hasten cognitive decline in dementia? Prospective study with necropsy follow up. *Br Med J*, 314:266–270.

Mega MS, Cummings JL, Fiorello T, Gombien J. (1996) The spectrum of behavioural changes in Alzheimer's disease. *Neurology*, 46(1):130–135.

Mishima K, Hishikawa Y, Okawa M (1998) Randomised, dim light controlled, crossover test of morning bright light therapy for rest-activity rhythm disorders in patients with vascular dementia and dementia of Alzheimer's type. *Chronobiol Int*, 15(6):647–654.

Mungas D, Weiler P, Franzi C, Henry R (1989) Assessment of disruptive behavior associated with dementia: the disruptive behavior rating scale. *J Geriatr Psychiatry Neurol*, 2(4):196–202.

Neal M, Briggs M (2003) Validation Therapy for Dementia (Cochrane Review). *The Cochrane Database of Systematic Reviews*, Issue 3.

O'Donnell BF, Drachman DA, Barnes HJ, Peterson KE, Swearer JM, Lew RA (1992) Incontinence and troublesome behaviours predict institutionalisation in dementia. *J Geriatr Psychiatry Neurol*, 5(1):45–52.

Paulsen JS, Salmon DP, Thal LJ *et al.* (2000) Incidence of and risk factors for hallucinations and delusions in patients with probable Alzheimer's disease. *Neurology*, 54(10):1965–1971.

Pinkney L (1997) A comparison of the Snoezelen environment and a music relaxation group on the mood and behaviour of patients with senile dementia. *Br J Occupational Therapy*, 60:209–218.

Politis AM, Vozzella S, Mayer LS, Onyike CU, Baker AS, Lyketsos CG (2004) A randomised, controlled, clinical trial of activity therapy for apathy in patients with dementia residing in long-term care. *Int J Geriatr Psychiatry*, 19(11):1087–1094.

Proctor R, Burns A, Powell HS *et al.* (1999) Behavioural management in nursing and residential homes: a randomised controlled trial. *Lancet*, 354(9172):26–29.

Rabins PV, Mace NL, Lucas MJ (1982) The impact of dementia on the family. *J Am Med Assoc* 248:333–335.

Rovner BW, Steele CD, Shmuely Y, Folstein MF (1996) A randomised trial of dementia care in nursing homes. *J Am Geriatr Soc*, 44(1):7–13.

Satlin A, Volicer L, Ross V, Herz L, Campbell S (1992) Bright light treatment of behavioral and sleep disturbances in patients with Alzheimer's disease. *Am J Psychiatry*, 149(8):1028–1032.

Schindler SD, Graf A, Fischer P, Tolk A, Kasper S (2002) Paranoid delusions and hallucinations and bright light therapy in Alzheimer's disease. *Int J Geriatr Psychiatry*, 17(11):1071–1072.

Schneider LS, Pollock E, Lyness SA (1990) A meta-analysis of controlled trials of neuroleptic treatment in dementia. *J Am Geriatr Soc*, 38(5):553–563.

Schrijnemaekers V, Van Rossum E, Candel M *et al.* (2002) Effects of emotion-orientated care on elderly people with cognitive impairment and behavioural problems. *Int J Geriatr Psychiatry*, 17(10):926–937.

Skjerve A, Holstein F, Aarsland D, Bjorvatn, Nygaard HA, Johansen IM (2004a) Improvement in behavioural symptoms and advance of activity acrophase after short-term bright light treatment in severe dementia. *Psychiatry and Clinical Neurosciences*, 58(4):343–347.

Skjerve A, Bjorvatn, Holsten F (2004b) Light therapy for behavioural and psychological symptoms of dementia. *Int J Geriatr Psychiatry*, 19(4):516–522.

Smallwood J, Brown R, Coulter F, Irvine E, Copland C (2001) Aromatherapy and behaviour disturbances in dementia: a randomised controlled trial. *Int J Geriatr Psychiatry*, 16(10):1010–1013.

Snowden M, Sato K, Roy-Byrne P (2003) Assessment and treatment of nursing home residents with depression or behavioural symptoms associated with dementia: a review of the literature. *J Am Geriatr Soc*, 51(9):1305–1317.

Spector A, Orrell M, Davies S, Woods B (2000) Reality Orientation for Dementia. *The Cochrane Database of Systematic, Reviews*, Issue 3.

Sumaya IC, Rienzi BM, Deegan JF, Moss DE (2001) Bright light treatment decreases depression in institutionalised older adults: a placebo-controlled crossover study. *J Gerontol A Biol Sci Med Sci*, 56(6):M356–M360.

Teri L, Logsdon RG, Uomoto J, McCurry SM (1997) Behavioural treatment of depression in dementia patients: a control trial. *J Gerontol B Psychol Sci Soc Sci*, 52(4):159–166.

Teri L, Logsdon RG, Peskind E *et al.* (2000) Treatment of agitation in AD: a randomised, placebo-controlled clinical trial. *Neurology*, 55(9):1271–1278.

Teri L, Gibbons LE, McCurry SM *et al.* (2003) Exercise plus behavioral management in patients with Alzheimer's disease: a randomised controlled trial. *J Am Med Assoc*, 290(15):2015–2022.

Teri L *et al.* (2005) Training community consultants to help family members improve dementia care: a randomised controlled trial. *Gerontologist*, (under review).

Thorgrimsen L, Spector A, Wiles A, Orrell M (2003) Aromatherapy for Dementia. *The Cochrane Database of Systematic Reviews*, Issue 3.

Vitiello MV, Poceta JS, Prinz PN (1991) Sleep in Alzheimer's disease and other dementing disorders. *Can J Psychol*, 45(2):221–239.

Woods R (2002) Non-pharmacological techniques In: Evidence-based Dementia Practice. Eds Qizilbash N, Schneider L, Chui H, Tariot P, Brodarty H, Kaye J, Erkinjunthi T. Blackwell Science. Oxford.

Woods B, Spector A, Jones C, Orrell M, Davies S (2005) Reminiscence Therapy for Dementia. *The Cochrane Database of Systematic Reviews*, Issue 2.

Worwood VA (1996) The Fragrant Mind: Aromatherapy for Mind, Mood and Emotion. Transworld Publishers, London.

14

Non-pharmacological Treatment of Severe Dementia: the Seattle Protocols

Rebecca G. Logsdon, Linda Teri and Sue M. McCurry

Introduction

Behavioural disturbances such as depression, agitation/aggression, physical inactivity, and sleep disturbances affect most patients at some point in progression of dementia, and are highly associated with greater functional impairment, higher levels of caregiver burden, and increased rates of nursing home placement. Management of behavioural problems in severe dementia typically emphasises pharmacologic intervention, but efficacy of such intervention is mixed and may be complicated by adverse side effects, interactions with other medications, and idiosyncratic responses. A consensus conference convened by the American Association for Geriatric Psychiatry, the Alzheimer's Association and the American Geriatrics Society concluded that non-pharmacological treatment is the most appropriate first step to treating behavioural disturbances in patients with dementia (Small *et al.*, 1997), and empirical data from clinical trials are accumulating to indicate that many behavioural problems can be effectively managed with behavioural or environmental interventions (Beck *et al.*, 2002; Bourgeois *et al.*, 1996; Forbes, 1998; Kasl-Godley and Gatz, 2000; Teri *et al.*, 2002). In this chapter we present an overview of the Seattle Protocols, which are empirically validated behavioural treatments for the most common behavioural problems seen in dementia: depression, agitation/aggression and sleep disturbance. In order to provide a broad overview, we will describe their use in community settings with family caregivers, and in residential care settings, with paid caregivers. We conclude with recommendations for clinical practice and for future research.

The Seattle Protocols: a comprehensive non-pharmacological intervention for reducing behavioural disturbances in patients with severe dementia

The Seattle Protocols for treatment of behavioural disturbances in dementia were based on an integrated model of social learning and gerontological theories. Social learning theory addresses how specific problems develop, are maintained and may be changed (Bandura, 1997). Gerontological theory addresses the importance of the psychosocial context of these problems for older adults (Lawton, 1990). The Seattle Protocols were derived from the experience of the authors, who are clinical psychologists experienced in working with older adults, their families and their care providers. Because of this clinical orientation the Seattle Protocols are clinically relevant, and are designed to provide a practical approach to a wide variety of dementia-related problems. The Seattle Protocols are ethically sensitive, developed with respect for the needs of the person with dementia and the caregiver and a commitment to supporting them both, with the ultimate goal of improving the quality of their lives throughout the course of dementia. Finally, the Seattle Protocols are empirically sound. They have been applied, tested and improved using an iterative process between

Severe Dementia. Edited by A. Burns and B. Winblad.
Copyright © 2006 John Wiley & Sons, Ltd.   ISBN 0-470-01054-1

the developers, other clinicians and the patients and caregivers for whom the treatments are intended. Each has been rigorously evaluated in controlled clinical trials to determine efficacy with patients and caregivers in diverse settings, and each has a standardised treatment manual to allow replication and evaluation by other clinicians and researchers.

The Seattle Protocols combine caregiver education and training with specific behavioural techniques. They emphasise practical skills that caregivers learn to employ to improve patient affective and behavioural health, and they teach caregivers to systematically approach problems so that they can continue to use this approach throughout the progression of dementia.

Each protocol begins by providing caregivers a rationale for the intervention, establishing mutually agreed-upon goals, and providing education and information about dementia, caregiving and community resources. The central phase of each protocol focuses on improving caregiver skills to reduce specific problems (depression, anxiety, agitation, sleep, etc.), increasing pleasant events, improving communication, and maximising patient cognitive function. Each protocol concludes with specific recommendations and plans for maintaining and generalising gains achieved during treatment.

To enhance caregiver skills in managing problem behaviours, caregivers are taught to: (1) identify specifics about the problem under consideration, (2) define the factors that lead up to and sustain their occurrence, and (3) systematically alter those factors to reduce problems. This process has been called the ABCs of behaviour change and we first applied it to dementia care in 1984. In this model, A is the antecedent or triggering event that precedes the problem; B is the behaviour of concern; and C is the consequence that follows a problem behaviour. Thus, ABC represents a chain of behaviours (or events) that occur and can be modified to reduce problems in care. This strategy of problem identification and treatment has been detailed elsewhere (Teri et al., 2002) and is available in a video training programme (Teri, 1990).

Empirical evaluation of the Seattle Protocols

Five randomised, controlled, clinical trials have been conducted to investigate the efficacy of the Seattle Protocols. Each examined the core protocol described above while targeting specific behavioural disturbances, including depression, agitation, sleep disturbance, physical inactivity and anxiety. All were conducted with community-dwelling persons with AD and their family caregivers, with the exception of the most recent study, conducted in assisted-living residences. Treatment was conducted by a variety of trained professionals, and employed specific treatment manuals and treatment integrity procedures, and interviewers blind to treatment condition conducted all assessments.

Depression

Depressive symptoms occur in 30% to 70% of individuals diagnosed with Alzheimer's disease (Lazarus et al., 1987; Teri et al., 1991; Weiner et al., 1994). Unhappiness, withdrawal, inactivity, fatigue, expressions of guilt and worthlessness, tearfulness and loss of interest can all signify depression. Patients with dementia gradually lose the ability to engage in enjoyable hobbies or activities and, owing to their cognitive impairment, may be unable to identify replacement activities. Consequently, they may spend much of their time in activities that are not gratifying or meaningful or, as the disease progresses, they may disengage from activity altogether (Brodaty et al., 1997).

The first Seattle Protocol was designed to reduce depression in persons with Alzheimer's disease (Teri and Gallagher, 1991; Teri et al., 1997). Although it is currently well established that depression is a debilitating yet treatable component of AD, at the time this study was conducted, few pharmacological trials had investigated the potential of treating depression in dementia and only one case report had addressed the potential of behavioural treatment. The Seattle Protocol for depression was tested in a randomised, controlled, clinical trial that compared two active behavioural treatments (Behavior Therapy–Pleasant Activities (BT-PA) and Behavior Therapy–Problem Solving (BT-PS)) to a usual care condition and a wait-list control. Treatment consisted of nine 60-minute sessions, conducted once a week. Caregivers assigned to both behavioural conditions followed the protocol described earlier; BT-PA emphasised pleasant events and a structured approach to the protocol while BT-PS covered protocol topics with a more flexible approach allowing caregivers to determine the flow of treatment.

Seventy-two AD patient–caregiver dyads were randomised and evaluated at pre-, post-, and six-months. All patients and 76% of caregivers met criteria for major or minor depressive disorder. Change in patient depression, the primary outcome, was measured by DSMIII-R diagnosis of depression, the Hamilton Depression Rating Scale, the Cornell Depression in Dementia Scale and the Beck Depression Inventory (modified for caregiver/patient report). Caregiver level of depression was measured with the Hamilton Depression Rating Scale.

Study results indicated that patients in both behavioural conditions showed significant improvement in depression symptoms and diagnosis as compared with patients in the two control conditions (Hamilton Depression Rating Scale: $F(3, 71) = 4.52$, $p < 0.001$). Sixty per cent of patients in the active conditions showed clinically significant improvement while only 20% in the control conditions did. Furthermore, none of the patients in the active conditions deteriorated while 10% of those in control did. Additionally, 70% of the controls showed no improvement over time ($F(6, 72) = 18.48$, $p < 0.005$). Caregivers in each behavioural condition also showed significant improvement in their own depression symptoms, while caregivers in the two control conditions did not (Hamilton Depression Rating Scale: $F(3, 66) = 4.73$, $p < 0.01$). These gains were maintained at six-month follow-up (patient HDRS ($F(60, 2) = 31.47$, $p < 0.001$); caregiver HDRS ($F(60, 2) = 4.28$, $p < 0.05$)).

Agitation

Agitated behaviours (such as irritability, restlessness, physical and verbal aggression, resisting needed assistance, pacing, and wandering) affect 70% to 90% of patients with dementia during the progression of the disease (Swearer et al., 1988; Teri et al., 1992) . Similar to depression, agitation may have a variety of causes, including physiological, environmental and interpersonal triggers. Furthermore, these causes often interact. For example individuals with dementia may have decreased tolerance for stimulation, or decreased inhibition of inappropriate behaviours due to neurological changes. They may exhibit agitation in response to environmental triggers such as overstimulation or activities they do not understand (e.g. being bathed by a caregiver they do not know or remember). The key to non-pharmacological intervention for episodes of agitation or aggression is to identify and avoid their triggers, thus reducing their frequency or impact.

We investigated the Seattle Protocol's efficacy in decreasing agitation in patients with dementia (Teri et al., 1998a; 2000). At the time this study was conducted, the predominant treatments for agitation in community-dwelling patients with AD were haloperidol, an antipsychotic, and trazodone, an antidepressant with sedating properties. Consequently, the Seattle Protocol for agitation was compared to both modes of pharmacotherapy in a randomised, placebo-controlled, multi-site clinical trial. Twenty-one sites around the country enrolled 149 agitated AD patients and their caregivers. Assessments were conducted at baseline and after 16 weeks (11 sessions) of treatment.

Results indicated that 34% of dementia patients improved relative to baseline. No significant differences were obtained between haloperidol (mean dose, 1.8 mg/d), trazodone (mean dose, 200 mg/d), Seattle Protocol, or placebo and no differences in specific symptom reduction were evident across active treatments. However, significantly fewer adverse events were evident in the Seattle Protocol arm. Consequently, although the Seattle Protocol was comparable to medications in outcome and yielded significantly fewer adverse events, the magnitude of improvement was small.

Subsequently, the Seattle Protocol was applied in a community home health setting, to investigate the extent to which community consultants could be trained to use it with family caregivers who were having difficulty because of agitation, anxiety and mood disturbances in their family members with moderate to severe dementia (Teri *et al.*, 2005). In this randomised, controlled trial, 95 family caregivers and care recipients with dementia were randomly assigned to the Seattle Protocol intervention or to control. Assessments were conducted at baseline, post-treatment, and six months by masked interviewers. Consultants were master's-level health care professionals who were currently practising in the community in settings serving older adults. The intervention was conducted in caregivers' homes, and each session was audio-taped and reviewed by the authors to ensure that consultants adhered to the behavioural treatment protocol. Caregivers receiving the Seattle Protocol showed significant improvements in caregiver depression, burden and reactivity to behaviour problems in the care recipient (all $p < 0.05$). There were also significant reductions in the frequency and severity of care recipient behaviour problems, and improved quality of life (all $p < 0.05$). Improvements were maintained at six-month follow-up. Thus, the Seattle Protocols appear to be a viable and reasonable approach to use with caregivers of individuals with moderate to severe dementia in a community home health setting.

Sleep disturbances

Wandering at night, bedtime agitation, disturbed sleep and night–day reversal are common problems for persons with dementia (McCurry *et al.*, 1999), and are often linked with nursing home placement (Hope *et al.*, 1998; Pollak and Perlick, 1991; Pollock *et al.*, 1990). There is general agreement that hypnotic treatments for sleep problems should be used sparingly in the elderly in order to minimise falls, impaired memory, drug-related sleep disorders, or aggravation of a preexisting sleep apnoea syndrome (Kripke, 2000; NIH, 1990). Behavioural approaches have been used effectively with older cognitively intact older adults, but they had not been applied to individuals with dementia. The Seattle Protocol for sleep disturbance in patients with dementia (NITE-AD) (McCurry *et al.*, 2005) was tested in a controlled clinical trial to determine whether patients receiving NITE-AD would show significant improvement on measures of sleep, depression and behavioural disturbances compared to subjects enrolled in a supportive contact control condition.

Treatment was provided in six one-hour sessions over a two-month period, with patients and family caregivers in their homes. In addition to the Seattle Protocol components discussed earlier, caregivers in NITE-AD were taught to develop an individualised sleep programme for their patient, which included daily walking and daily sessions sitting in front of a light box. Control caregivers received general information but no specific behavioural recommendations. Thirty-six AD patients were evaluated at baseline, post-treatment, and six-month follow-up. Sleep was measured using an Actillume wrist-movement recorder worn for one week at each sampling point. Caregivers also reported on patient daytime sleepiness (Epworth Sleepiness Scale), depression (Cornell Depression Scale) and behavioural disturbance (Revised Memory and Behavior Problems Checklist).

At post-test, significant ($p < 0.05$) differences were obtained between groups for Actillume estimates of patient time awake at night and sleep latency. For both outcomes, subjects in NITE-AD improved while contact control subjects declined. Compared to controls, NITE-AD patients at post-test spent an average of 36 minutes less time awake at night (a 32% reduction from baseline), and had 5.3 fewer nightly awakenings (also a 32% reduction from baseline). NITE-AD patients exercised significantly more days per week, and had significantly lower levels of depression on the RMBPC than controls. At six months, results were maintained and, in addition, NITE-AD patients had significantly fewer awakenings per hour than controls, their awakenings were for shorter durations, and there was a trend for NITE-AD patients to spend less time in bed. Thus, the Seattle Protocol for sleep disturbance appears to be an effective intervention for improving sleep in individuals with dementia, and had the additional benefits of increasing physical activity and decreasing depression.

Physical inactivity

It is widely recognised that individuals with dementia suffer from a cognitive disorder with significant behavioural impairments. However, they also suffer significant disability related to physical inactivity and frailty. Consequently, Reducing Disability in Alzheimer's Disease (RDAD), investigated a Seattle Protocol that was combined with exercise training. The goal of this study was to determine whether the Seattle Protocol was more effective than routine medical care in increasing physical activity and improving the physical and affective health in persons with AD (Teri et al., 1998b, 2003).

Treatment was provided twice a week for three weeks, followed by four weekly, two biweekly, and three monthly sessions. Caregivers assigned to the Seattle Protocol were taught: (1) to guide their demented patient through an individualised programme involving endurance activities (primarily walking), strength training, balance, and flexibility exercises and (2) behavioural management strategies as described above. One hundred and fifty-three AD patients and their caregivers were evaluated at baseline, post-treatment, and 6, 12, 18 and 24-month follow-up. Patient health status was measured with the Medical Outcomes Study Short Form (SF-36), the Sickness Impact Profile, the Cornell Depression Scale for Dementia, and caregiver reports of patients' restricted activity days, bed disability days, falls and exercise participation.

Results indicated that caregivers were able to learn and direct patients to follow scheduled exercise activities. Eighty-one per cent of active treatment patients attempted exercise recommendations. Significant differences between active and control conditions were obtained. At post-test, active treatment subjects exercised more (odds ratio (95% CI) 2.82 (1.22, 6.49)), had fewer restricted activity days (odds ratio 3.10 (1.08, 8.95)), and improved significantly more than controls on primary outcomes of physical activity (mean SF-36 Physical Role Functioning difference score 19.29 (8.75, 29.83)) and depression (mean Cornell Depression Scale difference score -1.03 (-0.17, -1.91). Over 24 months of follow-up, changes in physical activity and improvements in mobility were maintained. For patients entering the study with higher levels of depression, significant improvements in depression were also maintained at 24 months. There was also a trend among active treatment patients to have less institutionalisation due to behavioural disturbance throughout the 24-month follow-up period.

Staff Training in Assisted-Living Residences

The most recent Seattle Protocol is called STAR – Staff Training in Assisted-living Residences (Teri et al., 2002b, 2002c). Assisted living settings are the fastest growing residential option for older adults in this country, many of whom are demented. Consequently, STAR takes the Seattle Protocol into AL (assisted-living) residences to train direct care staff in methods to reduce the affective and behavioural disturbance of persons with dementia in AL residences.

STAR is conducted at the AL residence over two months. It consists of two half-day workshops, each followed by two on-site, one-on-one consultation sessions between trainer and trainee to enable on-the-job practice of strategies covered in the workshop. It also includes licensed staff training sessions to ensure that direct care staff receive the support and guidance necessary to sustain the programme once training is completed. Thus far, 15 AL residences, involving 114 staff and 120 residents, have participated in STAR training. Four additional residences, 25 staff members and 31 residents, participated in a small, randomised, controlled clinical trial to determine whether STAR was more effective in reducing resident distress and improving staff skill and satisfaction than routine in-service training conducted on site.

Results indicated that residents in the STAR condition improved on five out of six outcomes: they showed statistically significant reductions in their level of general behavioural disturbance (Neuropsychiatric Inventory (NPI) and Revised Memory and Behavior Problems Checklist (RMBPC) total), depression (Geriatric Depression Scale (GDS) and RMBPC–Depression Subscale) and anxiety (Clinical Anxiety Scale (CAS)). They showed no reduction in their level of agitation (RMBPC–Disruption). Residents in the control condition became worse on three of six outcomes, general behaviour problems (NPI), depression (GDS) and anxiety (CAS), and remained unchanged on the remaining three outcome measures. Differences between the two conditions were statistically significant. Staff receiving STAR reported significantly less impact from resident problems after training and staff in the control condition reported more (NPI-Staff Impact). Based on these successful outcomes, the star programme is currently being implemented and tested in other assisted living programmes in three states to evaluate its generalisability.

Conclusion

Behavioural problems in dementia are prevalent, pervasive and disruptive. They increase as dementia severity increases, and adversely affect patient and caregiver alike, often leading to patient institutionalisation and caregiver burnout. Although these problems are often difficult to manage, evidence is accumulating from rigorous, controlled clinical trials that many of them are responsive to behavioural intervention, both in community and institutional settings. Caregivers, whether they are family members, long-term care staff or health care professionals, are critical to the assessment and treatment of behavioural problems. Oftentimes, they are the sole providers of care for a patient with dementia and must learn how to manage the variety of problems that are experienced, including depression, agitation, sleep disturbance and inactivity. In this chapter, we have provided an overview of a theoretically and clinically based approach to teaching behavioural strategies to these caregivers, and reviewed the empirical basis for its application. Future research to more fully develop and test this approach in a variety of settings, including community home health, assisted living, adult family homes and nursing homes is needed to improve its efficacy and demonstrate its effectiveness in non-research settings.

Acknowledgements

Preparation of this chapter was supported in part by grants from the Alzheimer's Association (PIO-99-1800) and the National Institutes of Health (AG10483, AG10845). Portions of this chapter were presented at the 9th International Conference on Alzheimer's Disease and Related Disorders, July 17–22, 2004, Philadelphia, PA.

References

Bandura A (1977) Social Learning Theory. Englewood Cliffs, NJ: Prentice-Hall.
Beck CK et al. (2002) Effects of behavioural interventions on disruptive behaviour and affect in demented nursing home residents. Nursing Research, 51(4):219–228.
Bourgeois MS, Schulz R and Burgio L (1996) Interventions for caregivers of patients with Alzheimer's disease: a review and analysis of content, process, and outcomes. International Journal of Aging and Human Development, 43(1):35–92.
Brodaty H et al. (1997) Outline of a dementia caregivers' training program. In Research and Practice in Alzheimer's Disease, Vellas B et al. (eds). New York: Springer.
Forbes DA (1998) Strategies for managing behavioural symptomatology associated with dementia of the Alzheimer type: a systematic overview. Canadian Journal of Nursing Research, 30(2):67–86.
Hope T et al. (1998) Predictors of institutionalization for people with dementia living at home with a carer. International Journal of Geriatric Psychiatry, 13(10):682–690.
Kasl-Godley J and Gatz M (2000) Psychosocial interventions for individuals with dementia: an integration of theory, therapy, and a clinical understanding of dementia. Clinical Psychology Review, 6:755–782.
Kripke DF (2000) Chronic hypnotic use: deadly risks, doubtful benefit. Sleep Medicine Reviews 4(1):5–20.
Lawton MP (1990) Residential environment and self-directedness among older people. American Pschyologist, 45(5):638–640.

Lazarus LW *et al.* (1987) Frequency and presentation of depressive symptoms in patients with primary degenerative dementia. *American Journal of Psychiatry*, 144:41–45.

McCurry SM *et al.* (1999) Characteristics of sleep disturbance in community-dwelling Alzheimer's disease patients. *Journal of Geriatric Psychiatry and Neurology*, 12:53–59.

McCurry SM *et al.* (2005) Nighttime insomnia treatment and education for Alzheimer's disease: a randomized controlled trial. *Journal of the American Geriatrics Society*, 53:793–802.

NIH (1990) Consensus Conference: Treatment of Sleep Disorders of Older People. Washington, DC: National Institutes of Health.

Pollak CP, Perlick D (1991) Sleep problems and institutionalization of the elderly. *Journal of Geriatric Psychiatry and Neurology*, 4:204–210.

Pollock CP *et al.* (1990) Sleep problems in the community elderly as predictors of death and nursing home placement. *Journal of Community Health*, 15:123–135.

Small GN *et al.* (1997) Diagnosis and treatment of Alzheimer disease and related disorders: Consensus statement of the American Association for Geriatric Psychiatry, the Alzheimer's Association, and the American Geriatrics Society. *Journal of the American Medical Association*, 278:1363–1371.

Swearer JM *et al.* (1988) Troublesome and disruptive behaviours in dementia: relationships to diagnosis and disease severity. *Journal of the American Geriatrics Society*, 36:784–790.

Teri L (1990) Managing and Understanding Behaviour Problems in Alzheimer's Disease and Related Disorders. Seattle: University of Washington.

Teri L, Gallagher D (1991) Cognitive-behavioural interventions for treatment of depression in Alzheimer's patients. *The Gerontologist*, 31:413–416.

Teri L, Baer L, Reifler B (1991) Depression in Alzheimer's patients: investigation of symptom patterns and frequency. *Clinical Gerontologist*, 11:47–57.

Teri L *et al.* (1992) Assessment of behavioural problems in dementia: the Revised Memory and Behavior Problems Checklist. *Psychology and Aging*, 7:622–631.

Teri L *et al.* (1997) Behavioural treatment of depression in dementia patients: a controlled clinical trial. *Journals of Gerontology B: Psychological Sciences and Social Sciences*, 52B(4):P159–P166.

Teri L *et al.* (1998a) Treatment for agitation in dementia patients: a behaviour management approach. *Psychotherapy*, 35(4):436–443.

Teri L *et al.* (1998b) Exercise and activity level in Alzheimer's disease: a potential treatment focus. *Journal of Rehabilitation Research and Development*, 35(4):411–419.

Teri L *et al.* (2000) Treatment of agitation in Alzheimer's disease: a randomized placebo controlled clinical trial. *Neurology*, 55:1271–1278.

Teri L, Logsdon RG, McCurry SM (2002a) Nonpharmacologic treatment of behavioural disturbance in dementia. *Medical Clinics of North America*, 86:641–656.

Teri L, Young H, Huda P (2002b) STAR: Staff Training for dementia care in assisted-living residences, in Preconference workshop, 55th Annual Meeting of the Gerontological Society of America, Boston, MA.

Teri L *et al.* (2003) Exercise plus behaviour management in patients with Alzheimer disease: a randomized controlled trial. *Journal of the American Medical Association*, 290(15):2015–2022.

Teri L, McCurry SM, Logsdon RG, Gibbons LE (2005a) Training Community Consultants to Help Family Members Improve Dementia Care: a randomized controlled trial. *The Gerontologist*, 45(6):802–811.

Teri L, Huda P, Gibbons LA, Young H, Van Leynseele J (2005b) STAR: a dementia-specific training program for staff in assisted living residences. *The Gerontologist*, 45(5):686–693.

Weiner M, Edland S, Luszczynska-Halina (1994) Prevalence and incidence of major depression in Alzheimer's disease. *American Journal of Psychiatry*, 151:1006–1009.

15

Care by Families for Late Stage Dementia

Steven H. Zarit and Joseph E. Gaugler

Late stage care has generally received less attention than family involvement during middle stages of dementia. It is often assumed that by the late stages of dementia families have relinquished the care of their relative to an institution and meaningful involvement is significantly reduced. The reality of late stage care is different. A minority of caregivers of late stage patients continue to provide care at home, even after their relative has become bedridden. Those who place their relative usually remain involved in care, though the challenges they face have changed with placement and the progression of the disease. Spouses, in particular, are frequent visitors at nursing homes, sometimes coming every day to care for their husband or wife. These involvements of family at home and in institutional settings bear directly on the patient's quality of life, and have continuing implications for the carer's own wellbeing.

This chapter has organised the discussion of late stage care around four issues: (1) late stage care provided in the home; (2) involvement of family carers in institutional settings; (3) end-of-life issues; and (4) mourning and recovery. We draw upon the limited research available on late stage care, as well as clinical examples. The goal is to illuminate the main challenges faced by families and to identify the types of supports and services they need in the final stages of their relative's illness.

Late stage care in the home

Those carers who provide late stage care at home are clearly a select group who have a different kind of commitment, as well as physical, emotional and economic resources to allow them to carry out prolonged at-home care. There have been relatively few studies that characterise these individuals. For the most part, research has addressed the other side of this issue, that is, what are the predictors of institutional placement and who is likely to place a relative in a nursing home.

Most of the recent studies of placement have used event history analysis, proportional hazards models or similar statistical techniques that identify factors associated with the timing of an event, that is, whether carers place a relative sooner or later in the disease process. Thus, findings from these studies characterise carers who place a relative earlier compared to later in the disease, including those participants who have not institutionalised their relative during the observed time period. As a result, the available research provides only an indirect glimpse of the late stage carers who have not placed a relative.

The picture that emerges is that several characteristics of the person with dementia and the carer are associated with earlier placement, or conversely, maintaining someone at home longer. In studies which compare people with and without dementia, cognitive impairment and behaviour problems are typically a strong predictor of placement. Among carers assisting people with dementia, behaviour problems also emerge as a predictor (e.g. Phillips and Diwan, 2003), as does decline in performance of activities of daily living (Gaugler et al., 2003a), but these effects are often tempered by other characteristics of the caregiver and care context. Factors such as perceived burden, role captivity and family conflict are associated with continued residence at home (Gaugler *et al.*, 2000; Gaugler *et al.*, 2003a). Carers who receive help from family members, particular with activities of daily living and overnight care, are less likely to place their relative (Gaugler *et al.*, 2000). In a major longitudinal study, Aneshensel *et al.* (1995) found that poor health, a recent hospitalisation and role captivity were the strongest predictors of placement. Using paid help in the home had an effect opposite to what was expected. People receiving more paid help were more likely to place their relative. This finding may reflect a process of self-selection, that is, people who use paid help in the home are also more likely to turn to institutional care. Taken together, these findings suggest that behaviour problems create a context in which placement may occur, but the decision depends on a combination of factors in the situation.

Aneshensel *et al.* (1995) also asked carers to describe the factors that led to placement. Two main themes emerged from their responses. Approximately one-third of the sample reported that they had become concerned over their relative's safety at home, or that their relative might harm someone else. Almost as many carers reported that they were physically and/or emotionally exhausted, and were not able to continue providing help. The remaining third of the sample mentioned a variety of reasons, including their relative becoming incontinent or having failing health, or that the carer did not receive enough help to continue providing care at home. In response to open-ended questions, many carers reported that their families did not help enough, or that the patient was despondent or was left alone too much of the time.

It would be expected that kin relationship would also play a role in placement, specifically, that husbands and wives would be less likely to relocate a spouse than would children or other carers. Most studies, however, have not reported that spouses are more likely to remain at home (e.g. Aneshensel *et al.*, 1995; Gaugler *et al.*, 2000). In part, that may be due to the way studies have been conducted. Using samples of patients mostly in the middle to late stages of the illness, the researchers capture those carers who have made a strong commitment to keeping their relative at home. People with more fragile commitments have already moved their relative to a care facility. Some spouses are undoubtedly in that group, but it is likely that children and other carers turn to an institution earlier in the disease process.

One of the most likely immediate triggers of placement in middle and late stages is hospitalisation of the patient (Aneshensel *et al.*, 1995). A number of factors may come into play that lead to placement. Hospitalisation may represent a worsening of health, so that the carer decides that it is time to place. In turn, dementia patients have a difficult time in the hospital. They are prone to delirium, particularly when given anaesthesia for surgery or multiple medications. The associated behavioural and cognitive disturbances may convince some carers that placement is necessary. Doctors and family members may also use the occurrence of hospitalisation and any associated worsening of health and behaviour to persuade carers to consider placement. One other factor specific to the United States is that the old age insurance programme, Medicare, may pay for nursing home care for a short period of time (up to 120 days) following hospitalisation. Otherwise, people must pay for care privately, or qualify for indigent care under a different programme (Medicaid). One other factor that can lead to placement is when the carer's health declines or the carer dies. Usually in these cases, no other family member is able to step in to provide the care that is needed.

For carers who continue to provide assistance in the home, the possibility of placement undoubtedly looms large on their horizon. They have certainly wrestled with this decision many times, and have probably discussed it with family, friends and physicians. Advice to carers to place their relative with dementia is ubiquitous and often upsets carers without helping them think through the decisions facing them (MaloneBeach and Zarit, 1995). Some carers even place their relative in an institution, and then decide to take the person out again.

From discussions with late stage carers, several factors emerge which may contribute to the decision to continue home care. These carers may have made a promise to their relative or to themselves never to resort to a nursing home. Some carers find they can manage better in late stage care compared to earlier in their relative's illness (Zarit *et al.*, 1986). The turbulence of behaviour in the middle stages gives way to an increasing need for assistance with daily activities. These carers find that giving assistance is satisfying and that the resistance to helping with activities such as bathing and dressing also diminishes. End stage care may even be done at home. In fact, families may have an easier time finding trained nurses or nursing assistants to come into the home to help with a bedridden patient than to obtain assistance for an agitated and challenging middle stage patient.

The duration of care provided by families who continue care to the end is considerable. The median duration of dementia from the first onset of significant symptoms to death has been found to be 11 years, and the average period at home is almost seven years (Aneshensel *et al.*, 1995). Some patients live as long as 20 years after the onset of dementia, and a few remain at home during this whole period.

The effects of placement on carers

It is widely assumed that placing a relative in a care facility lowers stress of family carers. Physicians and other family members often argue that carers should institutionalise the patient to lower the stress they are experiencing.

The few longitudinal studies that look at carers' adaptation before and after placement present a different picture (Aneshensel *et al.*, 1995; Schulz *et al.*, 2004; Zarit and Whitlatch, 1992, 1993). While these studies do not single out late stage carers, most of the respondents are caring for someone with middle and late stage dementia. These studies report that placement relieves some stressors, especially those associated with daily care routines. Carers no longer feel the continual pressure to provide help or to be ready to help, and so feelings of overload and captivity decrease with placement (Aneshensel *et al.*, 1995). Work strain also decreases among employed carers. Not all caregivers, however, experience these benefits. Furthermore, new stressors emerge in the period leading up to placement or in the post-placement period. These stressors include worries about finding the right facility for one's relative and about paying for care, increases in family conflict both prior to and after placement, and difficulty accepting that staff in facilities would provide care in a different, and sometimes less optimal or acceptable, manner (Aneshensel *et al.*, 1995). Interestingly, wives and daughters who place, respectively, their husband or parent report an increase in emotional support during the process, while husbands placing their wives find that emotional support decreases (Gaugler *et al.*, 1999). Many carers experience considerable guilt or feel that they have failed or let their relative down. Carers may also feel socially isolated. Husbands and wives, in particular, may experience ambiguity in their role as spouse, that is, although legally married, they no longer live with their mate nor have companionship or other benefits of marriage (Rosenthal and Dawson, 1991). Social situations can become awkward when friends and relatives do not know how to discuss the institutionalisation or are too embarrassed to mention it at all.

The changing nature of caregiving stressors following placement is reflected in caregivers' wellbeing. On average, feelings of depression, anxiety and anger are stable across the transition from home care to institutionalisation (Aneshensel *et al.*, 1995; Schulz *et al.*, 2004; Zarit and Whitlatch, 1992, 1993). While the mean scores do not change on these measures, however, some carers experience an increase in emotional distress while others experience a decrease (Zarit and Whitlatch, 1992, 1993). Improvements in emotional status are associated with gaining more relief from stressors and receiving more emotional support (Aneshensel *et al.*, 1995).

One other factor associated with emotional wellbeing is mastery. The construct of mastery characterises the degree to which people believe that they have control over the events in their lives (Pearlin and Schooler, 1978). When providing care in the home, people with higher feelings of mastery report less depression and anxiety. After placement, however, high mastery is associated with higher levels of depression and anxiety (Aneshensel *et al.*, 1995). For people who like to be in control, turning care over to someone else is a difficult experience. We will return to this point below.

Feelings of emotional distress may persist long after placement has occurred. Three years after placement, about one-quarter of carers had significantly elevated symptoms of depression (Zarit and Whitlatch, 1993). Carers who experienced continued emotional distress were older, provided more care in the nursing home, and suffered an erosion of their own identity (Aneshensel *et al.*, 1995).

The family's involvement in late stage institutional care

One of the main reasons that carers continue to feel distress after placement is that they continue to be involved emotionally with their relative, and may even provide care in the institution on a regular basis (Aneshensel *et al.*, 1995). Contrary to expectations, most families do not abandon their relative at the institution's door. There are certainly people living in institutions who do not have family, or whose family do not visit and are not otherwise involved in their care; but in many cases they had few family supports in the first place, which put them at greater risk of placement. For carers who were involved in assisting their relative in the community, the transition to institutionalisation is characterised by continuity in their relationship.

Numerous studies have characterised how often family members visit relatives in residential long-term care settings, particularly nursing homes. Research throughout the 1970s sought to dispute the notion that families 'dumped' their relatives in nursing homes to relinquish responsibility, leaving residents in isolation. For example, data collected from the 1973–1974 National Nursing Homes Surveys indicated that most residents received visitors; 61% of residents were visited at least once a week, while 25% were visited less than weekly. Only 11% of residents received no visitors. The majority of residents (50.3%) received visits from children (National Center for Health Statistics, 1977, 1979). Other early studies suggested a similar frequency of nursing home visits (Gottesman, 1974; Spasoff *et al.*, 1978).

Later work tended to focus on family visits more explicitly. Efforts that focused on both qualitative (or narrative/open-ended information) and empirical/numeric data suggested that for many families visits tended to occur more than once a week and the quality of family–resident relationships remained strong (Smith and Bengtson, 1979; York and Calsyn, 1977). A considerable amount of research over the past 20 years has reiterated these findings; families tend to visit loved ones in nursing homes at least once a week, if not more. These findings remain similar, even for residents suffering from severe dementia (Bitzan and Kruzich, 1990; Hook *et al.*, 1982; Monahan, 1995; Moss and Kurland, 1979; Tornatore and Grant, 2002).

While the research cited above tended to be cross-sectional (or 'one-shot in time' research designs), other studies have examined family visits over time. Cross-sectional studies have suggested that length of stay is negatively related to family visits (i.e. the longer the resident has been in the nursing home, the less families visit). Studies that actually examine family visits over time have found a different pattern. Follow-up studies ranging from two weeks, to nine months, to two years, have observed either stability in visits or increases (Gaugler *et al.*, 2003b; Port *et al.*, 2001; Ross *et al.*, 1997; Yamamoto *et al.*, 2002). These visits also can be of considerable duration, lasting from 2 to 4 hours, on average.

Overall, the literature supports the notion that family members continue to remain involved in the lives of their relatives following institutionalisation. While the frequency and duration of visits vary somewhat, the data certainly dispute the perception that families leave their residents in isolation. However, several limitations are apparent in the existing literature. Most studies analyse data from a single informant (e.g. residents, family members or staff) on family visits, and issues such as social desirability, recall error, and an overall lack of reliability in hour estimates may influence the accuracy of this information. Considering multiple sources (i.e. family, residents and staff) on degree of family visits would offer greater insight into how often family involvement actually occurs.

Family involvement following placement often leads to tensions between families and staff that are evident in daily interactions, but usually are not discussed or addressed in any systematic way. The reasons for this conflict are obvious. Families believe that they want care to be provided in a certain way and precisely at the time that it is needed. The concerns expressed by families may in part be fuelled by guilt over having turned the care over to strangers. For their part, staff may resent the families' demands. They may also come to be attached to certain residents, and will bristle at suggestions by family members who they feel do not know the person or his/her needs as well as they do. Misunderstandings are sometimes the result of racial and social class differences between families and staff. These tensions sometimes erupt into overtly hostile behaviour, but positive and cooperative relationships can also develop between family and staff caregivers (Looman *et al.*, 2002).

Most facilities offer very little in the way of programmes to involve families in constructive ways, nor have they conceptualised how the assistance that families provide might complement or supplement the work done by paid staff. Usually, the extent of programming consists of a powerless family council, and an occasional conference on a patient's progress. The starting point for a family programme would be to educate family about how the facility operates (Zarit and Zarit, 1998). Specifically, families can benefit from learning what roles the various staff have and who to talk to if the family has concerns about the care their relative is receiving. Another element would be to welcome those family carers who visit often and to integrate them in an explicit way into their relative's care. Rather than being set in competition with the staff, the family carer can form a relationship with those staff who provide care to their relative, working together or in ways that complement each others' efforts. From the facility's perspective, involving families may mean becoming more flexible in rules about how things should be done. This type of involvement is also likely to be enhanced when staff do not rotate from one assignment to another, but are responsible for the same residents over time. Any programme to encourage appropriate family involvement would necessarily have to be flexible, since some carers will visit almost every day and others will come less frequently. Of course, even the frequent visitors will also vary in how they want to be involved, some mainly providing companionship and others giving hands-on care.

Several interventions have been developed to maximise family involvement in residential long-term care settings such as nursing homes (e.g. Anderson *et al.*, 1992; Maas *et al.*, 2000; Pillemer *et al.*, 2003). These approaches are built around the establishment of family–staff care plans designed to strengthen the responsibilities and standards of staff and family care in nursing homes. Specific approaches include the formation of care plans among family members and nursing staff (Anderson *et al.*, 1992), the establishment of formal and informal role behaviours between family and nursing staff (Maas *et al.*, 2000), and the provision of intensive education and training to family members and nursing staff to improve facility policies and practices (Pillemer *et al.*, 2003). Evaluations of these programmes suggest they have strong effects in facilitating family involvement (Maas *et al.*, 2000), improving staff job satisfaction (Pillemer *et al.*, 2003) and enhancing quality of care for residents (Anderson *et al.*, 1992). Until recently, many interventions designed to improve family involvement and family/staff relationships have not been subject to scientific evaluation; few evaluations utilise randomised, 'intention to treat' designs where treatment and control participants are randomly assigned prior to the intervention, allowing for more thorough assessment of programme effectiveness. Although a few interventions use fairly rigorous evaluation designs when determining efficacy, these programmes have been implemented in single facilities or within a limited geographic region. Given the diversity in resident populations in different facilities and regions, there is a need for replication programmes, as well as continued innovation. Finally, more rigorous evaluations are needed to determine the effectiveness of single approaches or compare various strategies and to assist practitioners and other stakeholders in identifying those programmes that would be most beneficial in their facilities.

Over time, the nature of care in institutional settings changes from managing an active, mobile resident to providing assistance for almost all the needs of an increasingly chair- or bed-bound resident. Special facilities that have been developed for the care of people with dementia have typically focused on the middle stages of the illness. With the transition to late stage care, the type of environment and programming of a special dementia care unit no longer is relevant. This transition is often handled by moving the resident from the 'special' unit to a regular nursing bed. The rationale for this move is that the late stage patient can no longer benefit from the facilities or programme on the special care unit and the space could be used by another resident. For families, this transition is often disturbing. It marks, of course, a new stage in the illness. Families also have to leave behind staff they have developed relationships with, and move their relative from a programme that was 'special', that is, focused on the specific needs of people with dementia, into an ordinary unit where they may be diverse demands on staff.

This dilemma can be addressed in different ways. In Sweden, which has developed an extensive network of small group homes for dementia (Malmberg and Zarit, 1993), the original plan was for residents to move to a more traditional nursing home for late stage care. Policy has changed in recent years, however, and residents now remain in the group home for the rest of their lives, unless there are medical reasons for a move. Late stage care is now provided in these settings, along with on-going care of people in the middle stages. No studies have been made of the effects of this change on staff or families, or of the potential benefits or drawbacks to residents themselves. Another approach that would address families' concerns would be to move the late stage resident from one 'special' dementia programme to a new type of 'special' unit specifically designed to provide late stage care. This unit could be structured around principles of hospice, and could provide assurance to families that their relative would be receiving expert care appropriate to the current circumstances.

End-of-life issues

Families of late stage patients will inevitably face end-of-life decisions. Most people with dementia experience a gradual decline in functioning over the last year of life, and to be completely dependent on care or nearly so at the time of death (Covinsky et al., 2003). Families are often asked to make difficult decisions about prolonging life, such as whether to administer antibiotics if the patient develops pneumonia or to authorise use of a feeding tube or other life-support measures. These decisions for families are understandably associated with considerable guilt and feelings of burden (Forbes et al., 2000). Although countries like the United States allow people to provide an advance directive about end-of-life medical care, most older people do not complete this document or may provide only vague guidelines for their families.

Overall, the quality of end-of-life care for people with dementia is poor, with too much use of feeding tubes and not enough management of pain or use of hospice services (Sachs et al., 2004). The impetus for life-support measures may come from the hospital or nursing home or from physicians. Families typically do not get enough information to understand the choices they are making or that implementation of a device such as a feeding tube can be an irreversible step; that is, there is a choice about initiating the procedure, but not stopping it. Physicians who recommend feeding tubes are often unaware of the limited therapeutic value for people with late stage dementia (Shega et al., 2003). Physicians' knowledge that dementia is a terminal disease and their understanding of the limited therapeutic benefits of feeding tubes for nutrition or for healing ulcers were related to lower use of this procedure (Shega et al., 2004).

End-of-life care often is one more in a line of events that families face without adequate information or resources for making decisions. Physicians and nursing homes may or may not share the same values about death and dying as the patient or family, and may not provide optimal care. A consensus and guidelines about end-of-life decisions that emphasise comfort and not needless prolongation of life might be helpful for families, and limit the use of unnecessary and painful procedures to dying patients.

Post-care adaptation

The death of the patient is the end of a long journey for the family. When death occurs in the late stages of dementia, families are often prepared and view it as an end to the patient's suffering. The well-established cultural rituals surrounding death can be a source of support and comfort to carers. People who may have drifted away from a carer who had placed a spouse in a nursing home now rally around.

The immediate reactions of carers to their relative's death is varied. About one-half report that they experienced little or no grief, while 17% report considerable grief (Aneshensel *et al.*, 1995; see also Schulz *et al.*, 2003). Grief reactions include preoccupation, longing for the person, painful emotions, a feeling of lack of connection with everyday events, and sensory illusions (visual, auditory) that the deceased is present. The frequency of grief emotions decreases over time, but even a year after the death, some carers continue to experience strong feelings. By three years after the death, most carers show recovery in their psychosocial functioning though a minority of people continue to experience significant depressive feelings (Aneshensel *et al.*). People who have emotionally let go of the patient in the period prior to his/her death generally show better adaptation following death.

Conclusions

One unintended consequence of improvements in health care is that people with dementia now frequently survive for long periods of time. The proportion of people living in nursing homes and suffering from severe dementia has grown, and many others are cared for at home. The main focus of support to families has been in early and, particularly, middle stages of their relative's illness, but there is clearly a need for education and support in the later stages. The stresses on the family continue after nursing home placement, and may become particularly pronounced around the end of the patient's life. The quality of the patient's death may be integrally tied to the wellbeing of families.

References

Anderson KH, Hobson A, Steiner P, Rodel B (1992) Patients with dementia: involving families to maximize nursing care. *Journal of Gerontological Nursing*, 18:19–25.

Aneshensel C, Pearlin LI, Mullan JT, Zarit SH, Whitlatch CJ (1995) Profiles in Caregiving: The Unexpected Career. New York: Academic Press.

Bitzan JE, Kruzich JM (1990) Interpersonal relationships of nursing home residents. *Gerontologist*, 30:385–390.

Covinsky KE, Eng C, Liu LY, Sands LP, Yaffe K (2003) The last 2 years of life: functional trajectories of frail older people. *Journal of American Geriatric Society*, 51(4):492–498.

Forbes S, Bern-Klug M, Gessert C (2000) End-of-life decision making for nursing home residents with dementia. *Journal of Nursing Scholarship*, 32(3):251–258.

Gaugler JE, Zarit SH, Pearlin LI (1999) Caregiving and institutionalization: perceptions of family conflict and socioemotional support. *International Journal of Aging and Human Development*, 49:1–25.

Gaugler JE, Edwards AB, Femia EE, Zarit SH, Stephens MAP, Townsend A, Greene R (2000) Predictors of institutionalization of cognitively impaired elders: family help and the timing of placement. *Journal of Gerontology: Psychological Science*, 55B:P247–P255.

Gaugler JE, Kane RL, Kane RA, Clay T, Newcomer R (2003a) Caregiving and institutionalization of cognitively impaired older people: utilizing dynamic predictors of change. *The Gerontologist*, 43(2):219–229.

Gaugler JE, Zarit SH, Pearlin LI (2003b) Family involvement in nursing homes: modeling nursing home visits over time. *International Journal of Aging and Human Development*, 57:91–117.

Gottesman LE (1974) Nursing home performance as related to resident traits, ownership, size, and source of payment. *American Journal of Public Health*, 64:269–276.

Hook WF, Sobal J, Oak JC (1982) Frequency of visitation in nursing homes: patterns of contact across the boundaries of total institutions. *Gerontologist*, 22:424–428.

Looman WJ, Noelker LS, Schur D, Whitlatch CJ, Ejaz FK (2002) Impact of family members on nurse assistants: what helps, what hurts. *American Journal of Alzheimers Disease and Other Dementia*, 17(6):350–356.

Maas ML, Swanson E, Buckwalter KC, Lenth R, Specht JP, Tripp-Reimer T, Tranel D, Reed D, Broffitt B, Brenneman D, Peters J, Rose D, Kelley L, Pottinger J, Ramler C, Schutte D, Sung C, Park M (2000) Nursing Interventions for Alzheimer's Family Role Trials: Final Report (No. RO1NR01689). Iowa City, IA: University of Iowa.

Malmberg B, Zarit SH (1993) Group homes for dementia patients: an innovative model in Sweden. *Gerontologist*, 31:682–686.

MaloneBeach EE, Zarit SH (1995) Dimensions of social support and social conflict as predictors of caregiver depression. *International Psychogeriatrics*, 7:39–50.

Monahan DJ (1995) Informal caregivers of institutionalized dementia residents: predictors of burden. *Journal of Gerontological Social Work*, 23:65–82.

Moss MS, Kurland P (1979) Family visiting with institutionalized mentally impaired aged. *Journal of Gerontological Social Work*, 1:271–278.

National Center for Health Statistics (1977) Characteristics, social contacts, and activities of nursing home residents, United States, 1973–4. Vital and Health Statistics. Series 13, No. 27, DHEW Publishing No. (HRA) 77–1778. Washington, DC: United States Government Printing Office.

National Center for Health Statistics (1979) The national nursing home survey: 1977 summary for the United States. Vital and Health Statistics. Series 13, No. 43, DHEW Publication (PHS) 79-1794. Washington, DC: United States Government Printing Office.

Pearlin LI, Schooler C (1978) The structure of coping. *Journal of Health and Social Behavior*, 19:2–21.

Phillips VL, Diwan S (2003) The incremental effect of dementia-related problem behaviors on the time to nursing home placement in poor, frail, demented older people. *Journal of the American Geriatric Society*, 51(2):188–193.

Pillemer K, Suitor JJ, Henderson CR, Meador R, Schultz L, Robison J, Hegeman C (2003) A cooperative communication intervention for nursing home staff and family members of residents. *The Gerontologist*, 43 Special Issue II:96–106.

Port CL, Gruber-Baldini AL, Burton L, Baumgarten M, Hebel JR, Zimmerman SI, Magaziner J (2001) Resident contact with family and friends following nursing home admission. *The Gerontologist*, 41, 589–596.

Rosenthal C, Dawson P (1991) Wives of institutionalized elderly men: the first stage of the transition to quasi-widowhood. *Journal of Aging and Health*, 3:315–334.

Ross MM, Rosenthal C, Dawson P (1997) Spousal caregiving in the institutional setting: visiting. *Journal of Clinical Nursing*, 6:473–483.

Sachs GA, Shega JW, Cox-Hayley D (2004) Barriers to excellent end-of-life care for patients with dementia. *Journal of General Internal Medicine*, 19(10):1057–1063.

Schulz R, Mendelsohn AB, Haley WE, Mahoney D, Allen RS, Zhang S, Thompson L, Belle SH (2003) End-of-life care and the effects of bereavement on family caregivers of persons with dementia. *New England Journal of Medicine*, 349:1936–1942.

Schulz R, Belle SH, Czaja SJ, McGinnis KA, Stevens A, Zhang S (2004) Long-term care placement of dementia patients and caregiver health and wellbeing. *Journal of the American Medical Association*, 292(8):961–967.

Shega JW, Hougham GW, Stocking CB, Cox-Haley D, Sachs GA (2003) Barriers to limiting the practice of feeding tube placement in advanced dementia. *Journal of Palliative Medicine*, 6(6):885–893.

Shega JW, Hougham GW, Cox-Haley D, Sachs GA, Stocking CB (2004) Advanced dementia and feeding tubes: do physician factors contribute to state variation? *Journal of the American Geriatrics Society*, 52(7):1217–1218.

Smith KF, Bengtson VL (1979) Positive consequences of institutionalization: solidarity between elderly patients and their middle-aged children. *Gerontologist*, 19:438–447.

Spasoff RA, Kraus AS, Beattie EJ, Holden DEW, Lawson JS, Rodenburg M, Woodcock GM (1978) A longitudinal study of elderly residents in long-stay institutions. *The Gerontologist*, 18:281–292.

Tornatore JB, Grant LA (2002) Burden among family caregivers of persons with Alzheimer's disease in nursing homes. *The Gerontologist*, 42:497–506.

Yamamoto MN, Aneshensel CS, Levy-Storms L (2002) Patterns of family visiting with institutionalized elders: the case of dementia. *Journals of Gerontology: Psychological Sciences*, 57:S234–S246.

York JL, Caslyn RJ (1977) Family involvement in nursing homes. *Gerontologist*, 17:500–505.

Zarit SH, Whitlatch C (1992) Institutional placement: phases of the transition. *The Gerontologist*, 32:665–672.

Zarit SH, Whitlatch C (1993) Short and long term consequences of placement for caregivers. *Irish Journal of Psychology*, 14:25–37.

Zarit SH, Zarit JM (1998) Mental Disorders in Older Adults: Fundamentals of Assessment and Treatment. New York: Guilford.

Zarit SH, Todd PA, Zarit JM (1986) Subjective burden of husbands and wives as caregivers: a longitudinal study. *The Gerontologist*, 26:260–270.

16

Person-centred Care for People with Severe Dementia

Murna Downs, Neil Small and Katherine Froggatt

A person is a person because of other people

South African proverb

Introduction

The care of people with dementia has undergone a radical transformation in the last 10 years. We now know that much can be done to support people to live a quality life. We now know the kinds of supports that assist family members and practitioners. Much as cancer has lost some of its dread, the inevitable link of suffering with dementia has been severed. *Living* with dementia is not only possible but can be asserted as a human right.

Much of the change in how we approach the care of people with dementia is captured in the term 'person-centred care'. While there is no recognised national or international definition of person-centred dementia care, it is a term that is commonly used both within the UK (e.g. Department of Health, 2001) and elsewhere (e.g. Alzheimer's Australia Western Australia). As an approach to care, person-centred care does not represent any one technique or therapeutic intervention. Rather, it is first and foremost a philosophy of care (Brooker, 2004; Epp, 2003; Kitwood, 1997a; Morton, 1999), espousing a group of core values which have implications both for *what* we do and *how* we do it.

The person-centred approach is as applicable to those with severe dementia as it is for those recently diagnosed with a dementing condition. The opportunities and challenges posed may differ as the condition progresses, but the aims and values of such an approach remain the same – the promotion of quality of life and the recognition of the essential humanity of all people, regardless of the degree of impairment or illness they experience.

Brooker (2004) provides a useful breakdown of the person-centred approach into four key elements:

(1) Affirms the value of the person and their life, regardless of degree of impairment
(2) Treats everyone as an individual
(3) Adopts the perspective of the person with dementia
(4) Provides a supportive social environment

The person-centred approach has much in common with the palliative care approach (Hughes, 2004; Small *et al.*, in press). Palliative care stresses the need to live well until death, emphasising the attainability of a good quality of life. Hughes (2004) outlines the comparability of the two approaches to care arguing that, at their heart, both are concerned with the inherent moral value of the person, regardless of their diagnosis.

Severe Dementia. Edited by A. Burns and B. Winblad.
Copyright © 2006 John Wiley & Sons, Ltd. ISBN 0-470-01054-1

The purpose of this chapter is to examine the key elements of a person-centred approach applied to those with severe dementia. Each of Brooker's (2004) four key elements of person-centred care will be discussed in relation to people with severe dementia. The therapeutic potential of providing a supportive social environment to people with severe dementia will be explored in some detail. The chapter ends with a section outlining strategies for ensuring that people with severe dementia are provided with a supportive social environment to maximise their wellbeing.

Affirms the value of the person, regardless of degree of impairment

The person-centred approach seeks to affirm the person as a living human and social being, regardless of degree of impairment or illness (Brooker, 2004; Kitwood, 1993; Woods, 2001). This affirmation has particular salience for those with severe dementia. People whose cognitive capacities are severely compromised, who have difficulty using language and whose functional capacities have diminished are at risk of being considered not fully alive, being somehow already dead, and/or of not being fully human, being a non-person or object. The sense of people no longer being fully alive is captured in phrases that have been associated with severe dementia both in professional and lay discourse, phrases such as 'the death that leaves the body behind' or 'social death' or 'the funeral that never ends' (Sweeting and Gilhooly, 1997).

People with dementia experience stigma and discrimination (Graham *et al.*, 2003). Jennings (2004) explains that dementia undermines those qualities which we in the West consider to be distinctively human – coherent communication, memory, being socially oriented, and having behavioural self-control. A person with dementia who has lost their memory for their past is assumed to have lost connection with their former selves; because they cannot communicate coherently it is assumed they have stopped being a person. The depersonalising manner in which care is delivered illustrates the view that people with dementia are viewed as non-persons or objects.

Brooker (2004) describes 'dementism' as the form of discrimination experienced by people with dementia. She notes the inverse care law where those with the least ability to communicate or advocate for themselves receive the least attention (Bruce *et al.*, 2002). In addition, most people with severe dementia are cared for in care home environments by unqualified staff who have little preparation for providing such care. In this way one can argue that people with severe dementia are even more discriminated against than people with a more recently diagnosed dementia.

Moral personhood, respect and acknowledgement of the individual as a member of the human community, is the moral basis of our caregiving. It leads us to maintain a sense of connection with the other person for as long as possible, out of a sense of the moral importance of that connection per se (Jennings, 2004).

> We need more than safe, comfortable warehouses for persons with advanced Alzheimer's. We need to demand caregiving environments that provide some measure of rehabilitation in terms of human relationships, modes of interaction and communication, and the sustaining of semantic agency (making meaning) and moral personhood (being treated with respect).
>
> (Jennings, 2004, p. 10)

Affirming the value of the person regardless of the degree of impairment involves engaging with questions about what constitutes humanity, personality and with questions about the worth of a life. For example we can ask:

(1) How far is there a recognisable connection between the person that was and the person that is now (Parfit, 1984)?
(2) To what extent do we view severe dementia as manifesting an inevitable disintegration of personality? (See the position of Winblad *et al.* (1999) and the evidence provided by Norberg *et al.* (2003)).

(3) To what extent is severe dementia compatible with quality of life or the experience of pleasure? Is it a condition inevitably synonymous with suffering (Graham *et al.*, 2003)?

(4) Even if a life is dominated by suffering can we deny its humanity (Jennings, 2004)?

The answers to these questions will determine the nature and degree of effort extended to improve quality of life for people with severe dementia.

Treats everyone as an individual

The person-centred approach recognises that each person with dementia is a unique human being with their own biography, personality, likes and dislikes (Brooker, 2004; Kitwood, 1997a). While general statements can be made about symptoms and treatment regimes, the experience of living with dementia will differ depending on the person's psychological make-up, life experience and current social and economic circumstances. This aspect of person-centred care, individualised care, is promoted in UK government directives on care of the elderly, such as the Department of Health's National Service Framework for Older People (Department of Health, 2001).

Providing individualised care requires a thorough knowledge of the person, both their past and their present. Understanding the person's biography can be achieved by engaging in life history reviews, directly with the person while they still retain language and/or with their close family members. Life histories need not be written records only but can include photographs and music (Aldridge, 2000). Engaging in, and applying the knowledge gained through, life story work is one mechanism for ensuring individualised care. For people with severe dementia it is more difficult to build an in-depth picture of their uniqueness. This requires close liaison with key informants, most commonly family.

Individualised care starts with individualised assessment. Within a person-centred and palliative care approach such assessment is multidisciplinary. It is concerned with the physical, emotional, social and spiritual wellbeing of both the person with dementia and their family carer. Kitwood (1997a) argues that people with dementia have psychological needs for comfort, attachment, occupation, inclusion, identity and love.

Critics of person-centred care cite this emphasis on the individual with dementia as flawed. Nolan *et al.* (2004) referring to the Department of Health's (2001) use of the term person-centred care, suggest that an emphasis on autonomy and individualism is untenable for some older people, including people with dementia. Nolan and colleagues propose a model of relationship-centred care emphasising interdependence rather than 'lionising' individualism. Here the milieu is the appropriate focus and the furthering of supportive social conditions is the aim. While at once seeming to 'move beyond' person-centred care, relationship-centred care in essence argues for the need to broaden such concerns to include all key parties – people with dementia, their families and care staff – in our concern with meeting psychological needs. They offer the 'Senses framework' to equip caregivers to ensure that all participants have a sense of security, continuity, belonging, purpose, fulfilment and significance.

While relationship-centred care and the 'Senses framework' offer staff useful guides and valuable ways to assess the value of their work, it is not difficult to see more points of similarity with Kitwood's approach than Nolan and colleagues would allow. This only replaces person-centred care if we set that up too narrowly. Person-centred care does not ignore context – indeed Kitwood refers to social environments which fail to meet psychological needs as 'malignant' and recognised the need to create, 'environments in which caring feels natural, and so, eventually bringing about a new culture of care' (Kitwood, 1997a, p. 3). Such supportive social environments, as we shall see in a later section, include supports for family and care staff, alongside people with dementia (Kitwood, 1997a).

Taking the perspective of the person as the starting point

Taking the perspective of the person with dementia is considered an essential component of person-centred care (Brooker, 2004; Cotrell and Schulz, 1993; Kitwood, 1997b). This involves recognising that each person's experience has its own psychological validity; and that people with dementia act from this perspective. Such an approach argues that people with dementia, no matter how severe their cognitive and functional impairments, retain the capacity for experiencing their world and seek to identify meaning in that experience (Berghmans, 1997; Sabat and Harre, 1994).

The importance of understanding the subjective experience is emphasised in research studies and personal accounts of the experience of dementia (see, for example, Harris, 2001; Snyder, 1999). Considerably less attention has been paid to the subjective experience of people with severe dementia (Downs, 1997). Certainly most of our recent efforts in understanding the perspective of people with dementia in both practice and research have tended to focus on people who are verbally articulate. It is questionable how much this experience represents the needs and experiences of those with advanced dementia. It has been assumed that people in this group have both limited experience and awareness of their experience. Further a lack of verbal expression and, for many, diminished nonverbal communication makes accessing this experience difficult.

A variety of approaches to assessing the person's perspective have been proposed. Approaches will differ along a temporal dimension, with certain approaches being better suited to different levels of impairment. As difficult as communication is with increased impairment, it is not impossible and, as we shall see, a significant body of empirical research testifies to the latent capacity for communication in people in advanced dementia (see Normann *et al.* (1998) for a review). These approaches draw upon different sources and types of knowing a person's perspective, from more objective measurements of preference, to presentational forms of expression from both the person with dementia and those that surround them.

Kitwood (1997b) offers six ways of accessing the subjective world of people with dementia. These have different applicability to people with severe dementia. They include: using accounts that have been written by people with dementia; careful listening to what people say when interviewed or in group work; careful and imaginative listening to what people say in the course of their everyday life; consultation with people who have experienced an illness with similar features; using poetic imagination; and finally, using role play or taking the part of someone who has dementia and living this experience in a simulated environment.

Behavioural measures exist including the Affect Rating Scale (Lawton, 1996), the Positive Response Schedule (Perrin, 1997a), and Dementia Care Mapping (Kitwood and Bredin, 1992) (see Brooker (1995) and Shue *et al.* (1996) for a review). Dementia Care Mapping (Brooker, forthcoming; Kitwood and Bredin, 1992) has as its explicit aim to increase empathy in care workers and professionals. Observations are made from the perspective of the person with dementia. Kitwood (1997a, p. 4) described DCM as 'a serious attempt to take the standpoint of the person with dementia, using a combination of empathy and observational skill'. Families and care staff that are familiar with the person can also provide valuable insights into the person's experience (Kane *et al.*, 2003).

Provides a supportive social environment

Perhaps the most significant contribution of the person-centred approach in promoting quality of life is its insistence on maximising the potential and possibility within both the person with dementia and their carer. Such an insistence results in there being an overriding sense of therapeutic optimism. Efforts are placed on providing people with dementia with an enriched social environment which both compensates for their impairment and fosters opportunities for personal growth, addressing all dimensions of a person's life. As such person-centred care is by its nature multidisciplinary care requiring an integrated approach to the multidimensional aspects of a person's life. Equally important it recognises that those providing care will also need a supportive environment.

People with dementia, especially those with severe dementia, have tended to be viewed in both academic and professional literature predominantly in terms of their cognitive and behavioural functioning – the physical, emotional, social and spiritual side of their lives has been largely neglected. For people with severe dementia whose cognitive functioning falls below that measured on most assessment scales, there has also been a neglect of retained abilities and relational aspects (Camp *et al.*, 1999; Winblad *et al.*, 1999).

Building supportive environments
We will now look at some of the components that might comprise a supportive social environment for people with severe dementia, recognising the needs and role for family and care staff. What can be offered is described along with how it might be delivered. Calkins (2005) describes the nature of a supportive physical environment which complements the discussion below.

Communication and relationships
Person-centred care, in common with the palliative care approach, recognises that all human life, including that of people with dementia, is grounded in relationships. The person-centred approach argues that the greatest threat to a person's wellbeing comes from their potential loss of personhood, or a withdrawal of recognition of their humanity (Kitwood, 1997a). It seeks to attain and maintain authentic engagement with a person with dementia whether that person is verbally communicative or not (Kovach, 1997).

Strategies for authentic engagement include being with (Kitwood, 1997b), confirming (Normann *et al.*, 2002) and being in communion (Norberg, 2001) with a person with dementia. For Kitwood (1997b) being with involves simply being present to a person with dementia. This he argued held great therapeutic potential. He stressed the difficulty for staff in simply being with a person when working in an environment which prioritised tasks over contact. Norberg *et al.* (2003) and Normann *et al.* (1998, 2002) have shown that people with severely reduced cognitive and functional capacities retain capacity for communication. This can be verbal or nonverbal. Normann and colleagues (1998, 2002) found that a supportive attitude in conversations with a person with severe dementia promoted lucidity. Such support included sharing the person's point of view, repeating and rephrasing what had been said, ignoring errors, and supporting the person's language. They found that such a form of engagement led to increased vocalisation and communication in people with severe dementia. Norberg (2001) describes the contact achieved between two people, whether with verbal communication or not, as communion. In many ways this form of interaction is resonant of Buber's (1937) 'I–Thou' basis for the meeting of two people.

Nonverbal communication is also possible, even in severe dementia (Roudier *et al.*, 1998). Magai *et al.* (2002) have demonstrated that staff can be trained to become more attuned to subtle behavioural cues of people with severe dementia.

Communication is not reliant on words alone but also comprises sound (Aldridge, 2000). People with severe dementia are capable of vocalisation, however quiet and sporadic. Therefore additional approaches to communication can be used. Music and music therapy offer contexts of expression and understanding 'where gesture, movement and vocalization make communicative sense' (Aldridge, 2000, p. 15). While language deteriorates musical abilities appear to be preserved (Swartz *et al.*, 1989). People who are otherwise not responsive, respond to music (Aldridge, 2000; Magee, 1999; Norberg *et al.*, 2003). Music can be used to create community for people at advanced stages of dementia (Rose and Schlingensiepen, 2000).

Validation therapy (Feil, 1993) recognises that passivity and withdrawal may be active coping responses. Feil (1993) argues that, no matter how severely impaired, people with dementia continue to seek meaning and resolution in their lives. Such attempts at reconciliation and resolution can be facilitated by knowledgeable and trained therapists. Much of this facilitation involves mirroring the actions and behaviours of the person with dementia. Such mirroring assists with developing empathy and communicates a form of understanding to the person with dementia (Killick and Allan, 2001).

While there are neurological reasons for a person's communication difficulties, there are also psychosocial factors which affect a person's opportunity and capacity for communication. Kitwood (1997b) described a variety of ways in which our interactions with people with dementia inhibit their capacity for communication and diminish their personhood. These he referred to as constituting a 'malignant social psychology'. Amongst these include our tendency to speak and act at our own pace thus 'outpacing' people with dementia. He advocated for the need for carers and staff to engage in 'positive person work' which includes holding, affirming and validating a person's experience (Epp, 2003).

Stimulation and engagement of the senses
A 'marked occupational poverty' for people with severe dementia living in hospital and residential settings has been noted (Perrin, 1997a, p. 938). This has been attributed predominantly to a failure on the part of staff to fully understand and share the person's experience. Perrin suggests that the person with severe dementia inhabits a shrunken environment, which she describes as a bubble. It is our task to attend to how we enter this bubble and to consider occupational strategies for engaging positively with the person. She stresses the importance of enriching the person's immediate environment through the nature of our interactions with them. Camp et al. (1999) argue for the need for a cognitive and functional assessment for those in advanced dementia in order to ensure the person is provided with appropriate stimulation and activity levels. Their Montessori-based functional assessment documents remaining abilities of people with severe dementia. Perrin (2004) similarly describes a need for therapeutic activities to be tailored to the individual's cognitive and functional capacity.

Physical care and comfort
Person-centred dementia care insists that optimal physical care is provided. People with dementia are at increased risk for dehydration and malnutrition, experience pain which they have difficulty expressing verbally and risk developing complications due to immobility. Appropriate care for people's physical needs requires attention to the person as a person, not an object. It will assist most with promoting quality of life if it is done by people who can affirm the essential humanity of the person's whose physical needs are being addressed. This requires that when assisting with physical care carers retain the sense of the person for whose body they are caring (Hellen, 1997; Twigg, 2000) and use these opportunities to promote their psychological wellbeing (Kihlgren et al., 1993, 1994).

Help with eating and drinking
People with severe dementia by definition will have difficulty eating and drinking without assistance. Nevertheless eating and drinking may well be a sensory pleasure for people with severe dementia. That potential source of pleasure should be maximised while at the same time ensuring optimum nutrition and hydration (Kulpa and DePaul, 1997).

Many people with severe dementia will ultimately experience difficulty with swallowing, dysphagia, which in turn is associated with aspiration pneumonia (Summersall and Wight, 2004). Personal accounts suggest that the person's interests are not always primary (Leveson, 2004) with professional interests or inter-professional disagreements reported (Leveson, 2004). Decisions about how to respond when someone develops swallowing problems are discussed elsewhere in this book.

Assistance with washing and bathing

Much has been written about the tendency for people with dementia to resist care. Indeed in some nomenclatures it is classified as a behavioural symptom of dementia (Finkel, 2000). Sloane *et al.* (2003) in the United States provide compelling evidence that the manner in which people are assisted with washing affects their response. They demonstrated that for many residents bed baths were preferable to shower facilities. Yet prior to the study most residents were showered daily. Adopting a person-centred approach to washing resulted in residents actively engaging with the comfort and stimulation derived from bed baths (Barrick *et al.*, 2001).

Help with positioning and transferring

People with severe dementia may need help moving from bed to chair and with repositioning themselves in their chair or bed. This requires a proactive approach to promote comfort and to avoid the development of skin breakdowns and associated bed sores. Help with repositioning and transfer provides carers and staff with the opportunity for engagement and communication. Families and staff may well need guidance and support in maximising these opportunities.

Assisting with incontinence

People with severe or advanced dementia will frequently be incontinent of urine and faeces. While incontinent they may well retain awareness both of its social meaning and of the burden of care it places on others. It is essential that in caring for this aspect of the person, they be afforded the highest degree of dignity and respect.

Pain detection and treatment

Untreated pain adversely affects quality of life and functional abilities and is linked to distressing behaviour (Volicer and Bloom-Charette, 1999). The assessment and treatment of pain is of concern in all people with dementia. There is a compelling need to improve the detection of pain for those with severe dementia who lack sufficient language with which to express their needs. For people with severe dementia a multidimensional approach including functional assessment as well as behavioural and physiological measures, along with family and carer input, is likely to be the best approach to assessing pain (Stolee *et al.*, 2005).

There is a need for increased awareness among physicians about pain experienced by people with severe cognitive impairments and a need to develop appropriate methodologies for its detection (Cohen-Mansfield and Lipson, 2002). Familiarity with the person with severe dementia is important to the detection of pain. There is some evidence to suggest that nursing staff in long-term care settings who know their residents well are more likely to identify pain in residents with severe dementia (Cohen-Mansfield and Creedon, 2002).

Feldt (2000) has demonstrated that while older people with cognitive impairment may not verbally report the experience of pain, they demonstrate pain behaviours during transfer and other personal care activities. She cautions that as much personal care is now delegated to non-professional care staff, such opportunities for detecting pain may be lost.

Spiritual care

The importance of spirituality in person-centred dementia care has recently been described in a special issue of *Dementia, the International Journal of Social Research and Practice*. Spirituality refers to our search for meaning and purpose in life and is not necessarily tied to any religious belief. Stuckey and Gwyther (2003) argue that spirituality has a place for the person with dementia, their family and the clinician. Thompson O'Maille and Kasayka (2005) offer creative approaches to spiritual care for people with severe dementia.

In the UK it is recognised that spiritual care is an essential part of care of older people and their families (Department of Health, 2001). Yet a recent survey of care homes within one geographic area in the UK suggests that staff have limited understanding of what spiritual care involves, lack resources internally and externally and need training in this area (Orchard, 2002).

Loss and grief

Grief is an integral part of the experience of dementia – for the person with dementia and their family. A person-centred approach to people with severe dementia argues that the provision of contact and comfort assists people to accept the coming of death (Kitwood, 1997a). Feil (1993) also argues for the need to support those in advanced dementia as they seek resolution of their life in preparation for death.

Families too may need help with adjusting to their relative's increasing frailty up to and including bereavement. Just as palliative care services offer family support with grieving and bereavement, so too a person-centred approach to people with severe dementia recognises the interrelationship between the person and their family (Kitwood, 1997a).

While most people with dementia are cared for at home by relatives in the community, most people with severe dementia live in residential or nursing home care settings (Albinsson and Strang, 2003). Therefore staff play a key role in the quality of life of both the person with dementia and their family. Despite the fact that many people die in nursing homes, death is a subject that is avoided in these settings (Moss, 2001). There are a variety of barriers to the expression of grief by care staff, including an assumption about what is appropriate 'professional distance' and a lack of legitimacy for grieving, referred to as disenfranchised grief (Moss et al., 2003). Disenfranchised grief is evident where losses are not legitimised or appreciated by others – where it is questioned how far the person has a right to mourn and where the loss is not openly acknowledged or socially sanctioned or publicly shared. In such situations others fail to validate and support grief (Doka, 1989, 2004).

Organisational and political strategies

The implementation of a person-centred care for people with severe dementia requires more than the generation and communication of ideas (Beck et al., 1999; Kitwood and Woods, 1996). While training and education are obvious components in ensuring person-centred care for people with severe dementia, we know from efforts to embed the palliative care approach that appropriate practice development and organisational frameworks are also needed (Froggatt, 2002; Hockley, 2002). It is only within a supportive practice development and organisational context that much-needed training and education initiatives will succeed in promoting quality of life.

Care homes, where a significant percentage of people with severe dementia live and die, present a critical zone for intervention. Political will is required to ensure adequate resources for the necessary supervision, induction and staffing ratios (Graham et al., 2003). High turnover, reliance on agency staff and part-time staff leads to discontinuity of care in these environments (Hockley, 2002). Furthermore the hierarchical structure, where those with the least training spend the most time with residents and yet have the least influence on care planning, does not promote quality of care. These organisational constraints limit the potency of person-centred care to promote quality of life.

Organisational structures, resources and values all affect the kind of care delivered. The care manager plays a key role in determining the kind of care that is provided. Integrated care pathways and available specialist services such as a gerontological nurse specialist, medical practitioners, pastoral support and palliative care services may help (Hockley, 2002). Furthermore, the expectations of regulatory agencies and of the broader society affect the experience of living and dying in care homes (Froggatt, 2004). Standard setting and monitoring of those standards is essential to quality of care. The Audit Commission (2000) and Brooker (forthcoming) describe the role Dementia Care Mapping can play is such audit cycles. It is essential that we address all of these elements to ensure that the necessary adjustments and reforms are made to health and social care practice to achieve the full potential of a person-centred approach in dementia care.

Conclusion

Person-centred care is a philosophy of care for people with dementia which seeks to promote well-being and quality of life, regardless of the degree of cognitive impairment. As such it is as applicable to people with severe dementia as it is to those recently diagnosed. In its application to those with severe dementia it has much in common with the palliative care approach. Both recognise that value of human life regardless of degree of impairment, both stress the importance of providing individualised care, both take as their starting point the person's experience, and both stress the need for a supportive social environment for both the person with dementia and their carers.

Nevertheless, despite having at least two philosophies to guide our care of people with severe dementia, we know that they often experience less than optimal quality of life. While quality of life includes physical, emotional, spiritual, and social wellbeing, the focus tends to be restricted to a person's cognitive and behavioural symptoms. Much of our current care fails to optimise the other areas of a person's experience. There is much that can be done to maximise the potential of people with severe dementia. This chapter has described how the person-centred approaches can be applied to maximise physical, emotional, social, and spiritual wellbeing.

Acknowledgement

Thanks to Professor Dawn Brooker for her comments on a previous draft of this chapter.

References

Albinsson L, Strang P (2003) Differences in supporting families of dementia patients and cancer patients: a palliative perspective. *Palliative Medicine*, 17:359–367.

Aldridge D (2000) Music Therapy in Dementia Care. London: Jessica Kingsley.

Alzheimer's Australia Western Australia. http://www.alzheimers.asn.au/index.php?page=viewStory&id=8208. Accessed Feb 17 2005.

Audit Commission (2000) Forget me not: mental health services for older people. London. www.audit-commission.gov.uk.

Ballard CG, O'Brien J, Reichelt K, Perry E (2002) Aromatherapy as a safe and effective treatment for the management of agitation in severe dementia: the results of a double blind, placebo controlled trial. *Journal of Clinical Psychiatry*, 63:553–558.

Barrick AL, Rader J, Hoeffer B, Sloane PD (eds) (2001) Bathing without a battle: Personal Care of Individuals with Dementia. London: Springer.

Beck C, Ortigara A, Mercer S, Shue V (1999) Enabling and empowering certified nursing assistants for quality dementia care. *International Journal of Geriatric Psychiatry*, 14(3):197–211.

Berghmans RLP (1997) Ethical hazards of the substituted judgement test in decision making concerning the end of life of dementia patients. *International Journal of Geriatric Psychiatry*, 12:283–287.

Brooker D (1995) Looking at them looking at me: a review of observational studies into the quality of institutional care for elderly people with dementia. *Journal of Mental Health*, 4:145–156.

Brooker D (2004) What is person-centred care for people with dementia? *Reviews in Clinical Gerontology*, 13:212–222.

Brooker D (2005) Dementia care mapping: a review of the research literature. *Gerontologist*, 45:11–18.

Bruce E, Surr C, Tibbs MA, Downs M (2002) Moving towards a special kind of care for people with dementia living in care homes. *NT Research*, 7(5):335–347.

Buber M (1937) I and Thou, translated by Ronald Gregor Smith. Edinburgh: T. & T. Clark; 2nd edn. New York: Scribners.

Calkins M (2005) Environments for late-stage dementia. *Alzheimer's Care Quarterly*, 6(1):71–75.

Camp CJ, Koss E, Judge KS (1999) Cognitive assessment in late-stage dementia. In Handbook of Assessment in Clinical Psychology. Lichtenberg PA (ed.). Chichester: John Wiley.

Cohen-Mansfield JK (1999) Measurement of inappropriate behaviour associated with dementia. *Journal of Gerontological Nursing*, 25:42–51.

Cohen-Mansfield JK (2003) Nonpharmacologic interventions for psychotic symptoms in dementia. *Journal of Geriatric Psychiatry and Neurology*, 16(4):219–224.

Cohen-Mansfield JK, Creedon M (2002) Nursing staff members' perceptions of pain indicators in persons with severe dementia. *Clinical Journal of Pain*, 18(1):64–73.

Cohen-Mansfield JK, Lipson S (2002) Pain in cognitively impaired nursing home residents: how well are physicians diagnosing it? *Journal of the American Geriatrics Society*, 50(6):1039–1044.

Cotrell V, Schulz R (1993) The perspective of the patient with Alzheimer's disease: A neglected dimension of dementia research. *Gerontologist*, 33:205–211.

Department of Health (2001) National Service Framework for Older People. Department of Health. London: Crown Copyright. www.doh.gov.uk/nsf

Doka KJ (ed.) (1989) Disenfranchised Grief: Recognizing Hidden Sorrow. Lexington, MA: Lexington Books.

Doka, K (2004) Grief and dementia. In Doka, K (ed.), Living with Grief. Alzheimer's Disease. Washington: Hospice Foundation of America, 131–144.

Downs MG (1997) The emergence of the person in dementia research. *Ageing and Society*, 17:597–607.

Epp TD (2003) Person-centred dementia care: a vision to be refined. *Canadian Alzheimer Disease Review*, April, 14–18.

Feil N (1993) The Validation Breakthrough: Simple Techniques for Communicating with People with 'Alzheimer Type Dementia'. Baltimore, MD: Health Professions Press.

Feldt KS (2000) The checklist of nonverbal pain indicators (CNPI). *Pain Management Nursing*, 1(1):13–21.

Finkel SI (2000) Introduction to behavioural and psychological symptoms of dementia (BPSD). *International Journal of Geriatric Psychiatry*, 15:S2–S4.

Finkel SI, Burns A, Cohen G (2000) Behavioural and psychological symptoms of dementia: a clinical and research update. *International Psychogeriatrics*, 12(s1):13–18.

Froggatt K (2002) Changing care practices: beyond education and training to 'practice development'. In Hockley J, Clark D (eds), Palliative Care for Older People in Care Homes. Buckingham: Open University Press, 151–164.

Froggatt K (2004) Palliative Care in Care Homes for Older People. London: The National Council for Palliative Care.

Graham N, Lidesay J, Katona C, Bertolote JM, *et al.* (2003) Reducing stigma and discrimination against older people with mental disorders: a technical consensus statement. *International Journal of Geriatric Psychiatry*, 18:670–678.

Hallberg IR, Edberg AK, Nordmark A, Johnsson K, Norberg A (1993) Daytime vocal activity in institutionalised severely demented patients identified as vocally disruptive by nurses. *International Journal of Geriatric Psychiatry*, 8(2):155–164.

Harris P (ed.) (2001) The Person with Alzheimer's Disease. Baltimore: Johns Hopkins University Press.

Hellen CR (1997) Communication and fundamentals of care: bathing, grooming, and dressing. In: Late Stage Dementia Care: A Basic Guide. London: Taylor & Francis, 113–125.

Hockley J (2002) Organizational structures for enhancing standards of palliative care. In Palliative Care for Older People in Care Homes, Hockley J, Clark D (eds). Buckingham: Open University Press.

Hughes J (2004) The practice and philosophy of palliative care in dementia. *Nursing and Residential Care*, 6(1):27–30.

Jennings B (2004) Alzheimer's disease and quality of life. In Doka K (ed.), Living with Grief. Alzheimer's Disease. Washington, Hospice Foundation of America, 131–144.

Kane RA, Kling KC, Bershadsky B, Kane RL, Giles K, Degebholtz HB, Liu J, Cutler LJ (2003) Quality of life measures for nursing home residents. *Journals of Gerontology Series A – Biological Sciences and Medical Sciences*, 58(3):240–248.

Kihlgren M, Kuremyr D, Norberg A, Brane G, Karlsson I, Engstrom B, Melin E (1993) Nurse–patient interaction after training in integrity-promoting care at a long term ward: analysis of video-recorded morning care sessions. *International Journal of Nursing Studies*, 30(1):1–13.

Kihlgren M, Hallgren A, Norberg A, Karlsson I (1994) Integrity promoting care of demented patients: patterns of interaction during morning care. *International Journal of Ageing and Human Development*, 39(4):303–319.

Killick J, Allan K (2001) Communication in the Care of People with Dementia. Buckingham: Open University Press.

Kitwood T (1993) Discover the person, not the disease. *Journal of Dementia Care*, Nov/Dec, 16–17.

Kitwood T (1997a) Dementia Reconsidered: the Person Comes First. Buckingham: Open University Press.

Kitwood T (1997b) The experience of dementia. *Ageing and Mental Health*, 1(1):13–22.

Kitwood T, Bredin K (1992) A new approach to the evaluation of dementia care. *Journal of Advances in Health and Nursing Care*, 1(5):41–60.

Kitwood T, Woods RT (1996) Training and Development Strategy for Dementia Care in Residential Settings. Bradford: University of Bradford.

Kovach CR (1997) Maintaining personhood: philosophy, goals, program development, and staff education. In Late Stage Dementia Care: A Basic Guide. London: Taylor & Francis, 25–43.

Kulpa JI, DePaul R (1997) Strategies for eating, swallowing, and dysphagia. In Late Stage Dementia Care: A Basic Guide. London: Taylor & Francis, 85–100.

Lawton MP (1996) Observed affect in nursing home residents with Alzheimer's disease. *Journals of Gerontology Series B–Psychological Sciences and Social Sciences*, 51(1):3–14.

Leveson R (2004) Lessons from the end of life. *British Medical Journal*, 329:1244.

Magai C, Choen CI, Gomberg D (2002) Impact of training dementia caregivers in sensitivity to nonverbal emotion signals. *International Psychogeriatrics*, 14(1):25–38.

Magee W (1999) Music therapy in chronic degenerative illness: reflecting the dynamic sense of self. In Aldridge D (ed.), Music Therapy in Palliative Care. London: Jessica Kingsley.

Morton I (1999) Person-centred Approaches to Dementia Care. Bicester: Speechmark Publishing.

Moss M (2001) End of life in nursing homes. In Annual Review of Gerontology and Geriatrics: End of Life: Scientific and Social Issues. Lawton MP (ed.), New York: Springer, 224–258.

Moss MS, Moss SZ, Rubinstein RL, Black HK (2003) The metaphor of 'family' in staff communication about dying and death. *Journal of Gerontology: Social Sciences*, 58B(5):S290–S296.

Nolan MR, Davies S, Brown J, Keady J, Nolan M (2004) Beyond 'person-centred' care: a new vision for gerontological nursing. *International Journal of Older People Nursing*, 13(3a):45–53.

Norberg A (1998) Interaction with people suffering from severe dementia. In Health Economics of Dementia, Wimo A, Jonsson B, Karlsson G, Wingblad B (eds). Chichester: John Wiley, 113–121.

Norberg A (2001). Communication in the care of people with severe dementia. In Hummert M L, Nussbaum J F (eds), Aging, Communication, and Health: Linking Research and Practice for Successful Aging. LEA's communication series, 157–173.

Norberg A, Melin E, Asplund K (2003) Reactions to music, touch and object presentation in the final stage of dementia: an exploratory study. *International Journal of Nursing Studies*, 40:473–479.

Normann HK, Asplund K., Norberg A (1998) Episodes of lucidity in people with severe dementia as narrated by formal carers. *Journal of Advanced Nursing*, 28(6):1295–1300.

Normann HK, Norberg A, Asplund K (2002) Confirmation and lucidity during conversations with a woman with severe dementia. *Journal of Advanced Nursing*, 39(4):370–376.

Orchard H (2002) Spiritual care in care homes: perceptions and practice. In Palliative Care for Older People in Care Homes, Hockley J, Clark D (eds). Buckingham: Open University Press.

Parfit D (1984) Reasons and Persons. Oxford: Clarendon Press.

Perrin T (1997a) The positive response schedule. *Ageing and Mental Health*, 1(2):184–191.

Perrin T (1997b) Occupational need in severe dementia: a descriptive study. *Journal of Advanced Nursing*, 25:934–941.

Perrin T (2004) (ed.) The New Culture of Therapeutic Activity with Older People. Bicester: Speechmark Publishing.

Rose L, Schlingensiepen S (2000) How do we make care-work more person-centred? An exploration through music for life project. Unpublished research for European Alzheimer's Clearing House.

Roudier M, Marcie P, Grancher AS, Tzortzis C, Stakstein S, Boller F (1998) Discrimination of facial identity and of emotions in Alzheimer's disease. *Journal of the Neurological Sciences*, 154(2):151–158.

Sabat SR, Harre R (1994) The Alzheimer's disease sufferer as a semiotic subject. *Philosophy, Psychiatry, Psychology*, 1:145–160.

Shue V, Beck C, Lawton P (1996) Measuring affect in frail and cognitively impaired elders. *Journal of Mental Health and Ageing*, 2(3):259–271.

Sloane PD, Hoeffer B, Mitchell CM, *et al.* (2003) Reducing disruptive behaviour: outcome assessment of a psychosocial intervention during bathing. Annual Meeting of the Gerontological Society of America.

Small N, Downs M, Froggatt K (in press) Improving end-of-life care for people with dementia: the benefits of combining UK approaches to palliative care and dementia care. In Caregiving and dementia Vol 4, Miesen B, Jones G (eds). London: Routledge.

Snyder L (1999) Speaking our Minds: Personal Reflections from Individuals with Alzheimer's. New York: Freeman.

Stolee P, Hillier LM, Esbaugh J, Bol N, McKellar L, Gauthier N (2005) Instruments of the assessment of pain in older persons with cognitive impairment. *JAGS*, 53:319–326.

Stuckey JC, Gwyther LP (2003) Dementia, religion and spirituality. *Dementia, the International Journal of Social Research and Practice*, 2(3):291–297.

Summersall J, Wight S (2004) When it's difficult to swallow: the role of the speech therapist. *Nursing and Residential Care*, 6(11):550–553.

Swartz K, Walton J, Crummer G, Hnatz E, Frisina R (1989) Does the melody linger on? Music cognition in AD. *Seminars in Neurology*, 9:152–158.

Sweeting H, Gilhooly M (1997) Dementia and the phenomenon of social death. *Sociology of Health and Illness*, 19(1):93–117.

Thompson O'Maille T, Kasayka R (2005) Touching the spirit at the end of life. *Alzheimer's Care Quarterly*, 6(1):62–70.

Thorgrimsen L, Spector A, Wiles A, Orrell M (2003) Aromatherapy for Dementia. In The Cochrane Library. Issue 4. Chichester: John Wiley.

Twigg J (2000) Carework as a form of bodywork. *Ageing and Society*, 20:389–411.

Volicer L, Bloom-Charette L (1999) Enhancing the Quality of Life in Advanced Dementia. New York: Brunner-Mazel.

Winblad B, Wimo A, Mobius HJ, Fox JM, Fratiglioni L (1999) Severe dementia: a common condition entailing high costs at individual and societal levels. *International Journal of Geriatric Psychiatry*, 14:911–914.

Woods RT (2001) Discovering the person with Alzheimer's disease: cognitive, emotional and behavioural aspects. *Ageing and Mental Health*, 5(1):7–16.

Palliative Care in Patients with Severe Dementia

Raymond T.C.M. Koopmans, H. Roeline W. Pasman and Jenny T. van der Steen

Introduction

Principles of palliative care (see Glossary box) apply to patients with life-threatening disease, which includes dementia (WHO, 1990). It is important that health care professionals need to be clear about dementia being a terminal disease like cancer. The course of the disease, however, differs in terms of disease progression and survival, typically a 'frailty pattern' with a slowly downhill and somewhat variable course rather than a steep downhill course in the last months of life as in cancer. Palliative care, with its focus on improving quality of life, arguably applies to all patients with dementia, but is particularly pertinent to patients with severe dementia. However, in the literature there is no consensus about the terminology and definition of severe dementia. Different terms are used, such as (very) advanced dementia, (very) severe dementia, end stage dementia, late (stage) dementia, final phase of dementia, and even vegetative state. We use the term severe dementia throughout this chapter, and this applies to patients who are fully dependent in activities of daily living, incontinent, and virtually non-communicative (see Glossary box).

There is much evidence that hospitalised older patients with advanced cognitive impairment often undergo inappropriate burdensome and non-palliative interventions despite having a limited life expectancy (Mitchell *et al.*, 2004). Nursing home patients with severe dementia more frequently receive non-palliative interventions such as tube feeding, laboratory tests, restraints and intravenous therapy than cancer patients. Furthermore, severe dementia patients are significantly less likely than those with terminal cancer to have advance directives limiting aggressive care. (Teno, 2000)

In 1995, a panel of experts in the field formulated eight recommendations to improve end-of-life (EOL) care in dementia (Hurley *et al.*, 1995). The recommendations were categorised in four areas where care needs improvement: palliative care, decision-making, acute care, and research and education. These areas are reflected in important issues of palliative care in severe dementia, which we discuss in this chapter. These include advance care planning, avoiding aggressive treatments, treatment of frequently occurring conditions and burdensome signs and symptoms such as pain, anxiety, shortness of breath, eating problems and pneumonia, and the issue of palliative sedation and euthanasia in dementia. Dutch clinical practice illustrates these issues; with data available, we contrast internationally different approaches. The chapter concludes with some general recommendations.

Advance care planning and shared decision-making

Ideally, advance care planning commences at the point of diagnosis, and when the person can still make his or her own decisions. Health care professionals caring for patients with severe dementia should enquire after the presence of a written living will and if available, they should discuss with

---

Glossary box

Palliative care (WHO, 1990)
An approach that improves the quality of life of patients and their families facing the problems associated with life-threatening illness, through the prevention and relief of suffering by means of early identification and impeccable assessment and treatment of pain and other problems, physical, psychosocial and spiritual

Palliative care in dementia (WHO, 1990)
• provides relief from pain and other distressing symptoms
• affirms life and regards dying as a normal process
• intends neither to hasten nor to postpone death
• integrates the psychological and spiritual aspects of patient care
• offers a support system to help patients live as actively as possible until death
• offers a support system to help the family cope during the patient's illness and in their own bereavement
• uses a team approach to address the needs of patients and their families, including bereavement counselling, if indicated
• will enhance quality of life, and may also positively influence the course of illness

Comfort care
This type of care avoids therapies entailing discomfort; life-prolonging treatments are contraindicated; and it directs efforts to relieve of suffering and to optimise quality of life and quality of dying.

Severe dementia (in this chapter)
Patients in which the dementia has progressed to the final phase. This means that cognitive testing is no longer possible, patients are totally impaired in their activities of daily living and totally incontinent, mobility is impaired and patients are wheelchair-bound or bedridden, and speech is limited to five words.

---

the proxy decision-makers (the relatives) the actuality of the text. Patients with severe dementia are no longer able to express their wishes and preferences. Relatives therefore need to pick up roles as substitute decision-makers respecting any known wish of the patients, or decide in the best interest of their family-member.

Living wills such as 'in case of severe dementia, which is when I don't recognise my children any more, I don't want to be hospitalised in case of a life-threatening disease such as pneumonia' should be respected whenever possible. Living wills requiring treatments withheld (a 'negative' wish), such as 'I don't want a feeding tube in case of severe stroke' are easier to respect than those with 'positive' wishes such as 'I want euthanasia in case of severe dementia'.

Living wills or advance care planning with substitute decision makers may reflect wishes pertaining to cardio-pulmonal resuscitation, hospitalisation, intravenous or subcutaneous administration of fluids, whether or not to insert a feeding tube, and whether or not to administer antibiotics. In severe dementia patients, the advisable primary goal of treatment is 'comfort-care' (see Glossary box).

This 'shared decision-making' with respect for the wishes of the family is essential for good care in severe dementia patients. The family needs to be informed that they will share the path of gradual deterioration together with the health care professionals and that it is important to keep in contact. The physician should repeatedly inform the relatives about prognoses and the course and anticipated complications. This prepares relatives for future events, and eases decision-making when a life-threatening illness develops with concomitant important end-of-life decisions. Of course, one cannot anticipate every possible complication. Therefore, the final treatment decisions are taken at the moment of the acute event. Treatment policies should be evaluated at least twice a year, and more frequently in case of rapid deterioration. In the Netherlands, the overwhelming majority of patients with severe dementia do not have a living will. In a Dutch study on starting or forgoing artificial nutrition and hydration (ANH) in nursing home patients with severe dementia, only 4% of the 190 included patients had a living will. By contrast, as much as in two-thirds of the cases, agreements were made with regard to starting or forgoing treatment in possible future situations. These agreements were more often about forgoing treatment (64% of all included patients) than about starting treatment (44% of all included patients). Most common types of treatment to forgo in future situations were: admission to a hospital, ANH, and resuscitation (48%, 42% and 42%, of all included patients respectively). (It is of note that many Dutch nursing homes employ a general do-not-resuscitate policy.) These agreements were most often made with the child(ren) of the patient (78%) and only 2% of the patients themselves participated in the agreement (Pasman et al., 2004). However, in the qualitative part of the study (participant observation in two nursing homes) it was found that when an ANH-decision had to be made, the advance care planning seemed of limited importance; policy agreements were useful in the decision-making process and for the dialogue with the family, but in the end the current medical condition of the patient, the wishes of the family, and the interpretations of the patients' quality of life by their care providers were the most important criteria for the decision to start or forgo ANH (The et al., 2002).

Avoiding aggressive interventions and treatment

Since 'comfort care' is the preferable treatment goal in severe dementia patients, aggressive interventions and treatments should be avoided whenever possible. In patients with serious swallowing problems, refusal of food and drinks or other eating problems related to the dementia, the decision whether or not to administer ANH becomes relevant. Tube feeding by a nasal tube or a percutaneous endoscopic gastrostomy is a very aggressive treatment, which should be discouraged and avoided whenever possible in these patients. Studies have found evidence that feeding tubes in this population do not prevent aspiration, nor prolong life, improve overall function, or reduce pressure sores (Finucane et al., 1999). The quality of life can be adversely affected when a feeding tube is inserted, and patients may require restraints to prevent them pulling out the tube. Despite the lack of evidence, it is estimated that 10% of US nursing home patients with severe dementia are tube-fed. However, the number of feeding tubes placed can be reduced by educational programmes on end-of-life care and on feeding management of severe dementia patients, as Monteleonie and co-workers found (Monteleonie and Clark, 2004). Nevertheless, there may still be legal, regulatory or cultural barriers in forgoing tube feeding. Chen et al. (2002), for instance, found that 63% of caregivers of Taiwanese severe dementia patients preferred highly aggressive care, whereas only 3% preferred solely palliative care at the end of the patient's life. Cultural differences in end-of-life attitudes were also found in a recent survey about forgoing treatment at the end of life in six European countries (Bosshard et al., 2005). Although this research-project was not particularly designed to study end-of-life decisions in dementia patients, the authors found that, for instance, physicians from the Netherlands, Switzerland and Belgium are more willing to distance themselves from an absolute duty to sustain life.

In the Netherlands, patients with severe dementia are rarely tube-fed. The primary aim of forgoing ANH according to most nursing home physicians is to avoid (unnecessarily) prolonging life, but not to hasten death (Pasman et al., 2004). When ANH is started, it is almost always in the case of an acute illness such as pneumonia and it is started in combination with other medical treatments, such as antibiotics, with a curative treatment.

Further, laboratory testing such as blood testing or urinalysis, and imaging and X-rays should consistently be avoided if there is no curative treatment goal. One could argue about the sense of controlling blood glucose in severe dementia patients suffering from diabetes. When patients develop severe eating difficulties, the intake of oral medication can become problematic. In this case palliative care entails acceptance of death and medication to relieve suffering.

Frequently occurring conditions and burdensome signs and symptoms
Pain

The limited ability of severe dementia patients to communicate and thus to express pain is a substantial barrier to pain assessment and management (Frampton, 2003). It is not clear whether dementia patients actually experience, or simply report less pain. It is hypothesised that patients with Alzheimer's disease would report less the motivational-affective aspects of pain compared to controls, and that they suffer more acute rather than chronic pain (Scherder *et al.*, 2005). These differences in pain expression are reflected in differences in medication prescription. Several studies have shown that dementia patients were prescribed fewer analgesics, even when they had more behavioural indicators of pain documented.

Visual analogue scales for pain assessment are not valid in these patients. Health care professionals are forced to rely on nonverbal or behavioural cues of physical and emotional pain such as motor agitation, repetitive shouting, sweating and facial expression. Manfredi *et al.* (2003) found that observation of facial expressions and vocalisations are accurate means for assessing the presence of pain, but not its intensity.

Despite the problem of adequate assessment of pain, the control of pain in severe dementia is crucial. The goal is to eliminate the pain. First, possible causes of the pain should be detected, such as pain caused by pressure sores, osteoarthritis, hypertonic muscles, angina and constipation. Any specific treatment of the cause of the pain is preferred above symptomatic treatment of pain. Despite efforts to detect the source of the pain, however, most severe dementia patients appear to suffer from generalised pain of unknown cause that is provoked by bathing and dressing.

The WHO analgesic ladder should be used to choose drugs on the basis of the severity of the pain. One should use a fixed-dose regimen to provide around-the-clock relief along with rescue-medication for break-through pain. In severe pain, opioids such as morphine are the treatment of choice. In the case of delirium caused by morphine, opioid-rotation is advised. When oral administration is impossible because of swallowing difficulties, a continuous subcutaneous infusion should be inserted.

Shortness of breath and death rattle

The most common causes of shortness of breath in severe dementia patients are aspiration, lower respiratory tract infection such as pneumonia, heart failure and, sometimes, anxiety. As in pain management, causal treatment of shortness of breath is preferred above symptomatic treatment. The issues of causal treatment of pneumonia and anxiety are addressed in separate sections of this chapter.

The first-line treatments of shortness of breath in severe dementia patients are oxygen-therapy, drainage of secretions, semiprone position and morphine. Morphine is probably the most effective treatment for relieving shortness of breath.

Shortness of breath can be complicated by death rattle (DR). DR is a term applied to dying patients to describe the noise produced by the oscillatory movements of secretions in the upper airways (Wildiers and Menten, 2002). The sound is particularly distressing for family members because it is associated with severe suffering or even choking to death. Therefore the physician should inform the relatives about the mechanism of DR and that it is different from severe shortness of breath. However, DR is a strong predictor for death. Physicians should be aware of the fact that artificial hydration increases the risk of DR. Withdrawing artificial hydration may reduce suffering and physicians should explain the pathophysiological process to the relatives. Several anticholinergic drugs are used to treat DR. Wildiers and Menten (2002) found that hyoscine hydrobromide, as a bolus of continuous infusion, is effective for DR and is comfortable for the patient and family.

Tracheal suction of secretions should be minimised, because frequent irritation of the pharynx by a tube can adversely stimulate secretion. A semiprone position encourages postural drainage.

Pneumonia

Pneumonia frequently occurs in patients with severe dementia, and it may be the ultimate cause of death of up to two-thirds of nursing home patients with dementia. Treatment may be curative, including use of intravenous or oral antibiotics to cure the episode of pneumonia and restore functioning to its previous level, or palliative. Palliative treatment relieves symptoms of pneumonia mostly without antibiotics, when, for example, death is imminent or there is a patient or proxy wish for comfort care. Although studies on prognoses after pneumonia have been published in recent years, and living wills have become increasingly popular in countries such as the USA, this end-of-life treatment decision is still frequently complex and emotion-laden for physicians and families.

Treatment approaches may vary dramatically internationally, which is particularly clear from studies among US and Dutch nursing home patients with dementia and pneumonia. In the 1980s, in one US nursing home, Volicer *et al.* (1986) pioneered a hospice approach for dementia patients including comfort care. Up till today, however, Volicer's approach is still exceptional in the USA, where patients with severe dementia who develop pneumonia are frequently transferred to the hospital and treated with intravenous antibiotics. By contrast, from two large prospective observational studies in the late 1990s in the Netherlands and in Missouri (van der Steen *et al.*, 2002, 2004a, 2004b, 2006; Mehr *et al.*, 2003; Kruse *et al.*, 2004, 2006), it appeared that Dutch nursing home patients with severe dementia are rarely hospitalised (0.3% versus 22% of patients with severe dementia in Missouri nursing homes). Related to this, they are more frequently treated with simple oral antibiotics (e.g. parenteral antibiotics are administered in only 16% of antibiotic treatments, and mostly intramuscular, in Dutch patients, versus 36%, and mostly intravenous, in Missouri patients). Further, antibiotics are more frequently withheld in Dutch patients with severe dementia: 33% versus 24% in comparable Missouri patients, respectively (van der Steen *et al.*, 2004a).

Treatment decision-making in individuals with severe dementia and pneumonia can benefit from outcomes of the prospective studies done in the USA and the Netherlands. First, specific prognostic models have recently become available to inform physicians and families on prognosis in terms of mortality and functional decline (van der Steen *et al.*, 2004b, 2006). Second, it appeared that hospitalisation might not be beneficial for many of these patients. The Missouri study showed that, after adjustment for differences in illness severity, hospitalisation of nursing home patients with lower respiratory tract infection – predominantly pneumonia – probably does not improve survival (Kruse *et al.*, 2004). Moreover, in general, hospitalisation and administration of intravenous fluids may burden severely demented patients, causing confusion and agitation, and increasing risk of pressure ulcers. Third, compared with oral antibiotics, use of intravenous antibiotics and multiple regimens may not improve survival, at least in the mid-to-long term, which appeared from analyses of the combined data of the prospective Dutch and Missouri studies. Although simpler antibiotics were used for Dutch patients and their mortality was higher, there was no difference in three-month survival after adjustment for Dutch patients being more ill. However, it is possible that more aggressive antibiotic treatment does provide a short-term survival benefit (up to one month after diagnosis) specifically in high-risk residents (Kruse *et al.*, 2005). Nevertheless, studies have poorly addressed patient's suffering at the end of life, family views, coping and grieving related to decision-making, and the course of the pneumonia after antibiotics are withheld. The latter is still unclear with conflicting results from US and Dutch studies. Volicer's single small classical study found no survival benefit from antibiotic treatment of febrile illness in nursing home patients with advanced dementia. Volicer and colleagues (Hurley, Volicer *et al.*, 1993) also observed higher levels of comfort in patients who received hospice care (without antibiotics, for febrile illness). By contrast, Dutch patients not treated with antibiotics almost all died within a few days, and despite more liberal use of treatments to relieve symptoms, they did not show less comfort than Dutch patients who were treated with antibiotics (van der Steen *et al.*, 2002). Further, overall discomfort levels were higher than in Volicer's study.

The few available studies – from the Netherlands and the USA – show that palliative care in nursing homes, with the exception of Volicer's studies (Volicer *et al.*, 1986; Hurley *et al.*, 1993) on effects of a hospice philosophy of care, may only partially address problems in patients dying with dementia.

Curative treatment of pneumonia without hospital transfer, and palliative treatment to relieve symptoms may be appropriate for patients with severe dementia, depending on the goals of treatment for the individual patient. A system fostering an on-going discussion between families, and physicians, and other involved (para)medical disciplines is needed for appropriate goal setting and to ensure a timely recognition of a need for palliative care, anticipating acute disease.

Anxiety

Anxiety is a distressing symptom in dying patients with severe dementia (Lyness, 2004). Anxiety may be a symptom of delirium and therefore the result of hallucinations and delusions, or it may present as a single primary condition or as secondary to medical illness or its treatments. Anxiety in severe dementia patients cannot easily be assessed. Sometimes facial expression or physical signs such as excessive sweating can provide a clue to the diagnosis. Family members who know the patient very well are able to interpret the patient's behaviour as anxiety. Sometimes the patient seems to be aware that he is going to die and 'fear of death' is observed. In the case of delirium, identification and treatment of the underlying cause may not always apply. The causes may not be remediable, or may be iatrogenic (for instance due to morphine use) in the service of palliation. The mainstay of therapy of symptoms of anxiety is a benzodiazepine such as diazepam or, in the presence of delirium, antipsychotic medication such as haloperidol.

Swallowing and chewing problems, including refusal of hydration and nutrition

Most patients with severe dementia need assistance with eating and drinking, and many show aversive behaviour when fed, such as turning away the head, pushing away the spoon, or spitting out the food. Food avoidance may be due to underlying physical, psychological and/or social problems such as swallowing problems, grief or an unpleasant environment. The cause often remains unclear because most patients have lost their speech (Pasman *et al.*, 2003). Studies show that nurses interpret the aversive behaviour of patients differently and, as a result of that, the type of assistance they provide, differs (stop or continue feeding, sometimes using force). Interpretations of aversive behaviour should be discussed with physicians, other involved disciplines and the patient's family. Their specific expertise can contribute to the understanding of the patient's behaviour, facilitating a well-balanced decision about how to deal with the aversive behaviour. Speech therapists can analyse swallowing problems and occupational therapists can look at posture and can, for example, be consulted for adjusting spoons and cups. Proper mouth-care is essential when eating problems arise. A dentist can specifically contribute in analysing eating problems, while the physician should look for treatable causes such as oral candidiasis. Finally, when problems with chewing or swallowing arise, the consistency of the food can be adapted in consultation with a dietician.

Other symptoms

Severe dementia is often accompanied by discomfort-causing problems such as constipation, skin problems such as pressure sores, paratonia, contractures and epileptic jerks. Immobile patients who have difficulties in eating and drinking and who are sometimes treated with anticholinergic medication or morphine are at risk for developing constipation. A diet with sufficient fibre and fluids in combination with laxatives prevents constipation.

The most frequently observed skin problems are itching, fungal infections and pressure sores. Itching is mostly caused by the dry (senile) skin and can improve by avoiding soap and moistening the skin with fatty oils. Sometimes antihistamines are indicated. Fungal infections, often the result of hypertonic flexions of the limbs, can be best treated with Miconazol. The first line of treatment of pressure sores is prevention by using special mattresses, and frequent turning and lifting of the patients. Paratonia, or 'gegenhalten' is a problem specific to dementia patients. In its most severe stage, paratonia can result in a total flexure posture and muscle contractures, with subsequent risk of skin problems and even pressure ulcers. Paratonia and contractures can cause considerable discomfort, especially during bathing and dressing. Treatment by physiotherapists sometimes results in a temporary relaxation of the muscle tone along with a reduction of discomfort in morning-care. Occupational therapists can provide specially designed ortheses to prevent further progression and to improve comfort in bedridden patients. A final option is surgical cutting of the tendons. Sometimes patients have severe epileptic jerks or even seizures, which best can be treated with valproate or benzodiazepines.

Palliative sedation and euthanasia

Although proper palliative care, in most cases, can eliminate physical suffering or reduce it to tolerable levels, there are some patients for whom the best efforts cannot produce an acceptable quality of life. An approach acceptable to many clinicians and families is the use of palliative sedation, that is the use of medication to produce an unconscious state in which the patient ultimately dies from the underlying disease or dehydration. Palliative sedation should be used as an option of last resort, when other treatments to relieve suffering to an acceptable level have failed. There is a debate on whether palliative sedation is a kind of 'passive' euthanasia, because, along with the administration of short half-life benzodiazepines, ANH is withheld.

However, the term euthanasia should be reserved for the physician-ordered intentional killing of a patient, by a lethal dose of a medication and on the explicit request of the patient. Euthanasia in severe dementia is prohibited. However, a few cases are reported in the Netherlands where euthanasia in (mild) dementia patients occurred and the doctor was not prosecuted. There is an on-going debate on this issue, since people request euthanasia in their living wills.

General recommendations

In the near future, the number of patients who will survive to the stage of severe dementia will increase dramatically. To date, the care for people with severe dementia is frequently poor, and palliative care principles are not commonly applied in clinical practice of care for dementia patients. Hughes *et al.* (2005) have suggested that people with dementia require specialist palliative care, and this care should take place in specialised dementia palliative care units. However, this approach has the disadvantage that patients have to move to such a unit, and this transfer and change of environment may be uncomfortable for patients and relatives. An alternative is outreaching palliative care for people living in the community, including in nursing and residential homes, as well as supporting hospitals and hospices (Hughes *et al.*, 2005). Since nursing homes are the place of death of many patients with severe dementia, the focus should be on improvement of palliative care in these institutions. A specially trained nursing home physician who is employed by the nursing home is essential for good continuous high-quality care for dementia patients in nursing homes (Hoek *et al.*, 2001). The nursing home physician should have outstanding skills and competency with regard to assessments, diagnostics, prognostics and interventions in dementia and be capable to deal with complex medical–ethical dilemmas and moral problems.

We conclude that palliative care is beneficial for patients with severe dementia, although there is a need for more research on this topic. The future challenge will be the proper training of health care professionals in the principles of palliative care and continuing the worldwide debate on cultural, legal and regulatory issues in the treatment of these complex patients.

References

Bosshard G, Nilstun T, Bilsen J et al. (2005) Forgoing treatment at the end of life 6 European countries. *Arch Intern Med*, 165:401–407.

Chen W, Wang S, Lu S, Fuh J (2002) Which level of care is preferred for end-stage dementia? Survey of Taiwanese caregivers. *J Geriatr Psychiatry Neurol*, 15:16–19.

Framptom M (2003) Experience assessment and management of pain in people with dementia. *Age and Ageing*, 32:248–251.

Finucane TE, Christams C, Travis K (1999) Tube feeding in patients with advanced dementia. *JAMA*, 282:1365–1370.

Hoek JF, Ribbe MW, Hertogh CMPM, Vleuten van der CPM (2001) The specialist training program for nursing home physicians: a new professional challenge. *JAMDA*, 326–330.

Hughes JC, Robinson L, Volicer L (2005) Specialist palliative care in dementia. Specialized units with outreach and liaison are needed. *BMJ*, 330:57–58.

Hurley AC, Volicer BJ, Mahoney MA, Volicer L (1993) Palliative fever management in Alzheimer patients: quality plus fiscal responsibility. *ANS Adv Nurs Sci*, 16:21–32.

Hurley AC, Volicer L, Rempusheski VF, Fry S (1995) Reaching consensus: the process of recommending treatment decisions for Alzheimer patients. *ANS Adv Nurs Sci*, 18:33–43.

Hurley AC, Volicer L (2002) Alzheimer disease: 'It's okay, Mama, if you want to go, it's okay'. *JAMA*, 288:2324–2331.

Kruse RL, Mehr DR, Boles KE et al. (2004) Does hospitalization impact survival after lower respiratory infection in nursing home residents? *Med Care*, 42:860–870.

Kruse RL, Mehr DR, van der Steen JT et al. (2005) Antibiotic treatment and survival of nursing home patients with lower respiratory tract infection: a cross-national analysis. *Ann Fam Med*, 3:422–429.

Lyness J (2004) End-of-life care. *Am J Geriatr Psychiatry*, 12:457–472.

Manfredi PL, Breuer B, Meier DE, Libow L (2003) Pain assessment in elderly patients with severe dementia. *J Pain Symptom Manage*, 25:48–52.

Mehr DR, Steen JT van der, Kruse RL, Ooms ME, Rantz M, Ribbe MW (2003) Lower respiratory infections in nursing home residents with dementia: a tale of two countries. *Gerontologist*, 43(Suppl2):85–93.

Mitchell SL, Kiely DK, Hamel MB (2004) Dying with advanced dementia in the nursing home. *Arch Intern Med*, 164:321–326.

Monteleonie C, Clark E (2004) Using rapid-cycle quality improvement methodology to reduce feeding tubes in patients with advanced dementia: before and after study. *BMJ*, 329:491–494.

Morrison RS, Siu AL (2000) Survival in end-stage dementia following acute illness. *JAMA*, 284:47–52.

Pasman HRW, The BAM, Onwuteaka-Philipsen BD, van der Wal G, Ribbe MW (2003) Feeding nursing home patients with severe dementia: a qualitative study. *Journal of Advanced Nursing*, 42:304–311.

Pasman HRW, Onwuteaka-Philipsen BD, Ooms ME, Wigcheren PT van der Wal G, Ribbe MW (2004) Forgoing artificial nutrition and hydration in demented nursing home patients: patients, decision-making and participants. *Alzheimer Dis Assoc Disord*, 18:154–162.

Scherder E, Oosterman J, Swaab D et al. (2005) Recent developments in pain in dementia. *BMJ* 330:461–464.

Steen JT van der, Ooms ME, van der Wal G, Ribbe MW (2002) Pneumonia: the demented patient's best friend? Discomfort after starting or withholding antibiotic treatment. *J Am Geriatr Soc*, 50:1681–1688.

Steen JT van der, Kruse RL, Ooms ME et al. (2004a) Treatment of nursing home residents with dementia and lower respiratory tract infection in the United States and the Netherlands: an ocean apart. *J Am Geriatr Soc*, 52:691–699.

Steen J van der, Ooms ME, van der Wal G, Mehr D, Ribbe M, Kruse R (2004b) Treatment strategy and risk of functional decline and mortality after nursing-home acquired lower respiratory tract infection. *Gerontologist*, 44(Spec No 1): 127–128.

Steen JT van der, Mehr DR, Kruse RL et al. (2006) Predictors of mortality for lower respiratory infections in nursing home residents with dementia validate transnationally. *J Clin Epidemiol*, in press.

Teno JM (2000) Advance directives for nursing home residents. Achieving compassionate, competent, cost-effective care. *JAMA*, 283:1481–1482.

The BAM, Pasman HRW, Onwuteaka-Philipsen BD, Ribbe MW, van der Wal G (2002) Withholding artificial fluids and food from elderly demented patients with dementia: ethnographic study. *British Medical Journal*, 325:1326–1330.

Volicer L, Rheaume Y, Brown J, Fabiszewski K, Brady R (1986) Hospice approach to the treatment of patients with advanced dementia of the Alzheimer type. *JAMA*, 256:2210–2213.

WHO (WHO World Health Organization) (1990) Cancer pain relief and palliative care. Report of a WHO expert committee (WHO Technical Report Series Nr 804). WHO, Geneva.

Wildiers H, Menten J (2002) Death rattle: prevalence, prevention and treatment. *J Pain Symptom Manage*, 23:310–317.

18

Narrative Ethics and Ethical Narratives in Dementia

Clive Baldwin

Prelude

Imagine a performance. At times the performer will be centre stage, at times at the back, to stage left or right. There will be occasions when the performer temporarily leaves the stage. On occasion the performer will draw attention to the backdrop, the scenery, the props; on other occasions all of these will be taken for granted.

Sometimes the performer will play to one part of the audience, at other times to another part. Sometimes the performer's voice will be loud, at others soft. Sometimes the words spoken will be poetic, at other times prosaic. At still other times the performer will be silent.

The lighting will affect and reflect the performer's moods; the actions and reactions of the audience will influence how the performer responds, sometimes with fear, sometimes with pleasure.

But the performer is never alone. There is always an accompaniment. People onstage, people offstage. Their words and actions sometimes louder, sometimes softer. Their characters sometimes lighter, sometimes fuller. Their relationships with the performer sometimes harmonious, sometimes discordant. Their role sometimes carrying the plot, sometimes silent. But the performer is never alone.

Imagine the performer centre stage, with gentle, unobtrusive accompaniment. The audience is drawn to the performer. The performer moves to the rear of the stage, the accompaniment moves centre. Still the audience is enwrapped in the performance. The performer moves centre once again.

The performance moves on, developing its themes, its plot, its characters. Major and minor leitmotifs emerge and recede. What happens next will be part of what happens next. The story is both well known and unique. The final act, the resolution, the last curtain.

And then others review, explain, reinvent. Were the characters believable and engaging or two-dimensional and lacking depth? Did the story demonstrate narrative strength or was it narratively weak? Was it consistent and coherent or fragmented and chaotic? Did the story resonate with other stories we already knew or was it so unique to be outside our ken? Did it invite us in or alienate? Did we care about what happened? The bottom line – was it a good story?

Introduction

Over the last 15 years or so there has been an exponential rise in the interest shown in narrative as a theory and a method across the disciplines. Narrative is, however, a somewhat nebulous term and its use is neither always clear nor consistent. For some, narrative provides a unique insight into the world and our experience of it (Astedt-Kurki and Heikkinen, 1994). In this view, narratives

Severe Dementia. Edited by A. Burns and B. Winblad.
Copyright © 2006 John Wiley & Sons, Ltd. ISBN 0-470-01054-1

are more or less accurate representations of 'what really happened' and our understandings of that reality (that is, data for subsequent analysis). Focus on such 'representational narratives' is an approach found in the works of writers such as Cortazzi (1993) and Riessman (1993), key authors and proponents of narrative analysis. For others, narrative forms reality, it is the world. Authors advocating such 'constitutive narratives' would include Bruner (1987, 1996), Polkinghorne (1995) and Barone (1995).

For the purposes of this chapter, and at the risk of setting myself a thankless, if not impossible, task, I want to examine what ethics might look like with regard to people with severe dementia if we start from the position of constitutive narrativity. To do this, we need to explore a number of general areas before we move to the specifics of severe dementia – if indeed severe dementia makes any significant difference to our narrative-based ethics.

In essence my argument is as follows:

(1) We, as human beings (let us leave aside for now the question of other species' narratives) are essentially narrative beings, our Selves and our world are narratively constituted. Consequently, we relate to one another in and through narratives.
(2) With the onset and progression of dementia, the ability to construct narratives is compromised, by both the underlying neuropathology and the reaction of others.
(3) A narrative approach to palliative care raises certain kinds of questions that help us focus on the types of narrative that are in play and the types of narratives that we want to construct towards the end of life.
(4) Ethics is fundamentally concerned with which narratives we choose to tell and how we choose to tell them (narrative ethics).
(5) Following this narrative understanding we can identify ways of enhancing narrative integrity and agency thus facilitating the construction of positive and meaningful (and thus ethical) narratives for people with severe dementia.

I realise that this is a somewhat ambitious project to be attempted in the confines of a single chapter. I would, therefore, crave the reader's indulgence if I am on occasion too brief for their liking or at times beg one too many questions. While full exploration of these, and related, complex issues must wait for another time, an outline of a different way of thinking is presented here for reflection and debate.

Narrative and the Self

The view that we are narrative beings is well-argued by authors such as MacIntyre (1984), Bruner (1987) and Taylor (1989). For these authors, among others, not only do we exist in a story-telling world but our very Selves are constituted by the stories we and others tell about ourselves. Our experience (of both the world and ourselves) is not reality put into narrative form but rather our narrative form made real. In other words, we are our stories. In these stories we constitute ourselves as persons in accordance with concepts of ourselves (Blustein, 1999). These self-concepts are not static (Blustein, 1999) and our identity is a combination of historical narrative and literary fiction (Ricoeur, 1987). The importance of narrative in the construction of identity is also becoming recognised in the field of dementia (Mills, 1997, 1998; Vittoria, 1998) though, as yet, the problem of the narrative identity of those who cease to be narrative agents (as currently understood in narrative theory) has not been addressed.

Lives, like stories, have a trajectory through time. What comes before affects and to some extent determines what happens next. This trajectory gives lives, and stories, a narrative coherence (Taylor, 1989) without which the story-line would give way to a mere assemblage of unrelated, episodic events. Maintaining this sense of coherence is an overarching feature of a life-project and productive of wellbeing (Androutsopoulou et al., 2004) and its loss is a feature of mental ill-health such as in schizophrenia (Lysaker *et al.*, 2003) or post-traumatic stress disorder (Hopper and van der Kolk, 2001).

The issue of narrative coherence is not, however, simply an individual matter. While it is generally true that we are the main protagonists of our own stories, we also feature more or less weightily in the stories of other people. Our narratives of them and their narratives of us are accompaniments to the primary narrative and primary narrator. These accompaniments may maintain, challenge, move forward, disrupt, strengthen or hinder the stories of the primary narrator (Nelson, 2001). In other words, narrative coherence is a function of the web of narratives of which we are all part.

Severe dementia and the compromising of the narrative enterprise

With the onset and progression of dementia there arise three challenges to the narrative enterprise. The first of these is the challenge to narrative agency – the ability and opportunity to author one's own narrative. Owing to cognitive difficulties or loss of language people with dementia may lose the ability to construct and articulate a coherent narrative (in terms of tellability, tellership, linearity and moral stance, see Ochs and Capps, 2001). Similarly their interactions with others may be lessened or restricted because of their condition, resulting in lessened opportunities to launch and maintain narratives (Ochs and Capps, 2001).

The second challenge to the narrative enterprise lies in the mobilisation of the meta-narrative of dementia on the part of others. Nelson (2001) argues that master narratives – stories that serve as summaries of socially shared understandings

> are often archetypal, consisting of stock plots and readily recognizable character types, and we use them not only to make sense of our experience (Nisbett and Ross, 1980) but also to justify what we do (MacIntyre, 1984).
>
> (Nelson, 2001)

With regard to dementia, the meta-narrative is the all-too-familiar one of irretrievable cognitive and functional decline and the loss of Self (for an extreme example of this see Brock, 1993). With the mobilisation of this meta-narrative the person with dementia becomes framed and imprisoned by an archetypal narrative of decline and poor prognosis and alternative narratives are marginalised or recuperated into the meta-narrative.[1] This meta-narrative is, however, being challenged by other models of dementia such as the psychosocial model (Kitwood, 1997), disability model (Baldwin, 2005; Downs, 2002) and citizenship model (Marshall, 2003).

The third challenge to the narrative enterprise is that posed by the response of others to narratives that do not fit the expected narrative norms and are thus classified as inadequate narratives or are not even recognised as narratives at all.

A narrative approach to palliative care

If we are narrative beings our death would seem to be an important part of our story and 'getting it right' in the sense of the end of the story being consistent and meaningful with what went before and what is happening now would seem to be essential. A narrative approach to palliative care would examine the types and roles of narratives in the person's life and look to constructing the most meaningful narrative for and with that person.

Palliative care is:

> devoted to achieve the best possible quality of life of the patient and family throughout the course of a life-threatening illness through the relief of suffering and the control of symptoms. Such relief requires the comprehensive assessment and interdisciplinary team management of the physical, psychological, social, and spiritual needs of patients and their families. Palliative medicine helps the patient and family face the prospect of death assured that comfort will be

a priority, values and decisions will be respected, spiritual and psychosocial needs will be addressed, practical support will be available, and opportunities will exist for growth and resolution.

(American Board of Hospice and Palliative Medicine, 2005)

In recounting their experiences of participating in educational policy reform, Clandinin and Connelly (2000) make clear that a narrative approach involves more than examining data in order to understand phenomena. A narrative approach involves asking questions about the phenomena from a particular standpoint. If we break down the above definition into its constituent parts and ask narrative-based questions we might have something like the following:

Palliative care	What are the narratives that are in play in this situation? (For example, the biomedical narrative of the person in general and the life-threatening illness/disease in particular; the organisational narrative of the hospital; the narratives of the person and the family with regard to their relationships to outsiders and authority)
The course of a life-threatening illness	What is the 'textbook' trajectory of the life-threatening illness/disease? What is the narrative trajectory desired by the person and/or their family? Are there alternative trajectories? How do alternative trajectories conflict?
Palliative medicine helps the patient and family face the prospect of death	How does the prospect of death fit into the person's narrative? What narratives support this and what stories disrupt this?
The relief of suffering and the control of symptoms	What roles and meanings do suffering and control have to the person? Are these external forces at work or are they integral to the person?
Such relief requires the comprehensive assessment and interdisciplinary team management of the physical, psychological, social and spiritual needs of patients and their families	Who are the primary, secondary and bit-part characters in the person's narrative? What roles do they play? How do their narratives support or disrupt the narrative of the person?
Values and decisions will be respected	How is the person actively engaged in the co-creation of the narrative that will realise these values and decisions? How do narratives about the person respect the person's values and decisions?
Opportunities will exist for growth and resolution	How does the chosen narrative maintain and develop the Self? How does the person's narrative affect those around him/her? What is a proper ending to this story?

In what follows I will attempt to address some of these issues, particularly those concerning narrative integrity and agency.

Narrative ethics

Narrative ethics, like narrative analysis, is interpreted in a number of ways. For some, narrative ethics is little more than utilising narrative as means of eliciting information on which to make decisions formulated within another ethical framework (Arras, 1997; Charon, 1994; Tomlinson,

1997). For others, narrative ethics is an ethical framework in and of itself, counterpoised against other ethical frameworks (Hauerwas and Burrell, 1989). The stance I will take here is very much in the latter camp, but will develop and deepen the formulation of ethics to stand alongside authors such as Newton (1995) who argue that:

> The fact that narrative ethics can be construed in two directions at once – on the one hand, as attributing to narrative discourse some kind of ethical status, and on the other, as referring to the way ethical discourse often depends on narrative structures – makes this reciprocity between narrative and ethics appear even more essential, more grammatical, so to speak, and less the accident of coinage.
>
> (Newton, 1995, p. 8)

Narrative is both the story being told and the telling of that story – the Said and the Saying, in Newton's words. This twofold nature embraces a twofold ethics: an ethics that is integral to the story being told, and an ethics of how that story is told, an ethics of the Said and an ethics of the Saying, of the narrated and the narrating. The term 'narrative ethics' binds the two indissolubly. Furthermore,

> narrative ethics implies simply narrative as ethics: the ethical consequences of narrating a story and fictionalising person, and the reciprocal claims binding teller, listener, witness, and reader in that process.
>
> (Newton, 1995, p. 11)

In this view ethics

> signifies recursive, contingent, and interactive dramas of encounter and recognition, the sort which prose fiction both crystallizes and recirculates in acts of interpretive engagement.
>
> (Newton, 1995, p. 12)[2]

Narrative ethics is thus concrete, personal and situated. It is, essentially, concerned with the stories we tell and how we tell them and 'since the vicissitudes of narrative situations do not easily submit to prescriptive or procedural norms of rationality' ethics is not 'a set of meta-theoretical ideas or pre-existing moral norms' (Newton, 1995). Rather, it is a moral response to the appeal of the other. This is the ethics that Illich refers to when he says

> we are creatures that find our perfection only by establishing a relationship, and that relationship may appear arbitrary from everybody else's point of view, because I do it in response to a call and not a category.
>
> (Cayley, 2005)

Ethical narratives

If we are entrusted to be co-authors of a person's story, as I believe we are in the palliative care of people with severe dementia, then it follows that we should endeavour to author the story in the best way possible. As a first step to developing a more comprehensive theory of narrative probity in relation to dementia care I want here to suggest four aspects of narrative that might form a basis on which to (co)authoring a narrative for and with a vulnerable Other:

(1) Narrative continuity: does the narrative emerge from and make sense against the backdrop?
(2) Narrative agency: maintaining the person's narrative agency as far as possible in terms of their own narrative and their contribution to the narratives of others.
(3) Countering the meta-narrative of dementia.
(4) Attention to small stories – although narrative theory is often concerned with longer rather than shorter tales (for example, life histories rather than what happened at breakfast) small stories can be important in the maintenance of Self.

Maintaining narrative continuity

By paying attention to the context and embodiment of the protagonist and to the significant others in the story it is possible to establish a backdrop against which to evaluate the narrative. Does the story emerge from this backdrop in a way that does not disrupt one's belief or does the story jar with the backdrop, a disruptive episode which does not appear to link with past or future? Do the choices and actions of the protagonist make sense against this backdrop? Do these choices and actions cohere with what we know of the protagonist? Is the narrative internally coherent in terms of its themes and the means utilised to relate events together? (Bennett and Feldman, 1981; Riessman, 1993). In other words, is the historical continuity of backdrop, story and protagonist maintained?

This element of narrative probity draws upon, but also extends, a number of biographical concepts and techniques already used in dementia care. In the dementia literature there is a good deal of debate about what happens to the Self with the onset and progression of dementia. Some authors, such as Post (1995) refer to the 'then' and 'now' selves – the 'then' Self being that before the onset of dementia, the 'now' Self being that of the person with dementia. The problem with this way of conceptualising the Self is that it is, essentially, biographically disruptive – like Gregor Samsa awakening from disturbing dreams to find himself transformed (Kafka: *Metamorphosis*). Unlike Gregor Samsa, however, any changes that occur for people with dementia rarely happen overnight and thus there is the possibility to prepare for and negotiate a less disruptive narrative of transformation. This, I believe, requires two things: first, an understanding of the 'now' in terms of the 'then'; second, a narrative trajectory for the future, informed by the past. Both of these need explanation.

It is common in dementia care for life histories to play a part in understanding and caring for individuals with dementia. Life histories move away from generalised assumptions to an appreciation of the uniqueness of the individual. In so doing, life histories can give us an insight into what is happening in the present, as can be seen in the following examples.

Example one

A gentleman in a nursing home would take all his clothes off in the sitting room every afternoon and the staff would scurry around collecting up his socks and his trousers and things. This behaviour, while appearing odd, makes perfect sense against the narrative backdrop of the gentleman having been a rower at university in his youth. Every day in the afternoon – because there would be no lectures in the afternoons – he would be stripping off and going off to practise on the river.

Example two

There was a lady who was forever running away with the tea trolley to the concern (and annoyance) of the staff at the residential home. Upon exploration of her history it turned out that she used to be in charge of the WRVS team at the local hospital. Given her history, the environment and the presence of a tea trolley, her behaviour becomes understandable.

In both of these examples, the 'now' becomes understandable in terms of the 'then'. In narrative terms, there is no biographical disruption. This is, of course, in opposition to the usual view of dementia as biographically disruptive.

The second challenge posed to narrative continuity by the onset and progression of dementia is to formulate and maintain a trajectory that emerges from the backdrop. In the Netherlands, for example, some attempt has been made to provide an environment that facilitates such narrative continuity. Hogeway, an innovative residential provision that attempts to bring the community into the home, caters for people with dementia on the basis of seven different lifestyles that are, in turn, based on a detailed study of cultural patterns and practices across the Netherlands (Notter *et al.*, 2004). Each group within Hogeway 'has its own pattern of daily life and activities which reflect what, for them, are the ordinary, everyday lives which individuals would have lived when in the community' (p. 450). Individuals are assessed and placed in the lifestyle group that most closely matches their pre-admission life: 'Emphasis is placed on establishing the type of work they did, their religious beliefs, their social class, their cultural patterns and practices, their hobbies and interests, and on finding ways to facilitate activities which help to keep them anchored in reality' (p. 450). This is more than simply understanding individual lives; it is maintaining those lives into the future, as far as is possible.

Maintaining narrative agency

If we are narrative beings and the primary narrative of our life is the one we construct for ourselves in relationship with others, then the maintenance of narrative agency takes on major importance. Narrative agency in this sense consists of two interrelated ideas: the ability and opportunity to construct one's own narrative; and the contribution one makes to the narratives of others.

The ability to construct one's own narrative

The importance of constructing one's own narrative is probably familiar to the majority of people involved in dementia care and is reflected in the emphasis on such things as life histories (Gibson, 1991; Goldsmith, 1996), values histories (Rich, 1996) and other therapeutic interventions (Bruce, 1999; Sutton and Cheston, 1997). Such activities are vitally important but the issue of the narrative agency of people with dementia goes deeper and prompts a reconsideration of what we think of as narrative.

Narrative, as it is generally conceptualised, is, amongst other things, fundamentally chronological (that is, there is a progression of events through time) and relies on language for its articulation, even when the language abilities of narrators are limited in some way (Booth and Booth, 1996; Goodley, 1996).

Such a conceptualisation of narrative, I would argue, restricts the possibility for narrative agency among certain individuals and groups of people. If an individual or group of people are unable to tell their story in a way that others recognise as a story, then they become what I will term 'narratively dispossessed'. This is a serious matter if we are, as I have argued, narrative beings as one loses the ability to construct one's Self and relate to Others. One way of addressing this issue is to reframe our understanding of narrative so as to include those who are currently dispossessed. This reframing would require that we give up, or at least loosen our hold upon, an insistence that all narratives should have a recognisably chronological basis. While this might seem to cut us adrift from our basis for understanding narrative, the skill required would be to discern how stories relate to other stories rather than to chronology. Narrative thus becomes related primarily to meaning rather than time. Thus, the chronologically fragmented stories or repetition of stories by a person with dementia can be understood as unaddressed, misunderstood, recurring meaning rather than merely as a result of forgetfulness. To understand the story we need to relate it to other stories this person has told and stories that have been told about this person. In so doing we are realising or enacting the sort of narrative competence that Montello refers to when discussing the benefits of engaging with literary narratives (Montello, 1997): 'joining one story with another, accurately to observe and make sense out of the chaos of suffering and loss' (p. 194). In so doing we can build up a narrative map both with and for the person with dementia, a map that may have little meaning or use for that individual but is essential for us in understanding the landscape of that person's experience:

> The person with moderate or moderately severe dementia may be able to present only fragments of a performance story. The more a nurse knows about narrative components or the different sections of a story, the more easily he or she can identify and follow up on a story fragment offered by a person with dementia.
>
> (Moore and Davis, 2002)

Similarly, in order to include people with limited language in the narrative enterprise it will be necessary to find ways of eliciting and constructing narratives making appropriate accommodation for the limited linguistic ability of the person (Booth and Booth, 1997). Moore and Davis (2002) report that normally ageing speakers use four narrative strategies to help the listener follow the story:

- estimating the listener's probable expectations for what the story will be about and how it will be told, alerting the listener to any unusual features;
- signalling the beginning of the narrative, providing some initial context;
- monitoring when the listener may need clarification or further detail;
- keeping the story on track and bringing it to an appropriate end.

People with dementia may lack the narrative capacity to utilise these strategies and Moore and Davis suggest quilting as a means of piecing together the narrative fragments of people with dementia. They point out, however, that more research is required on 'how caregivers, spouses, and family members might accommodate and facilitate the discourse by AD speakers to help construct a more sustained narrative' (Moore and Davis, 2002).

A further way of maintaining narrative agency for persons with dementia is to look to interpreting other symbolic means of expression in a narrative fashion. Dance, for example, can articulate a story as much as it can be a channel for self-expression. This is, of course, a familiar and common approach in the arts. Movement and artistic expression can also means of telling a story – if we as readers are sensitive enough to the narrative features of such media. Downs *et al.* (Chapter 16 in this volume) indicate the possibility of communication with people with severe dementia through sound, music, behavioural cues and mirroring. Similarly, observational techniques such as Dementia Care Mapping (Bradford Dementia Group, 1997) can provide us with some insight into the journey of individuals in context throughout the day. While the process of giving narrative form to these channels of self-expression is predominantly in the hands of caregivers, these means of communication and observation, coupled with the notion of narrative quilting (see above) and attention to small stories (see below) would seem to be means of facilitating narrative agency for people with dementia.

Contributing to the narrative of others

If we are narrative beings it follows that we will relate to others in and through narrative. This raises the issue of how others contribute to our own narratives. While this obviously includes stories others tell about us (and thus how we respond to those narratives) there is another equally important way that others can contribute to our narratives, that of how we 'read' the narrative of another.

In *In the Vineyard of the Text*, Illich (1996) makes a distinction between monastic and scholastic reading. Monastic reading, Illich says, was an embodied activity that required the reader to incorporate the reading into one's own life. The text was something that was approached as having something to say directly to one's own experience and existence ('What does this text say to my life?'). Over the course of history, around the twelfth century, monastic reading was replaced by what Illich calls scholastic reading. This form of reading, brought about by physical changes in the text such as spaces, paragraphs, punctuation and so on, came to focus on what the text itself was saying and thus the text became an object in its own right and a subject of debate ('What is this text saying?' or, 'What is the correct reading of this text?').

I want to suggest that a monastic approach to reading the text of another's life restores some degree of narrative agency to that person and thus displays more narrative probity than a scholastic reading that distances the other's narrative. In answering the question, 'What does this narrative say to and about my own life?' we are opening the door for others to contribute meaningfully and deeply to the construction of our life narratives.

It is my contention that we approach people with severe dementia, because of their vulnerability and dependency, as recipients of our care, service and narrative constructions rather than contributors to our own narrative constructions. In approaching a person with severe dementia in this way we are curtailing one aspect of his or her narrative agency and thus one aspect of the Self. Further-more, we are constraining our own development by limiting the range and nature of the narratives that we allow to affect us (Montello, 1997).

Countering master narratives

In order to challenge disabling master narratives, counter-stories that are individual, enabling and meaningful need to be both constructed and realised. The conceptual work of Kitwood (1997) has gone quite some way in challenging the master narrative of dementia as an inevitable decline into senescence and the 'new culture' of person-centred care is an attempt to make the conceptualisa-tion concrete. The stock plots of decline, rooted in the biomedical model of dementia and poor prognosis, are gradually being challenged by stories arising from psychosocial (Kitwood, 1997), disability (Baldwin, 2006; Downs, 2002) and citizenship (Marshall, 2003) models of dementia. These models of dementia, seek to open up a space in which the stories of people with dementia can be told (see Plummer, 1995) for a discussion of the nature of such stories) rather than seeking to recuperate those stories as further illustrations of the validity of the meta-narrative. For example, the embodied story of a person with dementia becoming aggressive because he or she is prevented from leaving the premises may be recuperated as evidence of dementia (wandering and aggression) rather than an appropriate response to the curtailment of freedom.

Attention to small stories

One other aspect of our current approach to narrative generally (and perhaps in dementia care particularly) that may actually serve to dispossess people with dementia is the tendency to focus on longer rather than shorter narratives. Concern with life history, for example, while essential for understanding the individual and the backdrop from which the current narrative emerges may, in its focus on the historical narrative construction of Self, fail to recognise the identity work that goes on in the here and now, both expressed and performed in what Bamberg (2004a) calls 'small stories'. In other words, past narratives may take precedence over current narratives even when the primary figure has forgotten the past and is functioning primarily in the present. In relying on past narratives, therefore, we may be both missing current ones and denying the individual the oppor-tunity to engage in identity work in the present.

In contrast to life histories that attempt to organise lives into coherent and consistent narratives over long periods of time, small stories are situated in chit-chat and are fundamental to the ongoing construction of local identities (Bamberg, 2004a). These small stories, unlike longer autobiographi-cal accounts, are not oriented towards coherency, authenticity and consistency but privilege the fleeting and fragmented as contributing to the performance of identity in everyday interactions (Bamberg, 2004a). A focus on small stories may, then, be highly appropriate in dementia care as such stories resonate more closely with the experience of the person with dementia and, perhaps, as Bamberg (2004b) has argued, to the experience of people in general. The skill required, therefore, is the ability to recognise these small stories, in all their complexity, collecting them in different times and settings so that we can learn to understand how they contribute to the development and maintenance of the Self.

Concluding remarks

Narrative, it seems, is essential in maintaining and creating our sense of Self. As narrative beings we construct our own lives in narrative fashion and accompany others in the construction of their narratives. The maintenance of narrative integrity and agency is, at root, an ethical activity as it is fundamentally concerned with how we live our lives in relationship with others. People with dementia may, however, be seen to lose both narrative integrity, in the sense of loss of coherence and consistency, and narrative agency in terms of losing the ability to author their own narratives. When we are called upon to accompany others in the (co)construction of their narratives, especially in the light of terminal or chronic illness, we need to focus upon both the narrative that is constructed and how the narrative is constructed. The first requires that we understand narrative ethics, the second that we commit ourselves to (co)authoring ethical narratives.

The loss of narrative integrity and agency for people with dementia results not only from cognitive decline and lessened opportunity for narration but also from how narrative is currently conceptualised. In order to restore narrative integrity and agency to people with dementia, in practice we need to find ways in which people with dementia can narrativise their lives such as living in environments that extend their narrative context such as Hogeway and ways of expressing narrativity in the face of limited language. In terms of narrative theory we need to reconceptualise the nature and role of narrative so as to avoid dispossessing those whose narratives do not conform to current views of what narrative is. In practice and in theory, a narrative approach is fundamentally supportive of a person-centred approach to dementia care. In the face of mortality, this narrative competence is fundamental to effective palliative care.

Notes

1. For an example of how narratives are marginalised and recuperated into other meta-narratives see Baldwin C (2000).
2. Newton, of course, is writing about the ethics of narrative fiction but this should not rule invalid the transposition of this form of narrative ethics to the realm of health care as it is well established that the interplay between literature and medicine is beneficial to the moral and professional development of health care practitioners (see, for example, Charon R and Montello M (1998). Indeed, given the somewhat imprecise boundaries between real life and fiction and the narrative nature of life (see later), developing a real-life ethics from the lessons of prose fiction seems entirely reasonable.

References

American Board of Hospice and Palliative Medicine (2005) Palliative care. http://64.85.16.230/educate/content/elements/abhpmdefinition.html Accessed 8th February 2006.

Androutsopoulou A, Thanopoulou K, Economou E, Bafiti T (2004) Forming criteria for assessing the coherence of clients' life stories: a narrative study. *Journal of Family Therapy*, 26(4):384–406.

Arras JD (1997) Nice story, but so what? Narrative and justification in ethics. In H. L. Nelson, Stories and their Limits: Narrative Approaches to Bioethics. London: Routledge, 65–88.

Astedt-Kurki P, Heikkinen RL (1994) Two approaches to the study of experiences of health and old age: the thematic interview and the narrative method. *Journal of Advanced Nursing*, 20(3):418–421.

Baldwin C (2000) Telling tales of illness. Unpublished PhD. Department of Sociological Studies, University of Sheffield.

Baldwin C (2005) Technology, dementia and ethics: rethinking the issues. *Disability Studies Quarterly*, 25(3). Online.

Bamberg M (2004a) Talk, small stories, and adolescent identities. *Human Development*, 47(6):366–369.

Bamberg M (2004b) Considering counter narratives. In M. Bamberg and M. Andrews, Considering Counter Narratives: Narrating, Resisting, Making Sense. Amsterdam: John Benjamins, 351–371.

Barone T (1995) Persuasive writings, vigilant readings, and reconstructed characters: the paradox of trust in educational storysharing. In J. A. Hatch and R. Wisniewski, Life History and Narrative. London: The Falmer Press, 63–74.

Bennett WL and Feldman MS (1981) Reconstructing Reality in the Courtroom: Justice and Judgment in American Culture. New Brunswick: Rutgers University Press.

Blustein J (1999) Choosing for others as a continuing a life story: the problem of personal identity revisited. *Journal of Law, Medicine and Ethics*, 27(1):20–31.

Booth T, Booth W (1996) Sounds of silence: narrative research with inarticulate subjects. *Disability and Society*, 11(1):55–69.

Booth T, Booth W (1997) Making connections: a narrative study of adult children of parents with learning difficulties. In C. Barnes and G. Mercer, Doing Disability Research. Leeds: The Disability Press, 123–141.

Bradford Dementia Group (1997) Evaluating Dementia Care: The DCM Method. 7th edition. Mapping manual. Bradford: University of Bradford.

Brock DW (1993) Life and Death: Philosophical Essays in Biomedical Ethics. Cambridge: Cambridge University Press.

Bruce E (1999) Holding onto the story: older people, narrative and dementia. In G. Roberts and J. Holmes, Healing Stories: Narrative in Psychiatry and Psychotherapy. Oxford: Oxford University Press, 181–205.

Bruner JS (1987) Life as narrative. *Social Research*, 54(1):11–32.

Bruner JS (1996) A narrative model of self construction. *Psyke & Logos*, 17(1):154–170.

Cayley D (2005) The Rivers North of the Future: The Testament of Ivan Illich as Told to David Cayley. Toronto: House of Anansi Press.

Charon R (1994) Narrative contributions to medical ethics: recognition, formulation, interpretation, and validation in the practice of the ethicist. In E. R. DuBose, R. Hamel and L. J. O'Connell, A matter of principles? Ferment in U.S. bioethics. Valley Forge, PA: Trinity Press International, 260–283.

Charon R, Montello M (1998) Literature and medicine: an on-line guide. *Annals of Internal Medicine*, 128(11):959–962.

Clandinin DJ, Connelly FM (2000) Narrative Inquiry: Experience and Story in Qualitative Research. San Francisco: Jossey-Bass.

Cortazzi M (1993) *Narrative Analysis.* London: The Falmer Press.

Downs M (2002) Dementia as disability: implications for practice. In S. Benson, *Journal of Dementia Care Conference Proceedings.*

Gibson F (1991) Working with People with Dementia: A Positive Approach. Jordanstown: University of Ulster Publication.

Goldsmith M (1996) Hearing the Voice of People with Dementia: Opportunities and Obstacles. London: Jessica Kingsley.

Goodley D (1996) Tales of hidden lives: a critical examination of life history research with people who have learning difficulties. *Disability and Society*, 11(3):333–348.

Hauerwas S, Burrell D (1989) From system to story: an alternative pattern for rationality in ethics. In S. Hauerwas and L. G. Jones, Why Narrative? Grand Rapids, MI: William Eerdmans, 158–190.

Hopper J, van der Kolk BA (2001) Retreiving, assessing and classifying traumatic memories: a preliminary report on three case studies of a new standardized method. In J. J. Freyd and A. P. DePrince, Trauma and Cognitive Science: A Meeting of Minds, Science and Human Experience. Binghamton, NY: Haworth Press, 33–71.

Illich I (1996) In the Vineyard of the Text: A Commentary to Hugh's Didascalicon. Chicago: University of Chicago Press.

Kitwood T (1997) Dementia Reconsidered: The Person Comes First. Maidenhead: Open University Press.

Lysaker PH, Wickett AM, Wilke N, Lysaker J (2003) Narrative incoherence in schizophrenia: the absent agent-protagonist and the collapse of internal dialogue. *American Journal of Psychotherapy*, 57(2):153–166.

MacIntyre A (1984) After Virtue: A Study in Moral Theory. Notre Dame, Indiana: University of Notre Dame Press.

Marshall M (ed.) (2003) Food, Glorious Food: Perspectives on Food and Dementia London: Hawker.

Mills MA (1997) Narrative identity and dementia: a study of emotion and narrative in older people with dementia. *Ageing and Society*, 17(6):673–698.

Mills MA (1998) Narrative Identity and Dementia: A Study of Autobiographical Memories and Emotions. Aldershot: Ashgate Publishing.

Montello M (1997) Narrative competence. In H. L. Nelson, Stories and their Limits: Narrative Approaches to Bioethics. London: Routledge, 185–197.

Moore LA, Davis B (2002) Quilting narrative: using repetition techniques to help elderly communicators. *Geriatric Nursing*, 23(5):262–266.

Nelson HL (2001) Damaged Identities, Narrative Repair. Ithaca, NY: Cornell University Press.

Newton AZ (1995) Narrative Ethics. Cambridge, MA: Harvard University Press.

Nisbet R, Ross L (1980) Judgmental heuristics and knowledge structures. In H. Kornblith, Human Inference: Strategies and Shortcomings of Social Judgment. Cambridge, MA: MIT Press, 17–42.

Notter J, Spijker T, Stomp K (2004) Taking the community into the home. *Health and Social Care in the Community*, 12(5):448–453.

Ochs E, Capps L (2001) Living Narrative: Creating Lives in Everyday Storytelling. Cambridge, MA: Harvard University Press.

Plummer K (1995) Telling Sexual Stories: Power, Change and Social Worlds. London: Routledge.

Polkinghorne DE (1995) Narrative configuration in qualitative analysis. In J. A. Hatch and R. Wisniewski, Life History and Narrative. London: The Falmer Press, 5–24.

Post SG (1995) Alzheimer disease and the 'then' self. *Kennedy Institute of Ethics Journal*, 5(4):307–321.

Rich BA (1996) The values history: restoring narrative identity to long-term care. *Journal of Ethics, Law and Aging*, 2(2, Fall-Winter):75–84.

Ricoeur P (1987) Time and Narrative III. Chicago: University of Chicago Press.

Riessman CK (1993) Narrative Analysis. London: Sage.

Sutton LJ, Cheston R (1997) Rewriting the story of dementia: a narrative approach to psychotherapy with people with dementia. In M. Marshall, State of the Art in Dementia Care. London: Centre for Policy on Ageing, 159–163.

Taylor C (1989) Sources of the Self. Cambridge: Cambridge University Press.

Tomlinson T (1997) Perplexed about narrative ethics. In H. L. Nelson, Stories and their Limits: Narrative Approaches to Bioethics. London: Routledge, 123–133.

Vittoria A (1998) Preserving selves: identity work and dementia. *Research and Aging*, 20(1):91–137.

Health Economics of Severe Dementia

Anders Wimo and Bengt Winblad

Introduction

Today, there is a great focus on the treatment of symptoms in mild and moderate dementia. However, several years in the course of dementia disorders take place in the stage of severe dementia, a devastating condition that causes great suffering for the patients and which is also very stressful for family members and staff (Winblad *et al.*, 1999). Even if dementia shortens life considerably (Aguero-Torres *et al.*, 1999) it is obvious that demented persons spend a much longer period in institutional care than non-demented. From the Kungsholmen project (Fratiglioni *et al.*, 1992) we know that demented spent about 22% of their remaining life from the age of 70 in institutional settings as compared to 15% for non-demented (Wimo, 2005). For those with severe dementia, the figure was 89%! Since the costs of institutional care is the major cost driver in the total costs of dementia, it is obvious that health economic aspects of severe dementia are of great importance. However, there is little written of it. A Medline search (March 2005) of 'economics' and 'severe dementia' resulted in only 20 hits, and of these very few were true health economical studies, in contrast to a general search on dementia and cost issues, which resulted in about a thousand hits.

Health economics – some basic notes

Health economics is the application of economic theory on health care (Drummond *et al.*, 1997). It has two basic components: descriptive theory and normative theory. In the descriptive studies factors that influence the demands for care, the relationship between economical growth and health and costs of care (so-called cost of illness) are analysed. Normative studies are evaluations of care interventions and aim to serve as a support for decision making.

Viewpoint

Any health economical study must define its perspective or viewpoint. Such a viewpoint may be a municipality, a county council, a private insurance company, a patient or the society as a whole. A societal perspective, which includes all costs irrespective of payer, is preferable. This is of particular interest in economical studies on dementia since it means that the costs of informal care should be included.

Costs and cost of illness

A key issue in all economics is the cost concept. The opportunity cost, which is recommended by most economists for use in descriptive studies and economic evaluations, is the value of a resource in its best alternative use. For an informal caregiver of working age who, because of the care

Severe Dementia. Edited by A. Burns and B. Winblad.

demands, is not in the working market, the opportunity cost is the value of the work forgone in the market that could have been done.

Costs can be divided into direct medical costs, direct non-medical costs and indirect costs. With a simplified approach, direct costs refer to the value of resources used and indirect costs to resources lost. Direct medical costs refer to resources used in the medical care system, such as costs of hospital care, drugs and visits to clinics. Direct non-medical costs are costs outside the medical care system, such as costs for formal community care and transport. Depending on the care system, costs of long-term nursing or home care can be regarded as a medical or non-medical direct costs. For direct costs, the cost is the product between a price vector p and a quantity vector q. The price vector depends on the viewpoint and it should refer to an opportunity cost. The source for quantity vector q is an assessment of resource utilisation in physical units, such as days of nursing home care or hours of home help. An example of an instrument to assess both formal and informal resource use is the RUD (Resource Utilisation in Dementia instrument) (Box 1), which we have used in several studies, both in the comprehensive (Wimo *et al.*, 1998a) and in the RUD Lite version (Wimo and Winblad, 2003).

Box 1.   Components of the resource utilisation battery in RUD (Wimo *et al.*, 1998a, copyright, John Wiley & Sons Ltd)

Patient	Caregiver
Accommodation/ long term care[*]	Informal care time (for patient)[*]
Work status	Work status
Respite care[*]	
Hospital care[*]	Hospital care
Out clinic visits	Out clinic visits
Social service[*]	Social service
Home nursing care[*]	Home nursing care
Day care[*]	Day care
Drug use[*†]	Drug use

[*]Included in RUD Lite (Wimo and Winblad, 2003). [†]Only study drug in RUD Lite.

Indirect costs are costs due to production losses (such as sick leave, early pension, impaired productivity) or mortality. Cost of informal care, which is a complicated issue itself (van den Berg *et al.*, 2004; Jonsson, 2003), is often classified as an indirect cost, but this is not always obvious. Informal care should be valued to its opportunity cost, which for a person of working age, as in the example above, is a production loss; but regarding leisure time and contributions by retired persons or persons without a position in the labour market, it is more complicated and there is no given answer.

Health economics studies

There are several approaches to the analysis of health economics (Box 2). In cost description and cost outcome description studies, no comparison between different treatment options is made. In a cost outcome description it is also possible to compare the costs and the results of a programme. Such studies may be of value to show how costs are distributed among different sectors and payers, but cannot be used to set priorities.

In cost of illness studies (COI), which aim to describe the costs of a disease/disorder in a country, for example, it is important to differ entiate between gross costs (costs for patients with a disease)

Box 2. Different kinds of health economical studies

Descriptive studies
CD   Cost Description
COD   Cost Outcome Description
COI   Cost of Illness

Evaluation studies
CA   Cost analysis (incomplete evaluation)
CMA   Cost–minimisation analysis
CEA   Cost–effectiveness analysis
CBA   Cost–benefit analysis
CUA   Cost–utility analysis

(CCA   Cost–consequence analysis)

---

and net costs (costs due to a disease). All costs related to a person with dementia are not related to the dementia disorder. Other medical conditions may contribute, such as diabetes, arthritis or cardiac disorders, and for those who live in an institutional setting a part of the costs relates to the needs that any person would have (for living and eating, so-called hotel costs).

There are also two ways to collect data. With a top-down approach, the sources are often register data of total costs on, for example, a national level; the costs are then apportioned to particular disorders. With a bottom-up approach, a representative sample of patients with a specific disorder, such as dementia, are carefully examined with a focus on resource utilisation and costs. In a next step, these costs are extrapolated to, for example, a nation's total population by a multiplication of the per person cost by the prevalence. Often these two methods are combined because of insufficiencies of data with just one of the approaches.

Cost of illness can also be described in terms of a prevalence or incidence approach. With the prevalence approach the total costs are estimated for all persons with a disease during an specified period (mostly a year), while with the incidence approach, costs are estimated from the beginning of a disease and on through the whole course of the disease.

Since cost of illness studies are descriptive, they cannot be used for setting priorities. They describe the economic burden and can describe how costs are distributed among different payers. In COI studies, the effects of a disease on caregivers are seldom included.

Economic evaluation

The purpose of an economic evaluation is to analyse 'value for money', that is the effectiveness in the use of resources. A complete economic evaluation includes at least two treatment options where both costs and consequences are analysed. Most health care systems in the welfare states include some kind of third-party payer (the two basic parties are the patient and the care supplier), since the costs of care are so high and irregularly distributed that a single person would not pay the whole cost. This third payer may be a municipality, a county council, the state, an insurance company, an HMO etc. The basic interest for this third payer is that the money is used as effectively as possible, not necessarily at the lowest cost. The interesting thing is the relation between costs and consequences. This can be expressed as the incremental cost effectiveness ratio (ICER):

$$\Delta C / \Delta E = (C_B - C_A)/(E_B - E_A),$$

where C is the cost, E is the effect, and A and B are different treatments.

The ICER expresses the costs of improving the effect versus the comparator by one unit (one unit may be a year of survival, an improvement of a score etc.).

It is important that the effects are clinically relevant, and this is an issue in regard to the dementia care that is under discussion. Traditionally, is has been regarded as important to postpone death (which means that the cost of prolonging life by, for example, one year is an interesting cost-effectiveness measure). Regarding dementia, this is not obvious. Other outcomes, such as quality of life, postponement of decline in severity or ADL can be regarded as more important than prolonging life per se. With quality-adjusted life-years (QALYs), both quantity and quality of life are included in an outcome measurement.

Since many of the factors that are included in a health economics analysis include variability and since the validity of sources may vary, it is also important to include a discussion of uncertainity in economic evaluations (Briggs and O'Brien, 2001). Uncertain important factors should be varied in a sensitivity analysis.

In a cost analysis (CA), only the costs of different therapies are compared (not the outcomes). Thus, a CA is an incomplete economical evaluation. With the cost-minimisation analysis (CMA) approach the effects of different treatments are assumed to be equivalent and the analysis is focused on identifying the cheapest therapy. However, the value of CMA is questionable, since the assumption of similar treatment effects is problematic (Briggs and O'Brien, 2001). In a cost-effectiveness analysis (CEA) the effect is expressed as a non-monetary quantified unit, such as the cost per extra year without progressing to a more severe state of dementia (with instruments such as CDR (Berg, 1988) and GDS (Reisberg et al., 1988) or multidimensional instruments such as GBS (Brane et al., 2001)). A cost-benefit analysis (CBA) expresses all costs and outcomes in monetary units, e.g. dollars or euros. Few attempts have been made to use CBA on dementia, but it has been argued that CBA approaches, such as 'willingness to pay', could be of value (Wimo et al., 2002). In a cost–utility analysis (CUA) the effect is expressed as utilities, such as QALYs (quality-adjusted life-years) (Torrance, 1997). CUA is based on the assumption that individuals exercise preferences to maximise their utilities. QALYs are expressed on a scale between 0 and 1, where 0 is death and 1 indicates perfect health. Examples of scales that are used for QALY assessments are the Health Utilities Index (HUI) (Torrance et al., 1996, Neumann et al., 2000), the EuroQoL/EQ-5D (Coucill et al., 2001) or the Quality of Well Being Scale (QWBS) (Kerner et al., 1998). QALYS can be applied to different diseases and different stages of diseases, but the use of QALY is not uncontroversial (Tsuchiya et al., 2003). Chronic, incurable, progressive disorders may be disfavoured when compared with, for example, curative surgical treatment, such as cataract surgery or hip-replacement surgery.

In a cost–consequence analysis (CCA), cost and outcomes are analysed and presented separately. The value of CCA is under discussion (Winblad et al., 1997), since results may be difficult to interpret and the selection of outcomes may be biased. More or less dementia-specific quality of life instruments such as DQoL (the Dementia Quality of Life instrument) (Brod et al., 1999), QOLAD (Quality of Life – Alzheimer's disease) (Logsdon et al., 2002; Selai et al., 2001) and QOLAS (Elstner et al., 2001, Selai et al., 2000) may be useful in CCA trials but are inappropriate for complete economic evaluations since these instruments are not preference-based (Torrance et al., 1996; Siegel et al., 1997).

Severe dementia and health economy
Cost of illness of severe dementia
Even if there is a comprehensive worldwide epidemiological database regarding dementia, there is no single study that fully covers the complexity of the health economics of dementia. From a theoretical point of view, it could appear to be ideal to longitudinally follow demented (incident) patients with regard to severity, gender and resource use/costs from the early stages to exit. However,

Table 1.   Annual costs according to severity (Swedish krona, SEK)

CDR stage	Annual cost	SD
0	39,000	52,000
0.5	56,000	82,000
1	108,000	109,000
2	248,000	171,000
3	374,000	118,000

such an approach would also have drawbacks. One reason is practical, since there are difficulties in recruiting a sufficient number of persons for such long-term studies. Care organisation as well as treatment also change over time, and during the potential lifespan with dementia (10–15 years) great changes will probably occur in society. Furthermore, since dementia care to a great extend relies on informal caregivers, the whole complex of informal care also influences, for example, women's position in the labour market etc. Therefore, much of our knowledge is based on cases in cross-sectional studies, even though on-going projects in the future probably will offer much more detailed information about the resource use and the costs of severely demented. Such a project is the Swedish national study of ageing and care (SNAC) (Lagergren et al., 2004), where about 9,000 Swedish elderly (60 years and older) will be studied longitudinally. SNAC includes, among other things, a comprehensive set of resource utilisation data.

From the Swedish Kungsholmen project (Fratiglioni et al., 1992) and its rural part, the Nordanstig project (Klarin et al., 2003), we have some cross-sectional results which highlight some of the cost of illness issues in severe dementia. We have in different ways tested different costing approaches, particularly regarding the costs of informal care and the costs of different kinds of institutional settings.

As can be seen in Table 1, there is a clear correlation between dementia severity and annual costs from a societal perspective, meaning that the costs of informal care are also included. The standard deviations are high, illustrating that there is a great variation in each severity stage (making statistical power calculations in intervention studies difficult).

If we compare the number of persons in each step with the summarised costs (Table 2), the influence of severe dementia is even more obvious. Even if those with severe dementia only constitute about 5% of the study population, they entailed about one-quarter of the total costs. As mentioned in the introduction to this chapter, the major cost driver in the total costs of dementia is the cost

Table 2.   Severity: relation between prevalence and costs

CDR stage	Percentage of population	Percentage of sum of costs	Ratio costs/ population
0	76.1%	39.5%	0.52
0.5	2.7%	2.0%	0.75
1	10.8%	15.4%	1.43
2	5.2%	17.2%	3.28
3	5.2%	25.9%	4.94
	100%	100%	1.00

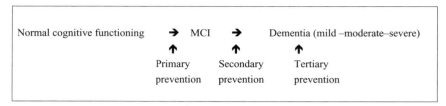

Figure 1.   Treatment approaches in dementia.

of institutional care. Of the total costs in the Kungsholmen cohort, 61% were costs of institutional care. In severe dementia, the institutional part of the costs was 91%!

We have also simulated the course of dementia in a progression model based on Swedish conditions with an estimated survival up to nine years for those who entered the model in mild dementia (Wimo *et al.*, 1998b). We found that about 75% of the total costs of dementia during the whole model period of survival were related to severe dementia (defined as MMSE <10).

Interventions in severe dementia

There are few studies published with a health economics approach in severe dementia, making it very difficult to present the state of the art.

Two basic approaches can be used, one focusing on economic evaluations of interventions in severe dementia, the other focusing on the whole course of dementia, e.g. interventions that may influence the transition from mild and moderate dementia to severe dementia. The latter approach is of course much more difficult to overview, but it is nevertheless important to have this dynamic approach in mind. Different treatment approaches in dementia can, in a simplified way, be described in terms of primary, secondary and tertiary prevention (Figure 1). This issue is of course also connected to the whole issue of survival and mortality as a result of interventions. Potential effects of different treatment interventions are illustrated in Figure 2, based on a hypothetical

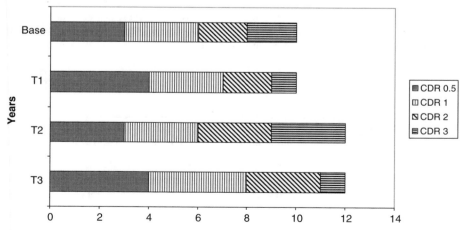

Figure 2.   Hypothetical course of dementia without treatment (base) and after three treatment interventions (T1, T2 and T3).

course of dementia. From a health economics viewpoint, it is the effects of interventions through the whole course of dementia that is of interest. In T1 life is not prolonged by the intervention but the length in different states of dementia is changed. If life is prolonged as a result of the intervention, it is of great interest to find out where in the course of dementia this possible effect on survival takes place (T2 and T3 in Figure 2). If the potential prolonged survival takes place in the early part of the disease (a potential cure of dementia is not discussed here since no such treatment yet exists), the long-run effect may be advantageous with regard both to costs and to consequences; but if a life prolongation mainly takes place in the stage of severe dementia, it is doubtful whether this effect is desirable. However, controlled clinical studies that make it possible to study such long-term effects are of course difficult to accomplish and thus economic evaluations of interventions cover only different segments of the course of dementia. With this in mind, economic models may be a useful tool in the simulation of long-term effects (Buxton *et al.*, 1997).

It is also important to realise that, even though the different severity related costs (as in Table 1) may illustrate potential cost savings, such effects need to be proved in controlled trials. As mentioned in the general health economics section of this chapter, a complete health economics evaluation must also include not only the costs but also the consequences. Simple cost-cutting projects may have negative effects on patients and caregivers which are missed if only costs are analysed.

Interventions in dementia can roughly be divided into three types: pharmacological interventions, 'programmes'/environmental interventions, and combinations. In 'programmes' and environmental interventions, a broad category, we include the different and often overlapping forms of case management, caregiver support, day care, housing/living arrangements (e.g. group living, special care units), caring strategies, and activation/stimulation approaches (e.g. reminiscence therapy, music therapy etc.). Often these kinds of treatment and management are referred to as 'non-pharmacological' treatment, which in our opinion is misleading since the daily care of the demented for much the most part consists of these 'programmes'.

We have identified eight economic studies of interest where patients with severe dementia are included (Table 3), four focusing on programmes and four focusing on drug treatment.

Drummond *et al.*'s study on caregiver support (Drummond *et al.*, 1991) also included patients with severe dementia. This study is very interesting from a methodological point of view even if the number of patients and caregivers is low. It has a cost-effectiveness design where the QALY-like

Table 3. Health economics studies where patients with severe dementia are studied

Source	Countries of intervention	Design	Treatment
Drummond *et al.*, 1991	Canada	RCT/CUA	Programme: caregiver support
Volicer *et al.*, 1994	USA	Quasi-experimental/ CCA	Programme: SCU
Rovner *et al.*, 1996	USA	RCT/CCA	Programme: AGE
Challis *et al.*, 2002	UK	Quasi-experimental/ CCA	Programme: case management
Wimo *et al.*, 2003	USA	RCT/CCA	Drug: memantine
Feldman *et al.*, 2004	Canada, France, Australia	RCT/CCA	Drug: donepezil
Jones *et al.*, 2004	UK	Model/CUA	Drug: memantine
François *et al.*, 2004	Finland	Model/CEA	Drug: memantine

outcome, caregiver quality of life instrument (CQLI), is caregiver related. The cost per QALY was Can$20,000, which can be regarded as cost-effective.

Volicer *et al.* (1994) compared, in a quasi-experimental study, costs of severely demented patients at special care units (SCU) ($n = 94$) with the demented in traditional long-term care units (LTCU) ($n = 43$). After three months, costs were significantly lower at the SCU unit. However, and surprisingly, after 24 months the mortality was significantly higher at the SCU (56%) compared to the traditional care (28%). This study had an incomplete health economics design and no statement regarding cost-effectiveness could be made. Furthermore, only direct medical costs were analysed, not the basic caring costs.

Rovner *et al.* (1996) studied a nursing home programme entitled The Activities, Guidelines and Educational Program (AGE) in the USA. The study was randomised but rather small (89 randomised patients). Compared to the ordinary programme costs were equal, but there were fewer behaviour disorders in the AGE group.

In a UK study, Challis studied a case management programme of home staying demented, where 70% suffered from severe dementia (Challis *et al.*, 2002). Although not significant, the costs in the intervention group were 21% higher. However, some outcomes, such as patient distress, social contacts and caregiver burden favoured the programme.

So far (March 2005) we have found four pharmaco-economic studies focusing on severe or moderate to severe dementia. Two studies are RCTs with resource use and costing data combined with outcomes, one on memantine (Wimo *et al.*, 2003) and one on donepezil (Feldman *et al.*, 2004). These studies can be characterised as cost consequence analyses. The other two studies are pharmaco-economic models on memantine (Jones *et al.*, 2004; François *et al.*, 2004).

The memantine study (Wimo *et al.*, 2003) included prospectively collected data on resource use and costs from a societal perspective, using the RUD instrument (Wimo *et al.*, 1998a). It is the pharmaco-economic part of the US memantine study by Reisberg *et al.* (2003). The monthly cost in the treatment group was 1,204 USD (inflated to 2003 US dollars) lower in the memantine arm compared to placebo ($p < 0.05$). The main cost drivers were costs of informal care and institutional care and the greatest reason for the difference in costs was the lower amount of informal care ($p < 0.05$) in the memantine group. The difference in institutionalisation was of borderline significance ($p = 0.52$). Combined with the results from the efficacy trial, it was concluded that the results indicate cost-effectiveness. Feldman *et al.*'s study (Feldman *et al.*, 2004), which took place in three countries (Canada, France and Australia), also included prospectively collected data from a societal perspective with the Canadian Utilization of Services instrument. The six month's costs were US$306 (2003 level) lower in the donepezil group (not significant), which in combination with the clinical data (Feldman *et al.*, 2001) suggests cost-effectiveness.

The two memantine models both use Markov modelling. The basic idea in a Markov model is that a person is always in one of a defined number of states (e.g. of severity of dementia) and to this state there is assigned costs and utilities or similar. The time horizon of the analysis is divided into cycles (e.g. a cycle may be of six months and a five-cycle analysis then has a duration of three years). During a cycle a person can make a transition to another state and for a population it will then be possible to identify transition probabilities between different states during a cycle. Based on, for example, empirical data from an RCT, it is possible in a Markov model to simulate the course with and without treatment, with different transition probabilities. One drawback is that the treatment results in the empirical core of a model (e.g. a clinical trial) are essential for the simulated course. In dementia, where aspects such as caregiver exhaustion may occur after several years and where behavioural problems often show an irregular pattern throughout the course of the disease, models may face problems. It is also often necessary to use several sources and assumptions for the model. Owing to the selection bias of study populations in dementia clinical trials (as compared to the general dementia population), data derived purely from within the trial may give results different from what would be obtained if the model also used external sources. This was clearly illustrated in a study by Jönsson *et al.* on donepezil (Jonsson *et al.*, 1999). To highlight the potential variability of results, a good model should include one basic option ('best guess'), but also a comprehensive sensitivity analysis where important inputs are varied. Even if the use of models is controversial, since it is difficult to run long-term RCTs, models can, with their limitations in mind, be useful to illustrate potential long-term effects.

Jones *et al.*, in the memantine model applied in the UK (Jones *et al.*, 2004) used QALYs as the outcome. The cost of informal care was not included. It had a total length of two years and the basic option suggested that treatment with memantine was cost-effective (costs were about 3% lower with treatment), but the range in the sensitivity analysis was rather large, from < 0 (results both regarding costs and QALYs favoured memantine treatment) to 2003 US$ 231,000/QALY. In the other memantine model, five year's treatment was simulated in Finland (François *et al.*, 2004) with dependency and years in community as the outcomes. This model also included costs of informal care, giving it a more societal perspective than the UK model. The cost savings were somewhat lower, by about 2%, and this model too indicated that treatment was cost-effective.

Conclusion

Although severe dementia is a devastating condition for both patients and caregivers and also a very costly stage in the course of dementia, little is known about resource use, costs and cost-effectiveness of treatment. There should be a greater focus on basic descriptive economic research as well as on studies of the cost-effectiveness of treatments.

References

Aguero-Torres H, Fratiglioni L, Guo Z, Viitanen M, Winblad B (1999) *J Clin Epidemiol*, 52:737–743.

Berg L (1988) *Psychopharmacology Bulletin*, 24:637–639.

Brane G, Gottfries CG, Winblad B (2001) *Dement Geriatr Cogn Disord*, 12:1–14.

Briggs AH, O'Brien BJ (2001) *Health Econ*, 10:179–184.

Brod M, Stewart AL, Sands L, Walton P (1999) *Gerontologist*, 39:25–35.

Buxton MJ, Drummond MF, Van Hout BA, Prince RL, Sheldon TA, Szucs T, Vray M (1997) *Health Econ*, 6:217–227.

Challis D, von Abendorff R, Brown P, Chesterman J, Hughes J (2002) *Int J Geriatr Psychiatry*, 17:315–325.

Coucill W, Bryan S, Bentham P, Buckley A, Laight A (2001) *Med Care*, 39:760–771.

Drummond MF, Mohide EA, Tew M, Streiner DL, Pringle DM, Gilbert JR (1991) *Int J Technol Assess Health Care*, 7:209–219.

Drummond MF, O'Brien B, Stoddart GL, Torrance GW (1997) Methods for the Economic Evaluation of Health Care Programmes, Oxford University Press, Oxford, UK.

Elstner K, Selai CE, Trimble MR, Robertson MM (2001) *Acta Psychiatr Scand*, 103:52–59.

Feldman H, Gauthier S, Hecker J, Vellas B, Hux M, Xu Y, Schwam EM, Shah S, Mastey V (2004) *Neurology*, 63:644–650.

Feldman H, Gauthier S, Hecker J, Vellas B, Subbiah P, Whalen E (2001) *Neurology*, 57:613–620.

François C, Sintonen H, Sulkava R, Rive B (2004) *Clin Drug Invest*, 24:373–384.

Fratiglioni L, Viitanen M, Backman L, Sandman PO, Winblad B (1992) *Neuroepidemiology*, 11 Suppl 1:29–36.

Jones RW, McCrone P, Guilhaume C (2004) *Drugs Aging*, 21:607–620.

Jonsson L (2003) *Pharmacoeconomics*, 21:1025–1037.

Jonsson L, Lindgren P, Wimo A, Jonsson B, Winblad B (1999) *Clin Ther*, 21:1230–1240.

Kerner DN, Patterson TL, Grant I, Kaplan RM (1998) *J Aging Health*, 10:44–61.

Klarin I, Fastbom J, Wimo A (2003) *Pharmacoepidemiol Drug Saf*, 12:669–678.

Lagergren M, Fratiglioni L, Hallberg IR, Berglund J, Elmstahl S, Hagberg B, Holst G, Rennemark M, Sjolund BM, Thorslund M, Wiberg I, Winblad B, Wimo A (2004) *Aging Clin Exp Res*, 16:158–168.

Logsdon RG, Gibbons LE, McCurry SM, Teri L (2002) *Psychosom Med*, 64:510–519.

Neumann PJ, Sandberg EA, Araki SS, Kuntz KM, Feeny D, Weinstein MC (2000) *Med Decis Making*, 20:413–422.

Reisberg B, Doody R, Stoffler A, Schmitt F, Ferris S, Mobius HJ (2003) *N Engl J Med*, 348:1333–1341.

Reisberg B, Ferris SH, de Leon MJ, Crook T (1988) *Psychopharmacol Bull*, 24:661–663.
Rovner BW, Steele CD, Shmuely Y, Folstein MF (1996) *J Am Geriatr Soc*, 44:7–13.
Selai C, Vaughan A, Harvey RJ, Logsdon R (2001) *Int J Geriatr Psychiatry*, 16:537–538.
Selai CE, Elstner K, Trimble MR (2000) *Epilepsy Res*, 38:67–74.
Siegel JE, Torrance GW, Russell LB, Luce BR, Weinstein MC, Gold MR (1997) *Pharmacoeconomics*, 11:159–168.
Torrance GW (1997) *Am J Manag Care*, 3 Suppl:S8–S20.
Torrance GW, Feeny DH, Furlong WJ, Barr RD, Zhang Y, Wang Q (1996) *Med Care*, 34:702–722.
Tsuchiya A, Dolan P, Shaw R (2003) *Soc Sci Med*, 57:687–696.
van den Berg B, Brouwer WB, Koopmanschap MA (2004) *Eur J Health Econ*, 5:36–45.
Wimo A (2005) Socialstyrelsen (The national board on health and welfare), Stockholm.
Wimo A, Wetterholm AL, Mastey V, Winblad B (1998a) In The Health Economics of Dementia, Wimo A, Jonsson B, Karlsson G, Winblad B (eds). Chichester, UK, John Wiley, 465–499.
Wimo A, Winblad B (2003) *Brain Aging*, 3:48–59.
Wimo A, Winblad B, Stöffler A, Wirth Y, Möbius HJ (2003) *Pharmacoeconomics*, 21:327–340.
Wimo A, Witthaus E, Rother M, Winblad B (1998b) *Clin Ther*, 20:552–566; discussion 550–551.
Wimo A, von Strauss E, Nordberg G, Sassi F, Johansson L (2002) *Health Policy*, 61:255–268.
Winblad B, Hill S, Beermann B, Post SG, Wimo A (1997) *Alzheimer Dis Assoc Disord*, 11:39–45.
Winblad B, Wimo A, Mobius HJ, Fox JM, Fratiglioni L (1999) *Int J Geriatr Psychiatry*, 14:911–914.
Volicer L, Collard A, Hurley A, Bishop C, Kern D, Karon S (1994) *J Am Geriatr Soc*, 42:597–603.

Index

accident risk in AD   77
acetylcholine   21, 22, 30, 31, 131, 132
activities of daily living (ADL)   8, 117
advance care planning   205–207
advance directives   205, 212
adverse events   127, 128, 135, 139–142, 145,
        152, 153, 158, 159, 161, 163, 168, 179
    donepezil   128, 135, 138, 141, 142, 145
    galantamine   139, 145
    neuroleptics   152
affective disturbances   4, 7, 11, 105
    vascular dementia   4, 7, 11
aggression   16, 52, 53, 58, 59, 61, 65, 68,
        71, 73, 125, 128, 133, 137, 141, 146,
        151–153, 155, 156, 158–161, 168, 173,
        177, 179, 223
    Alzheimer's disease   59, 125, 155, 158
    definitions   53
Agitated Behaviours Mapping Instrument
        (ABMI)   58
agitation   5, 7, 8, 11, 12, 16, 51–54, 56–61,
        65, 70–72, 77, 78, 104, 125, 128, 137,
        141, 144–146, 151–153, 155, 157–168,
        172–175, 177–180, 182, 183, 201, 208,
        209
    aetiology   51, 57, 58
    associations   51, 53, 125
    definitions   52, 53
    frequency   16, 51, 53, 155, 173, 179
    non-pharmacological treatment   177
    prevalence   11, 12, 58, 163
    Seattle Protocols   177, 179, 180
    therapy   7, 70, 72, 128, 141, 144, 145, 164,
        166, 167, 173, 179, 183, 201
agreements   207
alcoholism   8, 19
Alzheimer's disease (AD)   11, 21, 33, 43,
        51, 83, 84, 92, 99, 115, 117, 126, 131,
        148, 155

amyloid   148
behavioural symptoms/disturbances   4
cholinergic changes   22
cholinesterases   25, 133
cognitive features   11
cognitive function   11
definition   11, 33
depression   13
dopamine receptors   152
evolution   75
genes   126
glial cells   38
glutamate role   125
glutamatergic neurotransmission   125, 126
Lewy bodies   4, 6
medical follow-up   75, 78
microglia   21, 38
mixed vascular dementia   9
molecular pathology   33
mortality   77
motor disorders   12
muscarinic acetylcholine receptors   22
natural history   46, 75, 117
neurofibrillary tangles   21, 33, 36
neurological signs   12
neuronal loss   37
neuropathology   5, 27, 40, 113, 216
nicotinic cholinergic receptors   22
noradrenergic neurotransmission
pathogenesis   126
physical symptoms   76
psychiatric disturbance   11
serotonergic neurotransmission   26
staging   92, 99
time course   84
weight loss   76
Alzheimer's Disease Assessment Scale -
        Cognitive subscale (ADAS-cog)   16,
        133

Alzheimer's Disease Cooperative Study -
        Activities of daily Living Scale
        (ADCS-ADL)   16
ambulatory ability   91, 108, 118
amyloid (Aβ)   126
    Alzheimer's disease   11, 33, 75, 110
amyloid precursor protein (APP) gene   34
analgesics   208
Antecedents, Behaviours and Consequences
        (ABC) technique   58, 168
antibiotics   190, 206, 207, 209, 210
anticholinesterases see cholinesterase
        inhibitors   133
antidepressants   70, 151
antipsychotics   144, 147, 152–156, 159–161,
        173
    atypical   144, 152–155, 159–161, 173
        efficacy/safety   152
        sleep-wake disturbances   159
    typical   144, 152–155, 159–161, 173
anxiety   4, 8, 11–13, 16, 51, 52, 56, 65, 71,
        72, 77, 78, 105, 125, 137, 155, 164–166,
        173, 178, 180, 182, 187, 205, 208, 210
    shortness of breath   205, 208
apathy   7, 9, 13, 15, 16, 51, 54, 56, 63, 65, 71,
        72, 125, 137, 147, 155, 169, 174
    non-pharmacological treatment   68, 163,
        165, 177
ApoE gene   36
    E4 allele   36
apolipoprotein E (ApoE)   35
apoptosis, neuronal   38, 39
aripiprazole   152–154, 157, 159, 160, 162
aromatherapy   70, 72, 74, 164, 166, 169–171,
        173–175, 201, 204
    agitation   70, 72, 164, 166, 173, 201
artificial nutrition and hydration
        (ANH)   207
assessment instruments   3, 15
    depression   15
    functional ability assessment   8
associated features, course   4
audit cycles   201
autonomic dysfunction   14
autonomy   117, 120, 195
aversive behaviour   210
axes of evaluation   3, 4, 17

Babinski reflex   106, 108
Balancing Arousal Controls Excesses
        (BACE)   167

bathing, assistance with   86
bedridden patients in AD   75, 78, 185
Behavior Therapy-Pleaseant Activities
        (BT-PA)   179
Behavior Therapy-Problem Solving
        (BT-PS)   179
Behaviour Pathology in Alzheimer's Disease
        (BEHAVE-AD) scale   16, 155, 158
behavioural and psychological symptoms of
        dementia (BPSD)   103, 105, 151, 202
    aetiology   164
    assessment   51, 53, 57, 58
    atypical antipsychotics   152, 155, 159
    frequency   51
    interventions   58, 163, 166, 168
    measurement   58
    neuroleptic treatment   13, 151, 152
    non-pharmacological treatment   151
    symptom clusters   51, 52, 54, 57, 155
    see also agitation   51, 52, 155
behavioural education programmes   164,
        165
behavioural management techniques
        (BMT)   168
behavioural symptoms/disturbances   4, 6,
        11, 16, 103, 177
    Alzheimer's disease   9, 11, 33, 75, 133
    assessment instruments   15
    disinhibition   14, 15, 16, 51, 65, 155
    donepezil efficacy   138
    evaluation   6
    fronto-temporal dementia   14, 15, 39, 112
    misdiagnosis   7
    Seattle Protocols   177, 178, 179, 183
    understandable   63, 220
    vascular dementia   21, 22, 26, 129
benzamides   152
benzodiazepines   211
Binet intelligence test measure   103
breath, shortness of   205, 208
Brief Cognitive Rating Scale (BCRS)   16,
        99, 100, 114
bright-light therapy   70
butyrylcholinesterase (BuChE)   25

care in dementia   202, 205, 206, 212
    advance care planning   205, 206, 207
    caregivers' needs   71
    comfort   198
    end-of-life   146, 185, 190, 207
    families   206

help 206
management of patients 15
person-centred 57, 193, 195
physical 198
relationship-centred 195
social environment 196
spiritual 206
caregiver quality of life instrument
(CQLI) 234
caregivers 16, 17, 60, 71, 73, 83, 113, 117,
119–121, 125, 127, 129, 138, 139, 145,
151, 161, 165, 168–174, 177–182, 185,
187, 189, 192, 195, 203, 207, 212, 222,
231, 233, 235
ABC techniques 168
donepezil efficacy 138
family relationships 44, 180
grief expression 200
needs 71, 120, 189, 195
placement effects 140, 187
Seattle Protocols 177, 179, 180
sleep hygiene 171, 174
stressors 187
support for 79, 172
causes of dementias 15, 155
cerebral atrophy in fronto-temporal
dementia 39
cerebral blood flow (CBF) 57
cerebrovascular adverse events 152, 153,
158, 161
challenging behavior, definition 53
chewing problems in palliative care 205,
206, 209, 217
cholesterol serum levels 145
choline acetyltransferase (ChAT) 22
cholinergic neurotransmission 22, 25,
125
cholinesterase inhibitors 13, 25, 70–72, 83,
129–131, 133, 141–146, 148
add-on therapy 146
efficacy studies 100, 133, 145, 146
end-stage dementia therapy 146, 205
head-to-head studies 144
response predictors 145
trials 83, 131, 133, 141, 143, 144, 146
cholinesterases 25
clinical assessment tools see assessment
instruments 15
Clinical Dementia Rating scale (CDR) 16
clozapine 152, 153
cognitive behavioural therapy 170

cognitive deficit 5, 8, 11, 13, 25, 44, 47, 83,
131, 151
assessment instruments 15
donepezil efficacy 138
evaluation 16
fronto-temporal dementia 14, 15, 39
nicotinic acetylcholine receptor loss 22
cognitive function 11, 24, 38, 40, 43, 45, 46,
57, 59, 66, 76, 126–128, 130, 151–153,
178, 197, 232
pain detection/treatment 199
Cohen-Mansfield Agitation Inventory
(CMAI) 52, 58, 155, 158, 166
comfort 190, 191, 195, 198–200, 206, 207,
209–211, 217
comfort care 206, 207, 209
communication 11, 43, 63, 165, 166, 168,
178, 192, 194, 196–200, 202, 203, 222
components 197, 200
pain expression 208
supportive environment 197
see also language 15
community residences 81
confusion, Alzheimer's disease 77, 81
constipation 78, 80, 152, 208, 210, 211
constitutive narratives 216
contractures 12, 78, 91, 93, 105, 108–110,
115, 210, 211
coping responses 197
Cornell Scale for Depression in Dementia
(CSDD) 64, 170
cortical vascular dementia 9
cost analyses 229, 230
cost of illness (COI) studies 228, 229
costs 75, 121, 127, 139, 204, 227–235
direct/indirect 228
interventions 227, 231, 233
medical/non-medical 228
severity of dementia 3, 9, 21, 33, 41, 43,
63, 83, 117, 163, 177, 193, 205, 227
Creutzfeldt-Jakob disease, prion-associated
sporadic 6, 8, 14, 112
cultural issues in end-of-life care 185, 190

date collection 11, 44
death 19, 22, 24, 25, 27, 28, 37, 38, 64, 67,
69, 75, 76, 78, 79, 97, 98, 126, 139,
143, 154, 160, 183, 187, 190, 191, 193,
194, 200, 203, 204, 206–211, 213, 217,
218, 225, 230
acceptance 208

death rattle   208, 213
decision-making, shared   205
definition of severe dementia   43, 83
delirium   3, 5, 9, 10, 13, 19, 71, 158, 186,
      208, 210
delusions   7, 11–13, 16, 18, 29, 51, 52, 54,
      56–58, 61, 65, 73, 104, 153, 155, 157,
      158, 163, 174, 210
   AD   12, 13, 16, 18, 51, 52, 57, 58, 65, 104,
      153, 155, 158, 163, 210
   dementia with Lewy bodies   29
Dementia Care Mapping (DCM)   196, 222
dementia with Lewy bodies   10, 12, 13,
      18–21, 28–31, 39, 40, 43, 67, 68, 72,
      131, 148, 162, 166
   cholinergic changes   22
   cholinesterases   25, 131
   clinical features   13
   depression   13, 18, 67, 68, 72, 74
   differential diagnosis   14
   disease spectrum   39
   dopaminergic neurotransmission   13, 24
   glutamatergic neurotransmission   24, 125,
      126
   investigations   14, 15
   molecular pathology   33
   muscarinic acetylcholine receptors   22
   neuroleptic hypersensitivity   152
   neuropathology   5, 27, 40, 113, 216
   nicotinic cholinergic receptors   22
   serotonergic neurotransmission   26
dementism   194
depression   6, 7, 9–13, 18, 20, 29, 30, 51–54,
      56, 59–61, 63–74, 78, 114, 137, 143,
      158, 163, 164, 168–175, 177–183, 187,
      188, 192
   AD   6, 7, 9, 12, 13, 51–53, 59, 63–68,
      70–74, 78, 114, 143, 158, 163, 164,
      168, 170, 172, 175, 177–182, 187, 188
   aetiology   63, 66, 68
   assessment   12, 53, 60, 64–66, 69, 72,
      174, 178, 180, 182
   caregivers after placement   187, 188
   diagnosis   7, 63, 65, 68, 70, 72, 73, 179
   epidemiology   66
   genetics   34, 35
   non-pharmacological treatment   68, 170,
      177
   phenomenology   63, 65
   physical inactivity protocol   75, 177, 181

prevalence   12, 66, 67, 72, 74, 163, 183
   rating scales   64, 67, 170
   Seattle Protocols   177, 180
   sleep disturbance protocol   180
   treatment   7, 63, 64, 68, 70–74, 142, 158,
      168, 170, 172–175, 177–183
Depressive Signs Scale   64
developmental reflexes   105–108
diazepam   210
diet   211
differential diagnosis   3, 11, 13–15, 17–20,
      44, 59, 112
diffuse plaques   33
disability, non-dementia-related   112
Disability Assessment in Dementia (DAD)
      scale   17
disease severity   21, 22, 26, 148, 183
   neurochemistry   22
disinhibition, behavioural   16, 51, 155
dispossession, narrative   215, 216, 217, 218,
      219–223
donepezil   18, 20, 46, 48, 71–73, 115, 117,
      119–121, 128–131, 133–149, 234, 235
   head-to-head studies   144
   long-term studies   143
   nursing homes   119, 141, 145
      admission delay   140
      study   18, 48, 71, 72, 119–121, 128–130,
         135–149, 234, 235
      use   46, 70, 119, 120, 128, 131, 138–142,
         145, 146, 234, 235
   pharmaco-economics   234
dopaminergic D2 receptor
      dysregulation   152
dopaminergic neurotransmission   24, 39
dopaminergic receptors   152
dopaminergic transporter   14
Down's syndrome   34, 36, 39
   APP gene   34
   Lewy bodies   39
drinking   15, 198, 210
   difficulties   198, 210
dysphagia see swallowing disorders   198

eating   7, 8, 65, 70, 76, 86, 119, 128, 155,
      198, 203, 205, 207, 208, 210, 229
   difficulties   198
economic evaluation   139, 147, 227, 229,
      230, 232, 233, 235
   donepezil   139, 147

electroconvulsive treatment 71
emotional distress of caregivers after
    placement 187, 188
end-of-life care 190, 192, 203, 207, 212
  cultural issues 190
  end-stage therapy 34, 146, 187, 205
end-of-life issues 185, 190
engagement 197–199, 219
  authentic 197
epilepsy in AD 77
ethical narratives 215, 219, 224
ethics, narrative 215, 218
EuroQoL/EQ-5D scale 230
euthanasia 205, 206, 211
exercise 164, 165, 167, 170–172, 175, 181,
    183, 230
  Seattle Protocol 181
  sleep disturbance management 180
extrapyramidal signs 6, 12, 13, 26
  Alzheimer's disease 6
  antipsychotic medication 154, 210
  dementia with Lewy bodies 13, 39
  motor symptoms 6

falls in AD 76, 77
families 52, 78, 79, 81, 177, 185–191, 195,
    196, 199–201, 206, 209–211, 217,
    218
  care staff relationships 181
  decision-making 191, 209
  end-of-life issues 185, 190
  grief reactions 191
  post-care adaptation 191
  shared decision-making 205
  substitute decision-making 206
family care 172, 177, 178, 180, 185, 187,
    189, 192, 195
  late stage institutional care 188
family-staff care plans 189
fantasy therapy 166
fibrillogenesis 36
fronto lobes, white matter hyperintensity 9,
    11, 68
fronto-temporal dementia 4, 6–8, 10, 12,
    14, 15, 35, 39, 43, 67, 112
  clinical features 13, 14, 17
  differential diagnosis 15
  molecular pathology 40
  staging 112
  subtypes 15

fronto-temporal dementia with
    Parkinsonism 35, 36
functional abilities 8, 87, 199
  assessment instruments 15
  decline 117, 190
  donepezil efficacy 138
  randomized controlled trial
    assessments 92
Functional Assessment Staging (FAST)
    system 84
  AD 84
  cognitive capacity 103, 194
  Creutzfeldt-Jakob disease 6, 8, 14, 112
  development reflexes 105, 106, 107
  fronto-temporal dementia 14, 15, 39, 112
  motor disorders 6, 72
  Parkinson's disease,139
fungal infections 78, 211

gait impairment 6, 9
galantamine 46, 132, 133, 139–141,
    144–146, 148, 149
  efficacy 46, 132, 139
  head-to-head studies 144
  response prediction 145
gastrostomy, percutaneous endoscopic,207
gegenhalten *see* rigidity, paratonic,211
gerontological evaluation 78, 79
Gestalt Scale 65
glial cells 33, 35, 38
Global Deterioration Scale (GDS) 16, 43,
    46, 74, 83, 84, 86, 100, 106, 107, 134
  Ad staging 111
  normal pressure hydrocephalus 110
glutamate 21, 125, 126, 129, 130
  receptors 125, 126, 129, 130
  transporters 125
glutamatergic neurotransmission 125, 126
glutamatergic overstimulation 126
grasp reflexes,106, 108
grief reactions 191
  disenfranchised 200
GSK-3β 37

hallucinations 4, 7, 11–13, 16, 18, 20, 30, 51,
    52, 54, 56, 57, 65, 73, 153, 155, 157,
    158, 173, 174, 210
  see also visual hallucination 4, 7, 12, 13
haloperidol 151, 153, 160, 161, 168, 179, 210
  Seattle Protocol comparison 180

health economics   203, 227, 228, 230,
    232–234, 236
  evaluation of drugs   5, 16, 79
  studies   227, 228, 232, 233, 235
heart failure, shortness of breath   154, 208
home care   185–187, 200, 228
  continuation   186
  duration   228
  late stage   185, 186
  management with increased support   79,
    80
hospice care   209
hospital admission   53, 80
hospitalisation   79–81, 186, 206, 209
  at home   76, 80, 81
  placement effect   187
hydration   198, 207, 208, 210, 212
  artificial   208
    death rattle   208
  refusal   210
hydrocephalus, normal pressure   110
5-hydroxytryptamine (5-HT)   21, 26
  receptor polymorphism   68
5-hydroxytryptamine 1A (5-HT1A)
    receptors   69
hyperactivity   53, 54

illness, cost of   227, 228, 230
Imbalance in Sensoristasis   167
incontinence   11, 12, 14, 15, 78, 89, 90, 93,
    95, 104, 106, 109, 110, 112, 114, 118,
    159, 174, 199
  AD   14, 78, 89, 93, 104, 106, 109, 110,
    112, 118, 159
  assisting with   199
  dementia with Lewy bodies   12
  incipient   89, 90, 95, 104, 109, 112
incremental cost effectiveness ratio
    (ICER)   229
individuals, treatment as   171
infections in AD, 78
institutionalisation   3, 19, 76, 77, 79, 80, 161,
    174, 181, 182, 187, 188, 234
  admission delay   79
  contracture development   105, 108
  family involvement   188
  late stage   187
  small group homes   190
  see also nursing homes; residential
    care   51, 131, 133, 145, 151

instruments see assessment instruments   151
integrated care pathways   200
interleukin 1 (IL-1)   37
interventions   40, 53, 58, 68, 70, 72, 83, 103,
    163–173, 177, 182, 183, 189, 192, 202,
    205, 207, 211, 221, 227, 232, 233
  avoiding aggressive   207
  costs   233
  economic evaluations   139, 229
  non-palliative   205
  non-pharmacological   68, 163, 164, 166,
    169, 171, 172, 177, 233
    types   164, 172, 233
  pharmacological   68, 70, 163, 164, 166,
    168, 169, 171, 172, 177, 233
    types   164, 172, 233
  see also named drugs
itching   211
language   4, 5, 11, 14–16, 44–46, 75, 146,
    164, 165, 194, 195, 197, 199, 217, 221,
    222, 224
  impairment   4, 5, 16, 44, 46, 75, 194
  limited   11, 221, 222, 224
  narrative   217, 221, 222, 224
  see also communication   197

late stage dementia, family care   185
laxatives   211
Lewy bodies   10, 12, 13, 18–21, 23, 25, 26,
    28–31, 39, 40, 43, 67, 68, 72, 131, 148,
    162, 166
  Alzheimer's disease   10, 18–20, 28, 29,
    31, 39, 67, 72, 131, 166
  subcortical   13, 39
  see also dementia with Lewy bodies   13,
    21, 39, 131
life, worth of   194
life history   52, 195, 223–225
life-support measures   190
lives, trajectory   4, 216, 218, 220
living wills   206, 209, 211
long-stay units   80, 81
loss, personal   61

management of patients   15
manic symptoms   7
Markov modelling   234
massage theraphy   70, 164, 166
master narratives   217, 223
  countering   223

mastery 187
mattresses 211
M-Best study 115, 121, 129, 130, 149
medical evaluation 8
memantine 20, 46, 48, 83, 92, 98, 100, 102,
    115, 117, 119–121, 125–130, 144, 146,
    148, 149, 234, 235
  add-on therapy 146
  clinical trials 46, 127–129, 234
  mode of action 126
  pharmaco-economics 127, 234
  pharmacokinetics 127, 130
MEM-MD-01 128
MEM-MD-02 128
memory 3–7, 9, 11, 14–17, 22, 28, 37,
    44–46, 60, 63, 73, 75, 78, 80, 84, 93,
    100–104, 125, 126, 130, 151, 164, 165,
    180, 181, 183, 194
  episodic 6, 11, 44
meta-narrative 217, 219, 223, 224
microglia 21, 37, 38
Mild Cognitive Impairment (MCI) stage 84
Mini Nutrition Assessment (MNA) 77, 78
Mini-Mental State Examination
    (MMSE) 12, 22, 43, 83
mirroring 197, 198, 222
mobility 76–78, 108, 165, 181, 206
  Alzheimer's disease 77
  ambulatory ability 108
Modified-Ordinal Scales of Psychological
    Development (M-OSPD) 46
moral personhood 194
morphine 208, 210, 211
mortality with neuroleptics
motor disorders 12
  AD 6, 12
  Alzheimer's disease 6, 12
  evaluation 6
  ritualistic 6, 7, 8
motor symptoms,
    extrapyramidal/subcortical 6
mouth-care 210
movements 6, 91, 111, 112, 208
  convulsive 7, 71
  stereotypic 6
  story-telling 216
MRZ9605 127
multi-infarct dementia 9, 18, 38
multi-informant caregiver-based
    assessment 17

muscarinic acetylcholine receptor
    (nAChR) 22
muscarinic cholinergic receptors 24
music therapy 164, 165, 167, 170, 171, 173,
    197, 201, 203, 233

narrative 188, 215–226
  agency 216–219, 221–224
  compromise 216
  continuity 219, 220
  ethics 215–219, 221, 223–226
  inadequate 217
  of others 216, 217, 219, 221, 222
  palliative care 216, 217, 219, 224
  probity 220, 222
  and self 216
nasal tubes 207
neuritic plaques 21, 33, 34, 110, 111, 125
neurofibrillary tangles 21, 33, 36
  FAST staging 86
  pathogenesis 34, 37
  sequential deposition 37
neuroimaging in vascular dementia 9, 38
neuroleptic therapy 151
neurological signs in AD 121
neuron loss 23, 33, 35, 37
neurophysiologic changes 105
Neuropsychiatric Interview 64
Neuropsychiatric Inventory (NPI) 16, 78,
    128, 138, 155, 159
  agitation 155
  Alzheimer's disease 16, 58, 141
  BPSD clustering 53, 57, 59
neuropsychiatric symptoms, donepezil
    efficacy 63, 71, 131, 137, 152, 159
neurotransmitter systems 21, 22, 27, 68,
    130
  changes 22
  cholinergic 21, 27, 130
  depression 68
New York University - Clinician's Interview
    Based Assessment of Change Plus
    Informant 105
interview (NYU-CIBIC-Plus)
    assessment 100, 102
nicotinic acetylcholine receptor
    (nAChR) 22
nicotinic cholinergic receptors 22
NITE-AD 174, 180
NMDA receptors 100, 125, 126, 129

nonverbal interventions   164, 166, 169–171
   agitation   164, 166
   apathy   169
   depression   164, 169, 170
   sleep disorders   164
noradrenaline   21
nursing homes   12, 60, 110, 131, 145, 155,
         164, 166, 174, 182, 185, 188–192, 200,
         203, 207, 209–211
   admission delay   140
   cholinesterase inhibitor use   131
   palliative care   210, 211
   see also residential care   131, 133
nutrition   76, 77, 82, 190, 198, 207, 210,
         212
   artificial   77, 207
   refusal   77, 210
nutritional status, Alzheimer's disease   75

obsessive-compulsive behaviour   7
occupational therapists   210, 211
olanzapine   152–154, 157–160, 162, 163
Older Adult Behavior Checklist
         (OABCL)   8, 17
Older Adult Self-Report (OASR)   17
opioids   208
opportunity costs   227, 228
organisational strategies   200

pain   12, 52, 78, 190, 198, 199, 202, 203,
         205, 206, 208, 212, 213
   detection/treatment   199
   palliative care   206, 213
palliative care   78, 193, 195, 197, 200–203,
         205–208, 210–213, 216, 217, 219, 224
   ethical narratives   224, 218, 219, 224
   narrative approach   216–218, 224
paratonia *see* rigidity, paratonic   105, 106
parkinsonian gait   77
Parkinson's disease   6, 8, 10, 13, 18, 21,
         28–31, 39, 43, 72, 77, 111, 113–115,
         152, 153, 161, 162
   Lewy bodies   13, 21, 28, 29, 31, 39, 43,
         162
   staging   111
Parkinson's disease dementia   21, 28, 152
   dopaminergic neurotransmission   13, 14,
         23, 24, 125, 152
   glutamatergic neurotransmission   24, 125,
         126, 130

muscarinic acetylcholine receptors   22,
         24, 25
neuropathology   6, 27, 113, 216
nicotinic cholinergic receptors   22, 23,
         132
serotonergic neurotransmission   26, 27
passivity   14, 197
person-centred care   193–197, 200, 201, 223
   affirmation of value   193, 194
   perspective of person   196
pharmaco-economics   234
physical activity   77, 167, 172, 180, 181
   Seattle Protocol   180, 181
   sleep disturbance   180
Pick's body inclusions, fronto-temporal
         dementia   4, 6, 7, 8, 12, 14, 15, 35,
         36, 39, 40, 43, 112, 166
placement   125, 140, 141, 147, 177, 180, 183,
         185–189, 191, 192
   carer effects   166
pneumonia   76, 78, 154, 190, 198, 205–210,
         212
   AD   78, 154, 190, 205, 208–210
   aspiration   78, 198, 208
   curative treatment   207, 210
   palliative care   78, 210
   shortness of breath   205, 208
   treatment   154, 205–210, 212
political strategies   200
positioning, assistance with   199, 210
presenilin 1   35, 36, 57
presenilin 2   35, 36
pressure sores   75, 77, 78, 207, 208, 210, 211
protein-calorie undernutrition in AD   77, 78
psychiatric disturbance in AD   7, 11, 64, 70
psychosis   4, 7–9, 12, 18, 20, 30, 52–54, 57,
         60, 71, 72, 114, 144, 146, 152–155,
         157–162
   agitation   11, 52–54, 60, 144, 146, 152,
         153, 155, 157, 159–162
   late-onset   9
   pathophysiology   57
psychosis of Alzheimer's disease
         (PAD)   158, 161
psychosocial approaches to care   57, 193
psychotic symptoms   7, 9, 57, 151, 153, 157,
         158, 202

quality adjusted life years (QALYs)   230,
         233, 234, 235

quality of life   52, 60, 68, 70, 71, 75, 81, 137,
   141, 151, 163, 166, 168, 169, 180, 185,
   193, 195, 198–202, 204–207, 211, 217,
   230, 234
Quality of Well Being Scale (QWBS)   230
quilting, narrative   215, 216, 217, 218, 222, 224

radiological examination   79
randomized controlled trials (RCT)   92, 117,
   119, 120, 155, 167, 170, 234
   functional assessments   119
   memantine   119, 120
reading, monastic/scholastic   15, 44, 222
reality orientation   164, 165, 168, 174
recognition loss   6
reflexes, developmental   105, 106, 107, 108
relationship-centred care   195
relationships, supportive environment   44,
   193, 196, 197, 201, 218
reminiscence therapy   72, 164, 165,
   168–170, 172, 175, 233
representational narratives   216
residential care   51, 131, 133, 139, 145, 151,
   177, 202, 204
   admission delay   66, 76, 133, 140
   audit cycles   201
   contracture development   12, 78, 108
   monitoring   64, 222
   placement   140, 185, 186, 187, 191
   political interventions   200
   small group homes   190
   standard setting   200
   see also nursing homes   12, 110, 131, 155,
      164, 166, 182, 185, 188, 190, 200, 207,
      209, 210, 211
Resource Utilisation in Dementia (RUD)
   instrument   228, 234
respite care   228
retirement homes   81
rigidity   15, 77, 105, 106, 108, 110, 111
   paratonic   105, 106
risperidone   141, 146, 152–155, 157–163
ritualistic behaviours   8
rivastigmine   20, 30, 46, 74, 100, 132, 134,
   140–143, 145, 147, 148
   efficacy   17, 70, 128, 129, 131, 133, 135,
      141, 145, 146, 151, 152, 158, 159, 179,
      234
   nursing home use   234
rooting reflex   106

schizophrenia   9, 10, 19, 29, 104, 154, 217, 225
SCIP scale   46
screaming episodes in AD   12
Seattle Protocols   177–181, 183
secretases   35, 36
sedation, palliative   205, 206, 211, 217
selective serotonin reuptake inhibitors
   (SSRIs)   70
self, narrative and   216
senile plaques   33, 36, 40
senses   195, 198
   engagement   198
   framework   195
serotonergic neurotransmission   26
serotonergic receptors   26
serotonergic transporter   27
serotonin *see* 5-hydroxytryptamine
   (5-HT)   21, 26
Severe Impairment Battery (SIB)   16, 45, 47,
   48, 103, 127, 135, 136
Severe Mini-Mental State Examination
   (SMMSE)   46
severity of dementia   12, 24, 26, 53, 158,
   171, 234
   related costs   233
shared decision-making   205, 206
Simulated Presence   70, 72
skin problems   210, 211
sleep disorders   13, 53, 164, 172, 180, 183
   dementia with Lewy bodies   13
   non-pharmacological treatment   68, 163,
      177
   Seattle Protocols   180
sleep hygiene   167, 171, 172, 174
sleep-wake disturbances   159
Snoezelen therapy   70
social environment   193–197, 201
   changes   196, 201
   supportive   193–197, 201
social psychology, malignant   198
speech and language problems   15
   see also communication; language   15, 197
speech therapists   210
spiritual care   199, 200, 203
Staff Training in Assisted-living Residences
   (STAR)   181
staging   15, 16, 20, 21, 37, 40, 43, 48, 69, 73,
   74, 81, 83, 84, 86, 87, 89, 90, 92, 93,
   96–100, 102, 104, 109–115, 117, 118,
   121, 129, 134

stimulation 25, 59, 126, 164, 165, 173, 179, 198, 199, 233
stories 215–219, 221–226
  fragments 215, 221
  small 219, 222–224
  telling 216, 222, 224, 225
strategic infarct dementias 9
stroke risk with neuroleptics 154
subcortical vascular dementia 9
Subjective Cognitive Impairment (SCI)
  stage 84
sucking reflex 106
swallowing disorders 78
  analgesic administration 208
  palliative care 78
α-synuclein 13, 21, 39

tacrine 131, 140, 147, 148
  nursing home admission delay 133, 140
Tanaka-Binet Intelligence Scale 103
tau protein 25, 40
  mutations 40
Test for Severe Impairment (TSI) 46
third-party payers 229
tiapride 152, 160–162
time course of severe dementia 84
transferring, assistance with 199
transporter gene polymorphisms 68
trazodone, Seattle Protocol comparison 168
treatment 3, 4, 7, 16, 17, 19, 20, 27, 29, 30, 48, 58, 63, 64, 68, 70–74, 76, 79, 83, 92, 99, 100, 102, 115, 119–121, 125, 127–131, 133, 135–149, 151–155, 158–168, 170–175, 177–183, 189, 192, 195, 199, 201, 205–213, 227–235
  avoiding aggressive 205, 207
  costs 127, 139, 227–231, 233–235
  forgoing 207, 212
  policies 189
  response 4, 71, 128, 145, 162, 163, 168, 177, 179
tube feeding 205, 207, 212

Unified Parkinson's Disease Rating Scale (UPDRS) 111
urinary tract infections in AD 159
utilisation behaviour 14

validation therapy 164–166, 169, 174, 197
vascular dementia 4, 6–11, 14, 15, 18–21, 28, 31, 38, 40, 61, 68, 72, 121, 129, 131, 146, 147, 152, 157, 166, 171, 174
  behavioural symptoms/disturbances 4, 7, 43, 125, 128, 142, 155, 199
  cholinergic changes 22
  depression 7, 61, 67, 68, 72
  dopaminergic changes 13, 14, 23, 24, 125, 152, 159
  glutamatergic neurotransmission 24, 125, 126
  mixed Alzheimer's disease 8
  molecular pathology 33, 40
  neuropathology 21
  serotonergic neurotransmission 26
vascular dementia-Alzheimer's disease, mixed 9, 38
vascular impairment 5
  medicinal evaluation 8
verbal interventions 164–166, 168–171
  agitation 164, 166, 168
  apathy 169
  depression 164, 168, 170
  sleep disorders 164
vesicular glutamate transporters (VGLUT)
visual hallucinations 4, 7, 12, 13, 18, 30
  AD 12, 13
  dementia with Lewy bodies 13, 39
washing, assistance with 199
weight loss in AD 76
white matter hyperintensity 68
WHO analgesic ladder 208
withdrawal 64, 71, 135, 146, 178, 197

Zarit scale 78